365 WAYS TO KEEP KIDS SAFE

How To Make Your Child's World Safer

By Don C. Keenan

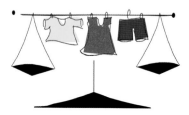

Keenan's Kids Foundation

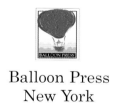

Balloon Press
New York

Copyright © 2006 by Don C. Keenan and Keenan's Kids Foundation
Published by Balloon Press, New York, NY

Printed by South China Printing Co. Ltd.

ISBN 0-9774425-3-5

First Edition
Printed and Bound in China

Book Design by Gretchen Steininger, Thunder & Lightning Image Group
Cover Design by Magnus Andersson, Innervision Design

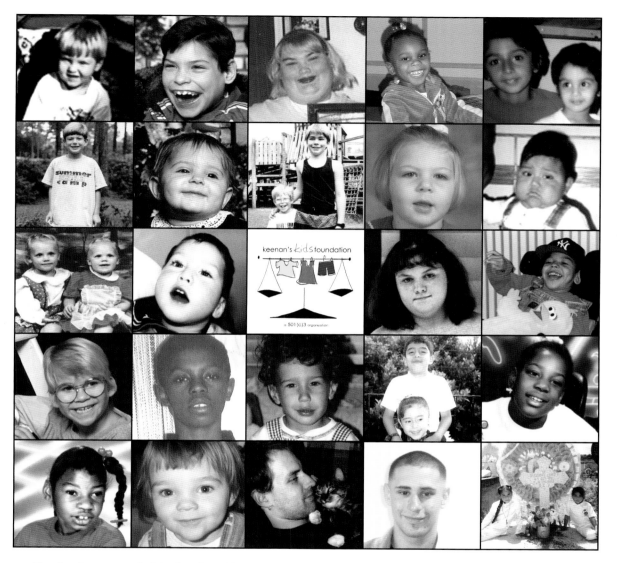

Each chapter of this book tells the painful true story of a child's death or serious injury. All of these children were my clients and many of their sweet faces can be seen here.

This book is dedicated to my children. From these tragedies and their family's suffering comes an understanding of how to prevent a repeat of this heartbreak.

Prevention is the purpose of this book.

All cases are actual cases; however, the names of the children have been changed to protect their privacy and the confidentiality of their settlements.

Acknowledgements

Preparation for this book began 30 years ago when, as a young lawyer, I was retained by a Kentucky family to represent their severely injured six-year-old boy. In that case and nearly all the other thousand plus children's cases I have represented, my law firm has hired experts to teach us how these injuries and deaths could have been prevented. From the preceding page, you know this book is dedicated to all the children and families I have represented. However, this is the proper place to acknowledge all the experts I have worked with over the years: the doctors, public health officials, safety advocates, politicians and others. They have taught me and ultimately the jury in our cases the simple truth, that all these tragedies could have been prevented. My heartfelt thanks to all of the experts.

Special thanks go to the jurors who sat in judgment on the cases I was privileged to represent. The juries' verdicts made clear that the injury or death was preventable and sent a strong message to the wrongdoers that if they did not accept responsibility for their actions, the jury would demand their responsibility. The verdicts went a long way to help preventing similar tragedies.

Thanks as well to my 99 brothers and sisters of the Inner Circle of Advocates (www.innercircle.org), whose assistance in the development of my lawyer skills has been immeasurable. The Inner Circle is the most elite of all trial lawyers groups. Membership is by invitation only and capped at 100. Although spread across the country, our intimate group functions often as a collective law firm in the pursuit of justice.

The local and national media deserves special credit. Many of my children's cases have appeared on every major news show, including *The Oprah Winfrey Show*, NBC's *Today Show*, *60 Minutes*, *60 Minutes II*, *Larry King Live*, *The O'Reilly Factor*, *Good Morning America*, *20/20*, *Dateline* and CNN specials. Without the media attention, many hazards would still pose danger.

Thanks go to Dave Schmeltzer, the former Director of Compliance for the U.S. Consumer Products Safety Commission (CPSC), for his laborious audit and confirmation of the correctness of our recommendations. Also special thanks to Arthur Kellerman, one of my safety heroes, director of the Center for Injury Control in the School of Public Health at Emory University (Atlanta, GA).

Finally, permit me to thank those that assisted in the preparation of this book. First, I would like to thank those who assisted in the writing of the book: Donna Ellingson, Nichole Schaffer, and Karen Miles. Thank you to Gretchen Steininger, who formatted the book and graphics, and Magnus Andersson of Innervision Design, for the design of the cover. I would also like to thank those persons who I work with everyday in either my law firm (www.keenanlawfirm.com) or children's foundation (www.keenanskidsfoundation.com), specifically Ben Wilcox and April Swanson.

My thanks do not end with this Acknowledgement section. You will find special thanks and congratulations to many safety groups, public leaders and associations throughout this book for notable outstanding advocacy and work in given areas. Since there have been many who have assisted in this text over 30 years, I am sure to overlook someone, for which I sincerely apologize.

Table of Contents

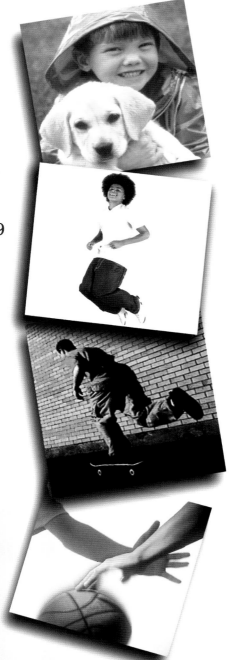

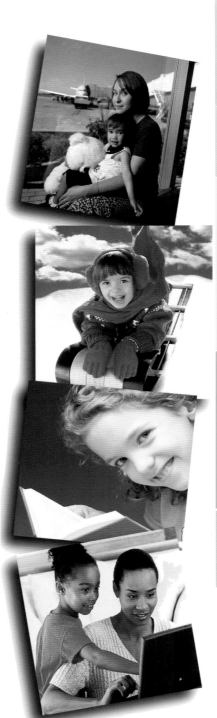

Introduction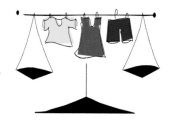

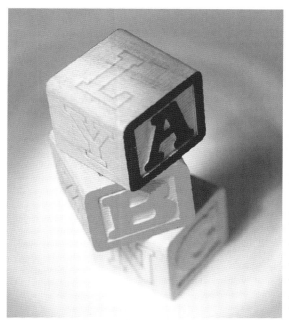

What business does a lawyer/child advocate have in writing a child safety/prevention book? After 30 years of representing catastrophically injured and deceased children, in 48 states and many foreign countries, I have unfortunately witnessed every possible way injury and death can happen to our children. Whether the tragedy happened at home, recreation, school/daycare, or during transportation, all of these tragedies were preventable. The 365 Hazards listed on the checklists and report cards throughout this book are REAL and preventable.

In the courtroom, whether the injury or death was preventable is not my opinion, but rather is established through experts' opinions. The ultimate decision on safety and prevention in all of my cases depends not on lawyers, experts or judges. People just like you are the people that decide the justice in our country; they are the people who serve on our juries. It's the lessons learned from these tragedies that form the backdrop of this writing.

The purpose of the book is two-fold: to open the eyes of parents and caregivers to the hidden hazards and dangers in the world of children, and most importantly, to provide easy-to-follow steps to prevention. We will use report cards and checklists, which are simple and bottom-line oriented.

My expertise has been driven by 30 years of successful litigation in hundreds of cases through jury verdicts and settlements. The work of Keenan's Kids Foundation, established in 1993 as a 501(c) (3) non-profit organization, has fueled my expertise as well.

The purpose of Keenan's Kids Foundation has been to research, with the aid of nationally recognized experts, how childhood injuries and deaths occur in not only our cases, but also everywhere. The purpose of this research is to develop rock-solid prevention guides. Public advocacy campaigns on a number of safety issues have been launched, i.e. toy safety, with our annual release of the 10 most dangerous toys, the playground safety report card project, featured on national media. We have also launched campaigns on stranger danger in the public elementary schools, the hazards of the neighborhood, day care and many other areas.

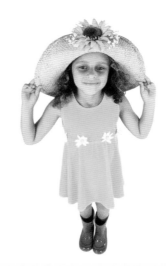

Keenan's Kids Foundation has also been instrumental in the passage of a number of state and federal child safety initiatives. Many on-going legislative initiatives are in this book. The litmus test on whether I have qualifications to write this book is best seen in the countless letters and emails received from thankful parents over the years. The following is an example:

Dear Mr. Keenan,

You saved our son's life. Our local playground had six life threatening conditions, none of which we or any of our neighbors were aware of before using your safety report card. Once we notified the city, they removed some of the hazards and the ones they didn't, we worked with our neighborhood association to make that playground safe. Thank you so much and please spread the word. We will.

Angie and Ralph Pendergrass

What motivates our passion for prevention? Our playground safety report card project originated because I had been the lawyer for over five childhood deaths and 22 brain damaged/blinded/paralyzed little children because of preventable playground injuries. As you will read later, 10 children die each year because of a playground injury; every two and a half minutes, a child is rushed to an emergency room with a playground injury. The Playground Safety Report Card was aimed at putting a stop to these senseless, preventable injuries and deaths. As you can see, at least one participant thought it saved their son's life.

My reasoning for this book is that I do not want to represent another family heartbroken from a preventable injury or death. The following pages document how, together, we can save children from preventable, catastrophic injuries and death in the home, recreation, school/daycare and during transportation.

With the power of knowledge and simple tools of prevention, we can accomplish a safe world for children. If my law firm's phone never rings again carrying the story of a grieving parent, I will be a happy man.

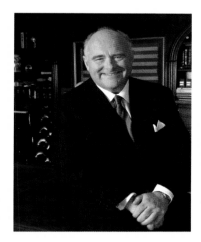

Don Keenan

Child Advocate/ Trial Lawyer
Atlanta, Georgia

DonKeenan@KeenansKidsFoundation.com

"Child Advocacy Lifetime Achievement Award"
Center For Injury Control
Emory University

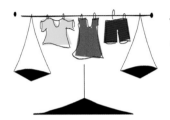

How to Use This Book

In order to be successful in the courtroom, I have used focus groups and mock juries for well over 20 years, first being featured on NBC *Nightly News* back in 1981. The format of this book is the result of dozens of focus groups conducted in the courtroom on the second floor of my office building. These focus groups were not conducted for benefit of our legal cases, but rather to discover how the average parent or caregiver approaches and deals with safety issues concerning their children. The results provided the roadmap for the book format.

The focus groups convincingly told us that the first step of safety is the parent or caregiver's awareness that harm and even death can and does occur. No awareness means you aren't on guard and thus have no power to recognize the hazards and therefore can not prevent the harm or death. Thus, to drive that point home, each of our chapters will begin by walking a mile in one of our past parent or caregiver's moccasins. You will read an overview of the case tragedy in a real case. In most cases, the names have been changed because the ultimate settlement dictated confidentiality. Those real-life cases will be indented and will have a yellow background.

Is Danger Lurking at Your Table?

"Hot dogs and beans, please," said four year-old Jeffrey when asked what he wanted for lunch one summer day. His mother, Jennifer Allen, had fixed that meal many times before but she had always fried and cut up the hotdogs separately before adding them to the beans she'd warmed up in another pot.

But this time Jennifer had bought a can of franks and beans manufactured by a major food company. It had both the hotdogs and beans already mixed together in the same can. As she cooked the contents of the can, Jennifer noticed that the hotdog pieces were a little bigger than the way she cut them but not so large as to alarm her. After the meal, Jeffrey happily ran out and resumed play in the backyard with his friends.

Thirty minutes later Jeffrey's friends came screaming, "Come quick, Mrs. Allen, come quick!" Jennifer was shocked to discover Jeffrey's lifeless body stretched out on the ground in front of her. After calling 9-1-1, she tried to rouse her son while waiting for the ambulance, but had no success. Neither did the EMS team. At four years of age, Jeffrey choked to death in his own backyard.

The autopsy revealed a partially chewed piece of hotdog that obstructed Jeffrey's airway, which caused his death.

LEGAL ACTION and OUTCOME

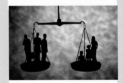

Jennifer Allen, a single parent, asked me to investigate to see if anyone was at fault and whether her son's death had been preventable. I had to inform her that, although such deaths are alarmingly common, under current case law, there was no case. My opinion is that, as public awareness increases in coming years, there will be a potential case.

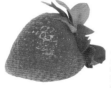

⇨ Approximately every five days a child in the United States dies from choking on food. More than 90 percent of these children are younger than age five, according to 2004 statistics from the Center for Science in the Public Interest (CSPI). (www.cspinet.org)

⇨ In 2001, more than 10,000 children were treated in emergency departments for choking on foods, according to the Centers for Disease Control and Prevention. (www.cdc.gov)

⇨ Nearly 2,000 people (with 62 percent being children) unintentionally swallow "button" batteries used to power hearing aids, watches and calendars, according to the National Capital Poison Center. (www.poison.org)

The focus group also told us that many parents and caregivers will react to the client's story with a feeling of "this couldn't ever happen to my child," or they will think "this tragedy is so rare that I don't need to worry." Therefore, the client's story will be followed immediately with a "STATISTICS" section to drive home the point that these injuries and deaths are not flukes but happen more often than you think. The book won't overwhelm you with statistics, but only the highlights.

Laws and Regulations

While there are some laws mandating the safety of sports equipment, there are no laws or government regulations directly pertaining to organized sports for children. The team on which your child plays may have its own set of guidelines; if so, read them and see if you agree with what's been outlined. It's up to parents and other concerned adults to see that children are safe when they participate in sports. Use the Report Card that follows to evaluate your child's sports program.

Recently, there has been a reemergence of the sport of dodgeball; a movie staring Ben Stiller is credited in part for the new found popularity. However, the National Association for Sports & Physical Education, a non-profit organization of 20,000 coaches, PE teachers, trainers and athletic directors, issued the following declaration:"dodgeball is not an appropriate activity for K-12 school physical education programs." Some school districts in Maine, Maryland, New York, Massachuetts, Texas, Virginia and Utah have banned dodgeball, according to an AP story of November 20, 2004. Noted recreation expert, Steve Bernheim, also advises against playing the sport of dodgeball. Although no statistics are available, there are many reports of serious injury. (www.aahperd.org/naspe)

Finally, the focus group sadly revealed to us that most people have a misplaced feeling that there are strong laws and regulations in place to protect their children. Unfortunately, this assumption is wrong. Thus, the next step in the format is an overview of existing laws and regulations. We will use the following "thumbs" symbols to help you:

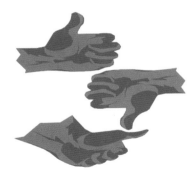

Thumbs up - In those rare instances where the law and regulations are indeed adequate.

Thumbs down -When the law provides little or no protection.

Thumbs to the middle - Where the laws and regulations are good in some areas and not in others.

Hopefully, the 82 percent registered voters in the 2004 election indicated an increased interest in participation in our democracy. With this hope, you will see a "capitol" symbol when you can be of help. There will then be a call to action section with a step by step on what you can do to help enact the laws and regulations to make things safe for children.

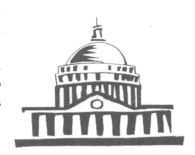

Taking Action

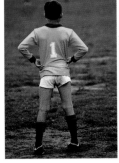

Most parents believe that there is nothing they could have done to prevent their child's sports-related injury, yet the National SAFE KIDS Campaign reports that half of all sports-related injuries ARE preventable.

In their 2003 study, the National SAFE KIDS Campaign found that more than half the parents (53 percent) surveyed expressed little concern about the possibility of their child getting hurt, despite the fact that one out of every three children is injured during team sports. Shockingly, four out of five parents surveyed whose child suffered a sports injury believe that it was part of the game and would have happened regardless of precautions. A third of the parents said they do not often take the same safety precautions during the child's practice as in the game, even though statistically most sports injuries occur during practice.

Parents need to take control and intervene when necessary in this injury-prone activity. They need to approach sports with the following REPORT CARD, designed to grade the coach and school with either a "pass" or "fail."

Sports 165

Now that you have walked the mile in the parent/caregivers' moccasins, seen the statistics, realized the laws and regulations that are inadequate, you will come to the real reason the book was written . . . the TAKING ACTION section. Each chapter has one, but we will use, depending on the chapter, one of two formats to help you TAKE ACTION as follows:

Report Cards

(From Chapter 14- Playgrounds)

Checklists

(From Chapter 4- Choking Hazards

REPORT CARD		
	SUBJECT	GRADE
1	Condition of equipment	
2	Surfaces must be smooth	
3	Trip hazards eliminated	
4	Tipping of equipment prevented	
5	Fall zones adequate	
6	Gaps or spaces absent	
7	Electrical wires secured	
8	Dangerous tree limbs removed	
9	Surface areas safe and uniform	
10	Hazards removed	

✓	⚠ CHECKLIST ⚠
1	Get to know the driver.
2	Know the specific driver-screening and audit system.
3	Know the specific drop off neighborhoods on the route and key people in the neighborhoods.
4	Make sure all pre-school children have seatbelts.
5	Make sure all vans have seatbelts.
6	Urge your school to modernize buses.
7	Check out the safety of any charter bus services used.

These "TAKING ACTION" steps are so important that the Keenan's Kids Foundation has compressed all of the Report Cards and Checklists found in this text to a CD, as well as the hyperlinks to all of the Web sites referenced. The CD can be obtained at NO CHARGE by calling 1-800-677-2025, or by email at office@keenanskidsfoundation.com. You can simply load the CD on your home computer, print out what you need, and with clipboard and pen or pencil in hand, take control of the safety of your child.

Remember, with every danger and hazard you recognize and remove, your child comes one step closer to a safer world.

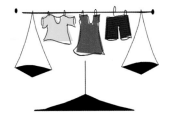

Risks Versus Hazards

IMPORTANT, PLEASE READ

You may think these terms, risk versus hazard, are technical, but as you will see in a moment, they are very simple, very easy to understand and very, very important to using this book.

RISKS are all around a child's world and most often, risks are just fine. Risks are part of the fun of being a child, i.e., the risk of getting wet at an amusement ride, the risk of getting hit while trying to catch a baseball or a twirling baton, or the risk of falling out of a tree or off a bicycle.

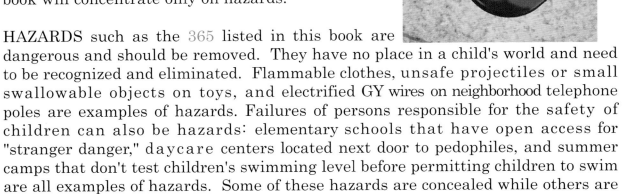

This book will not discuss nor propose any preventions for the normal risks of everyday child's life. Nor will the book even discuss the risks which are in the total control of the parent/caregiver i.e.: we won't discuss the need to give water to a child during play to avoid the risk of dehydration, the risk of playing with matches or the risk of talking with strangers. Instead, the book will concentrate only on hazards.

HAZARDS such as the 365 listed in this book are dangerous and should be removed. They have no place in a child's world and need to be recognized and eliminated. Flammable clothes, unsafe projectiles or small swallowable objects on toys, and electrified GY wires on neighborhood telephone poles are examples of hazards. Failures of persons responsible for the safety of children can also be hazards: elementary schools that have open access for "stranger danger," daycare centers located next door to pedophiles, and summer camps that don't test children's swimming level before permitting children to swim are all examples of hazards. Some of these hazards are concealed while others are known and all one has to do is recognize them.

The difference between risks versus hazards is best explained by a great question asked by *Today Show* host Matt Lauer, the second year I was a guest for our Keenan's Kids Playground Safety Report Card.

TODAY SHOW TRANSCRIPT

Matt Lauer: "Don, are you trying to make playgrounds risk-free? If kids are going to play and swing on swing sets, slide down slides, they are going to fall down and get cuts and scrapes. This isn't zero tolerance is it?"

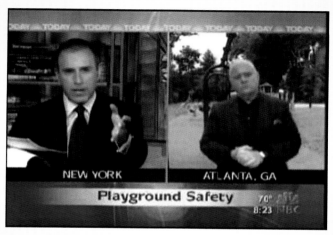

Don Keenan: "Matt, when you and I were kids we wanted to run full blast, we wanted to tackle each other, we wanted to somersault, and we want kids to do that today; have fun. What we don't want them to do is hit those hidden dangers, obstacles, the hazards that have no business being in the playground: the exposed nail, the high voltage electrical wires, and the dangers that we think would be gone but are hidden somewhere in almost every playground."

BOTTOM LINE: Most risks are okay, and risks in general are the exclusive control of the parents and caregivers and their responsibility. Hazards and dangers need to be recognized and immediately removed...this book identifies the hazards and gives parents and caregivers the tools to recognize and remove them.

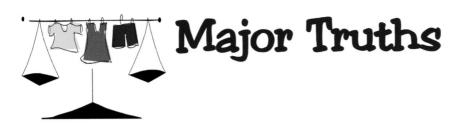

Major Truths

1. You can not remove all the risks in a child's world. You CAN remove all 365 hazards set forth in this book .

2. If it can happen (a hazard killing or injuring a child), it WILL happen.

3. Hope for the best, ALWAYS plan for the worst.

4. KIDS will often "misuse" before "using" a toy safely. The same is true for playground equipment, etc...its more fun.

5. Kids think like kids: NOT ADULTS!

6. Safety education of kids is not enough- they simply don't get it.

7. BOTTOM LINE: the parents and caregivers have the ultimate burden of removing the HAZARDS.

YOU ARE THE CHILD'S SAFETY NET!

Myths and Facts

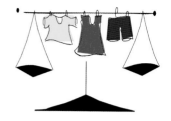

MYTH: The government, with its regulations and inspections, has removed the hazards in a child's world.

FACT: There is no such safety net provided by the government as you will consistently see in the Law/Regulation sections of this book. In most instances, there are no regulations or laws. When laws are present, *they are usually weak and rarely enforced.*

MYTH: All this talk about children's safety takes the fun out of a child's life.

FACT: The world has drastically changed since we were kids, and the rules have changed as well. We once were able to play in local neighborhoods without a worry about safety. Now, virtually no one lets their children play outside unsupervised. The purpose of this book is to remove the hazards from a child's world *so kids CAN have fun.*

MYTH: If a defective product is recalled, that means it's not available, and I won't have to worry.

FACT: Only a small portion of recalled products are returned to the manufacturer or destroyed. Instead, recalled products, such as toys, helmets and scooters, are simply handed down from one family member to another, get sold on Ebay, or get donated to a charity such as Salvation Army or Goodwill. They stay in a child's world forever. The only good thing about a recall is that the product is no longer manufactured.

MYTH: Simple safety education is all a child needs.

FACT: Safety education is important, but beyond the comprehension of children for two reasons. First, they lack the complex reasoning skills of an adult. They may understand the "don't" or "no" but do not comprehend the "why not." It is the understanding of the "why not" that solidifies safety education.

The second and most obvious reason is that kids are built to break rules, move boundaries and defy authority. And of course, sometimes they will do what they know is dangerous.

MYTH: To really remove the hazards from a child's life would require more time than I have.

FACT: The purpose of this book is to identify hazards so they can be removed simply and quickly. The report cards and checklists at the end of each chapter are straightforward and result-oriented.

MYTH: If I remove the hazards from our home and our car, this will make my child's world safe.

FACT: Unfortunately, statistics show a substantial number of children die or are seriously injured at the homes of neighbors, friends and family members. This is also true for toys in these other homes and automobiles. Everywhere your child goes needs to be hazard free.

MYTH: Statistically, the chances are small for my child to be injured from a dangerous hazard.

FACT: Every one of the parents I've represented in death and catastrophic injury cases probably said the same thing before tragedy struck. No matter how rare the occurrence, if you can easily remove the hazard, why not?

Just imagine you are in a football stadium of 50,000 people, and over the loud speaker you are told someone will fire a single bullet into the crowd. One person will be killed. Would you stay seated because your chances of dying are only one in 50,000, or would you leave?

Impact of Childhood Injuries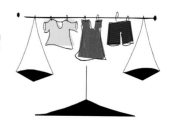

An important part of injury prevention and hazard avoidance is knowing the outcome from a failure of prevention or avoidance. If we know the depth of the consequences, the harm that can occur, we will try very hard to prevent or avoid them. So with that recognition, having represented injured children for over 30 years, I have learned some good news and some bad news:

⇨ THE GOOD NEWS

When a child breaks a bone, strains a muscle, or receives a severe laceration, the likelihood of permanent damage is quite remote. The resilience of the developing child up to late teens is simply remarkable. In a physical injury that would otherwise debilitate an adult, we will usually see the child rebounding quickly, often with little or no long-term effects.

⇨ THE BAD NEWS

THE BRAIN INJURY

Childhood brain injury has long-term effects, more so than adult brain injury. Sadly, when it comes to an injury to the child's brain, the effect is quite opposite to that on the adult's brain. The injury that has no permanent effect to an adult's brain because it is fully formed can often have catastrophic consequences to the child. This factor is the most overlooked area of injury prognosis. I have handled hundreds of cases where the child, at the time of the injury and immediately thereafter, appeared to rebound quickly and have no permanent deficits; yet, as the childhood years continued, the deficit became more pronounced and more debilitating.

The "why" to this phenomenon comes from recent advances in our knowledge of how and when the child's brain develops. The cover of *Time* magazine on May 10, 2004 proclaimed "Secrets of a Teenage Brain" (Vol 163, No. 19) and the PBS *Frontline* story "Inside the Teenage Brain," first aired in 2002, chronicled our new understanding and has reversed many ways we look at childhood injury prognosis. The following is a portion of the transcript:

NARRATOR: Dr. Giedd of the National Institute of Mental Health gets the use of this imaging machine one night a week to look at the brain structure of normal children. Teens come in and sometimes even sleep in this large magnet, so he can take a long, hard look inside their brains.

Dr. JAY GIEDD: Now, for the first time in our human history, we can actually start exploring the living, growing activity of the human brain.

Five, four, three, two, one, blast off.

NARRATOR: What he discovered in the all-important part of the brain that sits behind the forehead, in an area called the frontal cortex, was an unexpected growth spurt, an overproduction of cells just before puberty.

Dr. JAY GIEDD: This is a process that we knew happened in the womb, maybe even the first 18 months of life. But it was only when we started following the same children by scanning their brains at two-year intervals that we detected a second wave of over-production. And this second wave of over-production is manifest by an actual thickening in the gray matter or the thinking part in the front parts of the brain.

Dr. CHARLES NELSON, University of Minnesota: Many people mistakenly believed that most of the changes occurred in the first few years of life, and then after a child was about three there was actually relatively little change occurring. And we know now that's absolutely incorrect.

Dr. JAY GIEDD: Well, I think the most surprising thing has been how much the teen brain is changing. By age six the brain's already 95 percent of its adult size. But the gray matter or thinking part of the brain continues to thicken throughout childhood as the brain cells grow extra connections, much like a tree growing extra branches, twigs and roots.

NARRATOR: It's like this. The brain grows like a tree. First, there is a flurry of growth. Then, unused branches or pathways are pruned. And it is this pruning that gives the tree its shape for the future.

Full transcript at:
www.pbs.org/wgbh/pages/frontline/shows/teenbrain/etc/script.html

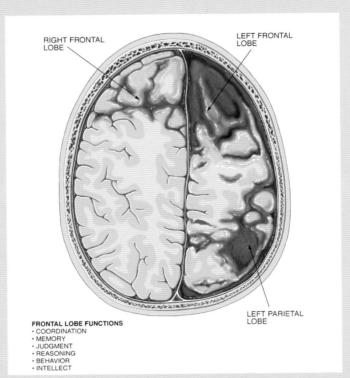

RIGHT FRONTAL LOBE

LEFT FRONTAL LOBE

LEFT PARIETAL LOBE

FRONTAL LOBE FUNCTIONS
· COORDINATION
· MEMORY
· JUDGMENT
· REASONING
· BEHAVIOR
· INTELLECT

The BOTTOM

The medical illustration above is from an MRI of a two-year-old with essentially normal functions. The area of damage (in black) clearly shows the damaged area of the brain which will prevent normal growth and development.

LINE is simple: Assume the child sustains a brain injury at age five, whether because of blunt trauma, oxygen deprivation/asphyxiation, or the spread of disease such meningitis. At age five, the brain is not fully developed; the child is incapable of complex reasoning and logical rationalizing functions. As the brain grows, so does its ability to function at higher levels of thinking and reaction. The current medical literature now holds that the child's brain experiences two major growth spurts rather than one major explosion. The first explosion at ages one and two have been well known for years, but the new advances tell us there is a second and even more profound "spurt" at roughly ages 16 to 17. It is this later spurt when the brain kicks in to a higher functioning capability.

When a child sustains a brain injury at the age of five, the child will often exhibit no deficits; normal developmental landmarks are seen up until the time he or she has the second spurt. The child's injury does not affect the lower reasoning functions of the brain, but when the brain is supposed to kick in to the high level later, because of the damage, it cannot. The deficits can be seen in diminished I.Q., anti-social behavior, reduction in self-esteem and sometimes physical disabilities.

Unfortunately, I have seen this tragedy unfold too many times. Often, when the deficit occurs later, the caregiver does not even suspect the earlier brain injury event because there have been so many "normal" years.

The example I can give is one given to me by one of my experts. He said, "Don, it is like the child can keep up with his peers from age five until age 15, but then because of the other children's advance development, the child falls further behind and the deficit is more pronounced. The child stands still while the peers continue to develop."

Another example is the rings of a tree, similar to that referenced in the PBS special previously noted. When a tree sustains a year of drought, which one can see on the rings of the tree, it may take many years before the damage is seen, the underdevelopment of limbs- even limb death.

As you can see, as a child's lawyer, I must be knowledgeable of this phenomenon because my job is to present the full injury and damage picture of the child to the jury for assessment of lifetime damages. You must know the phenomenon because what may seem to you like an inconsequential injury to the child in early childhood could, in fact, explode in to a nightmare in later life. Thus, with the knowledge of the potential damage, you can take steps as we will outline in this book to prevent the injury from ever occurring.

NEW KNOWLEDGE ON POST-TRAUMATIC STRESS DISORDER EFFECTS

The post-traumatic stress disorder (PTSD) first came to the forefront following the Vietnam War. The survivors, many exhibiting bizarre anti-social and self-destructive behavior, were studied by a number of medical and psychiatric disciplines. From that body of literature, much has been learned about the effect of PTSD, its potential treatment, and to some extent, prevention.

In recent years, the PTSD has been studied extensively in child abuse cases and found to have profound lifetime effects on the abused child. Recently, this same body of knowledge is being applied to children who have suffered extreme emotional injury, often, but not always, coupled with physical injuries.

I have had the privilege of working with two pioneers in this area: one being Dr. Philip Saigh, Ph.D., of New York, and Dr. J. Douglas Bremner, M.D. of Emory University, Atlanta, GA. Together, these two doctors have pioneered the understanding of post-traumatic stress disorder and its lifetime effects on children in all types of physical and emotional injury cases which I have handled.

Note: For further study: Bremner, J. Douglas and Philip Saigh. 1999. *Post Traumatic Stress Disorder*. Boston: Allyn and Bacon Publisher.

Simply stated, often the long-term emotional damage to the child far exceeds the effect of the physical injuries.

I discuss the PTSD because normally injury prevention and ultimate legislation and regulation is an outgrowth of outrageous, headline-grabbing cases that involve severe physical injuries. Unfortunately, because we have only recently been aware that emotional injuries can be as profound and, in many instances, more profound than physical injuries, the prevention recognition and protocol in legislation and regulation is lagging years behind.

THE CHILD DEATH

My responsibility to the reader would not be complete unless I said a word about the impact of the child death. Annually, we see the release of what events in life are the most traumatic. The number 1 on the lists has always been and always will be the death of a child. It's an act against the order of nature. No parent should be forced to bury their child. Those that study death and dying, the field of Teratology, give many reasons for the depth of the grief. I've witnessed that grief in many forms. A mother in West Virginia pleaded that I not visit her daughter's gravesite. I explained that, as her lawyer, it was my duty to see and feel the final resting place, its something I do in all child death cases. When I did visit on a snowy morning, I knew in an instant why Mom didn't want me to go...there on the ground next to the headstone were the child's unopened Christmas presents. Not only for the past Christmas, but for the prior two as well. You see, to the mother, her child was not dead.

For another set of parents, after dinner they did something each night that brought them comfort. Mom would go in the living room and insert a video cassette into the player and return to the dinner table for dessert and a cup of coffee with her husband. The house became full of their deceased seven-year-old son's voice...saying "watch me Mommy...I love you Dad." After the five-minute video was done playing, Mom would dutifully get up, go to the living room and remove the video cassette. Having shared dinner with them one night fully five years after the child's death, no expert was needed to tell me the level of grief in those parents heart. Larry Platt, Ph.D., the nation's leading Teratology expert and an expert I have used in many child death cases, reports that on several occasions, he has witnessed several families replaying video tapes at dinner or during the evening hours.

The devastation of a child's death knows no geographical boundaries. I was in rural Mexico with a client who lost their child, and just as with most of my American families, the deceased child's room was intact, nothing moved or disturbed since the day of the death. This was also true of the countless foreign families I have had the privilege to represent.

So, if the countless child tragedies told in this book, and the many hours of text preparation, can save just one child's life and spare a family of the deepest grief and heartbreak imaginable, this book will have served its purpose.

Part One
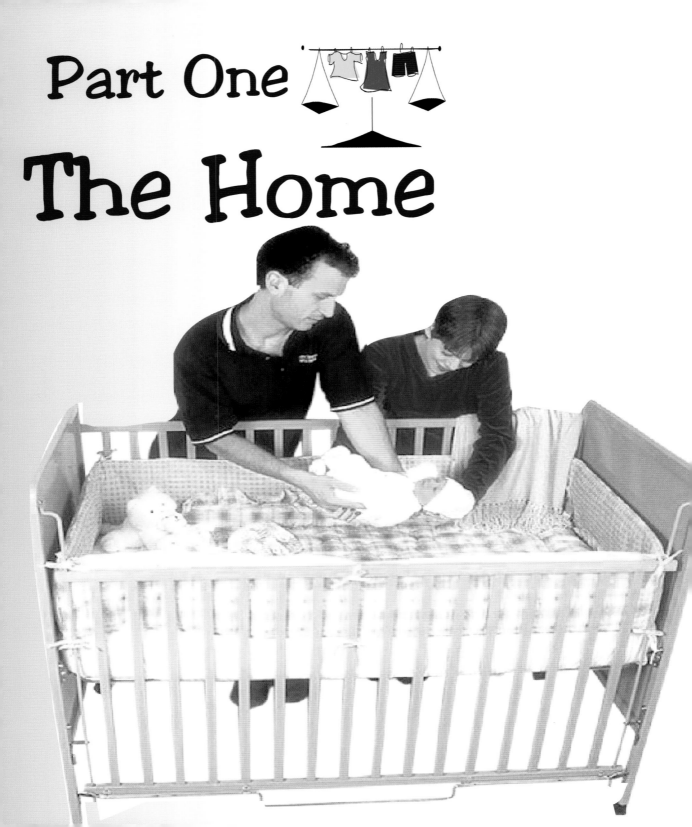
The Home

Preface

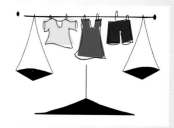

The following nine chapters of Part One discuss the home and how to recognize and remove hazards. But before we proceed, there are two widely used child products present in millions of homes that never should have been purchased, BABY BATH SEATS and BABY WALKERS.

If you possess either or both of these dangerous products, immediately put them in the trash. If you are considering purchasing either or both of these products, STOP...and read the following.

BABY BATH SEATS

According to industry statistics, over 700,000 to 1,000,000 infant bath seats are sold each year in the price range of $10.00 to $20.00 each. These products are primarily for children five to 10 months of age.

In January 2005, Consumer Reports, (www.consumerreports.org) a distinguished independent testing and safety rating national organization, determined there have been over 120 drowning deaths and at least 160 injuries since 1983 while baby bath seats are in use.

The manufacturers prefer that the baby seat be secured to the bathtub floor, and for years, they used suction cups. These suction cups would easily pop off, making the seat unstable so the child could fall over in the water and in the parent's absence could drown.

Beginning in 2000, Consumers Union, the publisher of Consumer Reports and several other prominent consumer organizations, petitioned the Consumer Products Safety Commission (www.cpsc.gov) to ban the seats because of the high death and injury rate.

The industry reacted by devising a new method of holding the seat to the bathtub floor. Instead of using a suction device, a spring clamp would be used to fit over the edge of the tub. This was an entirely voluntary industry safety standard, which took effect in February of 2005. The CPSC has made no effort to ban the bath seats.

Unfortunately, this so-called "safety reform" by the industry has made a bad situation even worse. Under the independent testing of Consumer Reports technicians, the new design failed. "We found that when the tub wall is wet, the seat tipped forward and backward and dislodged with less force than the revised safety standard specifies for suction cup seats,"according to Consumer Reports.

Please remember there is never any valid reason to leave an infant unattended in the tub, however, as urged by Consumer Reports such situations will happen, and therefore the child should not be put in harm's way. With 120 deaths and 160 serious injuries, the bath seat should not be used.

Safe Alternative: Rather than using the deadly baby bath seat, the child should be bathed either in a sink or a small bathing tub, which holds only a small amount of water curdling your child throughout the bath.

BABY WALKERS

According to the American Academy of Pediatrics (www.aap.org), a baby walker sent an estimated 8,800 children younger than 15 months to the hospital in 1999. In 2000, 6,000 children were injured by baby walkers according to the AAP. In 2002, 4,600 children ages four and 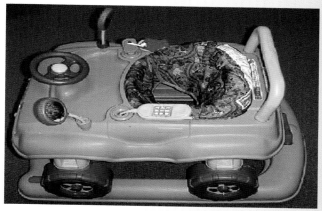 under were treated for baby walker falls, according to www.safekids.org.

Nearly 80 percent of the infants who suffer baby walker injuries are supervised at the time of the incident. More than half of the caregivers are in the same room as the child, according to www.safekids.org.

In 2004, the Canadian government banned the manufacture and sale of all baby walkers. Since 1995, the American Academy of Pediatrics, the largest group of doctors (over 60,000 nationwide) rendering medical care to children, has urged the Consumer Products Safety Commission to stop production and distribution of baby walkers. Joining with the AAP is the National Association for Children's Hospitals and Related Institutions (NACHRI).

The AAP outlines the several ways baby walkers account for serious injuries and deaths occur in the presence or close proximity of the parents:

⇨Rolling down the stairs, which often causes broken bones and severe head injury. This is how most children get hurt in baby walkers.

⇨Getting burned- a child can reach higher when in a walker. A cup of hot coffee on the table, pot handles on the stove, the radiator, fireplace or space heater are all now within a baby's reach.

⇨Drowning- the child can fall into a pool, bathtub or toilet while in the walker.

⇨Being poisoned- reaching high objects is easier in a walker.

As the statistics indicated most of these injuries occur in the presence or close proximity of the parents. The children can move so quickly in the walker (more than three feet per second) that even the best of supervision is not enough.

Safe Alternatives: The American Academy of Pediatrics suggests three alternatives:

⇨ <u>Stationary walkers</u>- these have no wheels, but have seats that rotate at the hip and bounce.

⇨ <u>Playpens</u>- great safety zones for children as they learn to sit, crawl and walk.

⇨ <u>Highchairs</u>- older children often enjoy sitting up in the highchair and playing with toys on the tray.

Although new safety standards were instituted in July of 1997, the injury and death rates have been unaffected.

Some parents and caregivers don't want to discard the walkers because of a mistaken belief that their child will be able to learn walking quicker with the walker. The AAP has dispelled these myths and has stated that walkers may slow a child's progress in walking.

<u>**BOTTOM LINE:**</u>

TOSS OUT THE BABY BATH SEATS AND BABY WALKERS.

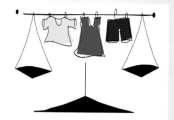

Cribs and Beds

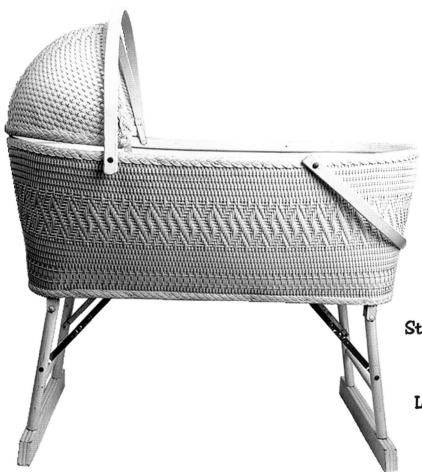

5

Deadly Cribs

The Dawsons had prayed for Josie, their 8 ½ month-old angel. Nora Dawson placed her baby daughter in a portable crib in a room adjacent to the living room. It had been a great day full of family fun, and things were winding down in front of the living room TV. The crib posed no danger because it had been purchased new at a major retail chain store. The Dawsons believed their sleeping baby was safe.

Josie's brother, six years old, was in and out of the baby's room playing with his toys and simply watching his little sister sleep. Nora went in to check on Josie and discovered the crib rails had collapsed. She frantically rushed to the baby only to find her lifeless and not breathing under the blankets.

Josie's father, Pete, called 911. Ironically, he was a volunteer firefighter who had worked with the paramedics, who arrived within minutes. Sadly, the paramedics realized instantly that there was nothing they could do, but tried valiantly nonetheless.

LEGAL ACTION and OUTCOME

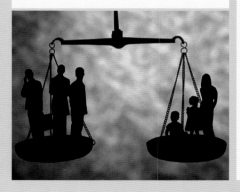

The distraught parents had so many questions about how this could have happened. They hired my law firm to find the truth. My suspicions were raised considerably when a database search found that another child had died in this very same crib. The circumstances of the death were identical- collapsing rails that caused asphyxiation of the baby. Even worse, we discovered that a month before Josie's death, the manufacturer had recalled this very crib, but the Dawsons never received the notice.

Although the crib had killed another baby and was recalled at the insistence of the government, the manufacturer and national retail chain fought the lawsuit for more than two years. First they contended that the death certificate listed the cause of death as Sudden Infant Death Syndrome (SIDS). But the coroner was unaware of the crib's involvement in the death or the past history of the crib. Once he was given this information, the coroner changed the certificate to "asphyxial death due to crib collapse."

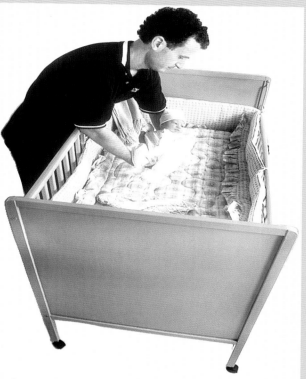

Still denying fault, the manufacturer called an out-of-state forensic pathologist who testified the crib had nothing to do with the baby's death. He could not explain why the baby died other than a SIDS death. Then the company made the most outrageous allegation- the locking mechanism was safe but Josie's six year-old brother had leaned on the rail, causing it to collapse. In other words, a six year-old had caused her death. The little boy said he never touched the rail, and the parents agreed they had never seen him even touch or lean on the rail.

After all the evidence was fully discovered with depositions, the case was settled on the eve of trial. A week before trial, we discovered that the crib's manufacturer had an automatic locking mechanism on all units sold in Europe. However, this very locking feature, which would have saved Josie's life, was absent on all U.S. cribs. Ironically, the company had earlier denied that an automatic locking mechanism was even possible to put on a crib.

Statistics Tell the Story

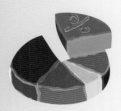

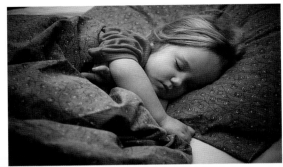

Asphyxiation is the most lethal outcome from a malfunctioning crib. However, there are many reported cases of brain injury and internal organ damage from babies getting caught in open slats. And a number of cases have involved head trauma and lacerations to babies from falling to the floor due to collapsing rails or wide open slats. The following statistics were provided by The Danny Foundation, a public advocacy group dedicated to child safety while sleeping. The Foundation does an outstanding job of awareness and legislative action. Visit the foundation at **www.dannyfoundation.org**.

CRIBS
⇨ Every year, approximately 26 infants die, and another 11,500 are hospitalized from injuries sustained in cribs.

⇨ Most crib deaths occur in second-hand or hand-me-down cribs. Nearly four million babies are born in the United States every year, but just over one million cribs are sold. Thus, many infants are placed in used cribs.

⇨ Cribs are the only baby products manufactured expressly for leaving a child unattended. Therefore, every necessary measure should be taken to ensure that the crib is the safest possible environment.

ADULT BEDS
⇨ Between 1999 and 2001, the Consumer Products Safety Commission (**www.cpsc.gov**) reported over 100 child deaths from suffocation in adult beds.

New Sales

Existing federal and voluntary crib safety guidelines have been effective in addressing most safety hazards associated with new cribs. The Consumer Products Safety Commission (CPSC) published mandatory standards for full-size cribs in 1973 and non-full-size cribs in 1976. CPSC estimates these standards prevent as many as 240 deaths annually.

⇨Voluntary standards were revised in 1986 and 1989 to address entanglement on cornerposts on all cribs and mechanical problems on full-size cribs.

⇨Ten states, AZ, AR, CA, CO, IL, LA, MI, OR, PA and WA, have adopted legislation that would make it illegal to manufacture or sell a crib that does not meet current safety standards.

Resales

In 2003, the *Infant Crib Safety Act* (S-2016) was introduced in the U.S. Senate and House of Representatives (H.R. 3371). The legislation would prohibit the sale, resale, lease or use of secondhand cribs in lodging facilities, daycare centers, etc.

It also adds secondhand cribs to the list of child products covered by the *Federal Hazardous Substances Act*, the law that already applies to new cribs and other children's products. Sadly, this excellent legislation is stalled in Congress.

Taking Action

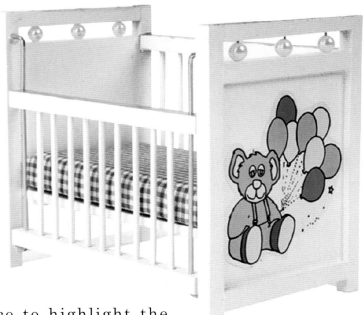

Do not depend on the government to protect, and do not assume the CPSC efforts to address crib hazards have focused on assembly and maintenance problems associated with older cribs. In August of 1995, CPSC was joined by representatives of the American Academy of Pediatrics, the Danny Foundation, the Juvenile Products Manufacturers Association, the Consumer Federation of America and others at a press conference to highlight the hazards of older, used cribs. These groups were also involved in a national campaign to promote safe cribs during Baby Safety Month in September of 1995. As part of this campaign, used crib roundups were held in San Francisco, Denver, Rochester, and Washington, D.C. The campaign received extensive national publicity and was extremely successful in alerting parents and caregivers to important crib safety issues.

Unfortunately, this doesn't change the bottom line: Do not depend on the government to protect and do not assume the crib is safe.

The following checklists will ensure your baby's safety:

⚠ CHECKLIST ⚠

✔	
	Crib Design
1	No older or used cribs with decorative cutouts.
2	Check for recalls.
3	Spaces between slats are safe.
4	No sharp edges.
5	No missing slats.
6	Corner posts no more than 1/6 inch higher than the end panels.
7	No cutout areas on the headboard or footboard.
8	Top rails must be high.
9	Height needs to be addressed with growth.
10	No missing screws or bolts.

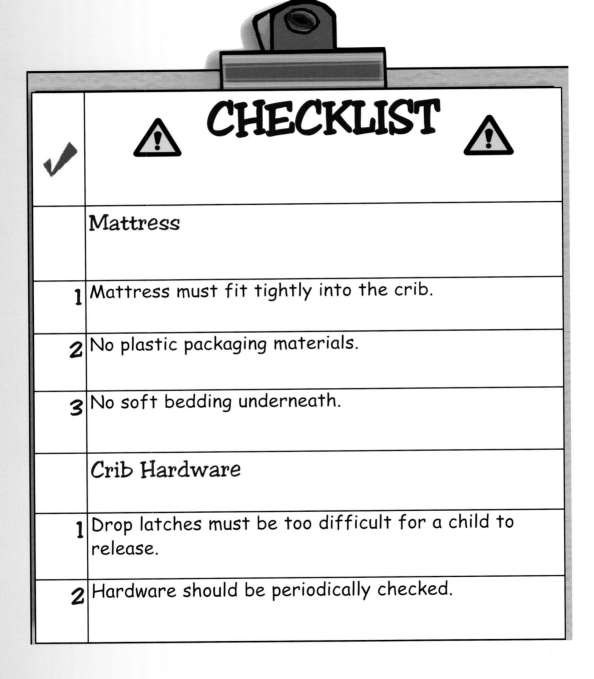

CHECKLIST

✔	⚠	⚠

Mattress

1. Mattress must fit tightly into the crib.

2. No plastic packaging materials.

3. No soft bedding underneath.

Crib Hardware

1. Drop latches must be too difficult for a child to release.

2. Hardware should be periodically checked.

CRIB DESIGN

1. NO OLDER OR USED CRIBS WITH DECORATIVE CUTOUTS.

Grandparents love to provide such cribs for family visits to their home: however, many of these older cribs are unsafe, and many contain lead paint.

2. CHECK FOR RECALLS.

Even if a crib is still on the market, it does not mean it is safe. Go to **www.cpsc.gov/cgi-bin/recalldb/model.asp,** and you will find a directory of products, including cribs. Well over 40 cribs have been recalled since 1986 and three in 2004.

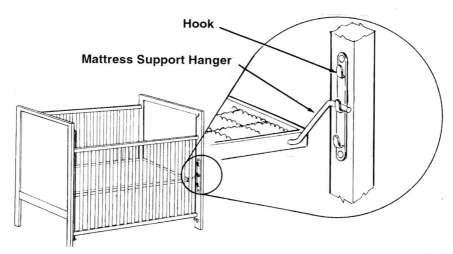

Hook

Mattress Support Hanger

3. SPACES BETWEEN SLATS ARE SAFE.

Slats should be no more than 2 3/8 inches apart. All cribs manufactured after 1974 should meet this strict safety requirement, but measure, nonetheless.

4. NO SHARP EDGES.

Each year, a number of children are found profusely bleeding in their cribs due to sharp edges.

5. NO MISSING SLATS.

Missing slats can cause the child's head to become stuck, creating a lack of oxygen causing brain damage or death.

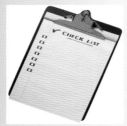

6. CORNER POSTS NO MORE THAN 1/6 INCH HIGHER THAN THE END PANELS.
Children's clothes can easily get caught on anything higher.

7. NO CUTOUT AREAS ON THE HEADBOARD OR FOOTBOARD.

8. TOP RAILS MUST BE HIGH.
When in position, they should be at least 26 inches above the top of the mattress. This assures the child will not be able to climb or fall out.

9. HEIGHT NEEDS TO BE ADDRESSED WITH GROWTH.
As soon as children can pull themselves up to a standing position, set and keep the mattress at its lowest position. Stop using the crib once the height of the top rails is less than three-fourths of the child's height.

10. NO MISSING SCREWS OR BOLTS.
This problem can cause cuts and abrasions.

MATTRESS

1. MATTRESS MUST FIT TIGHTLY INTO THE CRIB.
No more than two fingers should fit between the edge of the mattress and the crib.

2. NO PLASTIC PACKAGING MATERIALS.
Do not use any artificial coverings such as dry-cleaning bags. Plastic can cling to the child's face and should never be used anywhere near the crib.

3. NO SOFT BEDDING UNDERNEATH.
Put your baby to sleep on his or her back or side in the crib with a firm mattress.

CRIB HARDWARE

1. DROP LATCHES MUST BE TOO DIFFICULT FOR A CHILD TO RELEASE.

2. HARDWARE SHOULD BE PERIODICALLY CHECKED.
Parts will often become broken, disengaged or loose.

The following checklist should be used to help prevent child deaths and serious injuries while sleeping on **ADULT BEDS**, as follows:

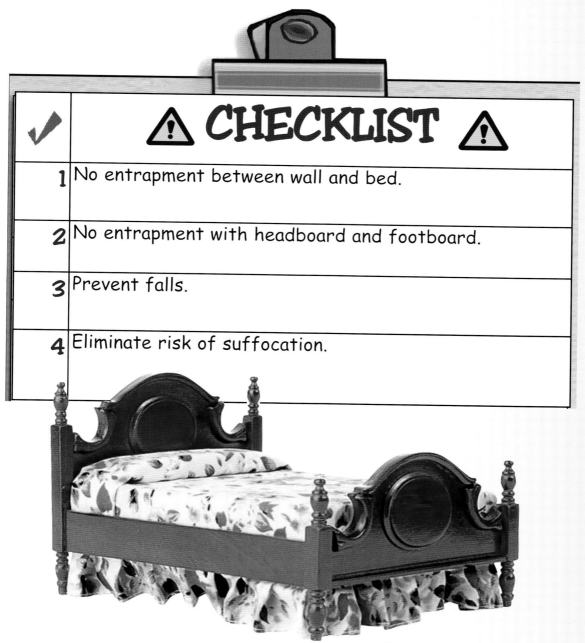

✔	⚠️ CHECKLIST ⚠️
1	No entrapment between wall and bed.
2	No entrapment with headboard and footboard.
3	Prevent falls.
4	Eliminate risk of suffocation.

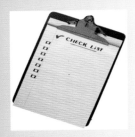

1. NO ENTRAPMENT BETWEEN WALL AND BED.

Most parents believe that if the bed is pushed next to the wall or pillows are placed along the sides of the bed, the small child will be safe. However, further investigation reveals that a child can wedge themselves in very small gaps between the bed and the wall, and a pillow may contribute to suffocation.

2. NO ENTRAPMENT WITH HEADBOARD AND FOOTBOARD.

As discussed in the preceding section, any gaps or decorative cutout on a crib can provide a way for the baby's head to become entrapped thus causing suffocation or brain injury.

3. PREVENT FALLS.

In the blink of an eye, a baby can move from the safe middle of the bed to a tragic fall on the floor. A fall from an adult bed can cause serious injury to a small child, thus the child should be in arm's reach at all times. Creating a barrier of pillows will not work because the inquisitive child views the pillows as a play area to conquer.

4. ELIMINATE RISK OF SUFFOCATION.

While most parents would never put plastic dry cleaning bags near a crib, each year several children are suffocated from dry cleaning bags left on the adult bed with a sleeping child. Also, laundry baskets are often close to a bed and pose an adventure that could cause death by suffocation to a young child.

SPECIAL NOTE ON SOFT BEDS

In the summer of 2002, the American Academy of Pediatrics (www.aap.org) and the Consumer Products Safety Commission (www.cpsc.gov) revised their recommendations on safe bedding practices for children under 12 months of age.

The following checklist should be used to help prevent child deaths and serious injuries while sleeping on **SOFT BEDS**, as follows:

✔	⚠️ CHECKLIST ⚠️
1	Place baby on his/her back on a firm tight-fitting mattress that meets current safety standards.
2	Remove pillows, quilts, comforters, sheepskins, pillow-like stuffed toys and other soft products from the crib.
3	Consider using a sleeper or other sleep clothing as an alternative to blankets, with no other covering.
4	If using a blanket, put baby with feet at the foot of the crib. Tuck a thin blanket around the crib mattress, reaching only as far as the baby's chest.
5	Make sure your baby's head remains uncovered during sleep.
6	Do not place baby on a waterbed, sofa, soft mattress, pillow, or other soft surface.

*Cited verbatim from the Joint Recommendation, CPSC.

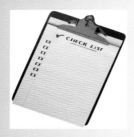

SAFETY ON THE ROAD

For a number of years the hotel industry was oblivious to the need for safe cribs in their hotels. One of the biggest problems continues to be the use of regular bed sheets on the cribs, which become loose-fitting and can strangle a child.

The National SAFE KIDS Campaign, (**www.safekids.org**) has been instrumental in promoting new cribs for hotels. The Starwood Hotel Group, purchased more than 2,000 cribs at a cost of over $1 million for its Westin, Sheraton and Four Points hotels. While the effort of Starwood is commendable, the rest of the industry lags behind. To be absolutely safe, parents and caregivers should bring their own portable cribs. Use the Checklist on these, too!

As a final reminder, please be aware that grandparents, friends and relatives may not always pay the same attention to safety as you do. Therefore, make sure that you take your own crib on the trip or that the crib they provide is as safe as yours.

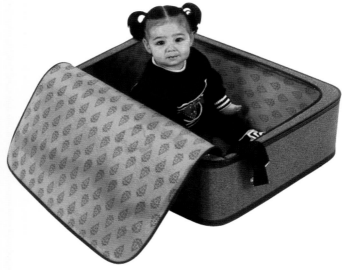

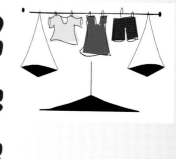

2

Flammable Clothes and Drawstrings

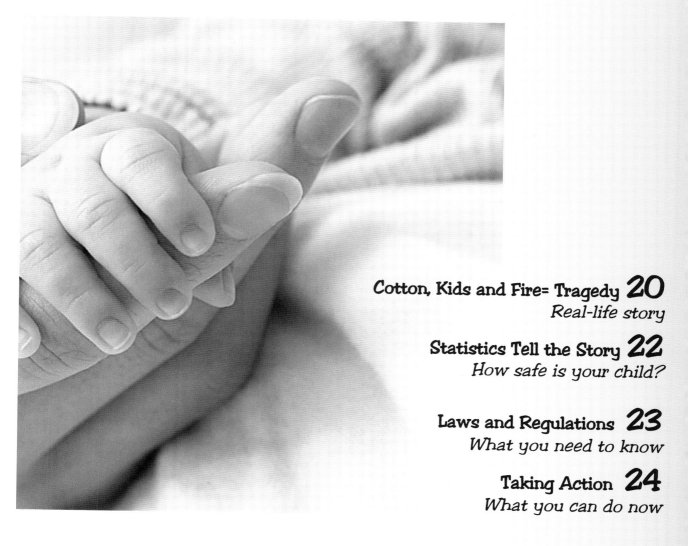

Cotton, Kids and Fire = Tragedy

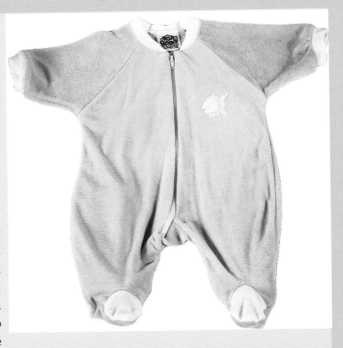

The McElroys were excited to spend the weekend at a rented cabin in the mountains. The cabin was complete with all kitchen utensils, games for the children and just about anything the family needed to have fun. On the first night, the weather turned chilly. Max, the father, started a fire and placed the screen tightly around the fireplace. The family played Monopoly at the table until the parents went on the back porch to watch the sun go down. Emily, the six year-old, and Billy, eleven years old, moved the game board to the floor right in front of the fireplace. Both children had dutifully put on their sleepwear in preparation for bed.

The fire felt good on the cold night and provided excitement for the children, watching the fire burn brightly. Although Emily was a three-foot distance from the guarded fireplace opening, the burning logs shifted suddenly and a burning ember shot out through the opening of the guard. Within an instant the amber landed on the back of Emily's cotton sleepwear and according to Billy, it exploded. Emily's back was instantly in flames. Billy yelled and acted quickly throwing a blanket from the couch on his sister's back. Max and Emily's mother were instantly smothering the flames. The child received superior medical treatment and underwent two surgeries for her burns creating large medical bills and a permanent disfigurement. The family wanted to know if this was preventable.

LEGAL ACTION
and
OUTCOME

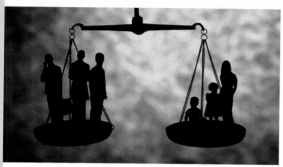

The key fact for the family was how quickly Emily's cotton bedclothes ignited, according to Billy, her brother "exploding." The first task my law firm performed after being retained by the family was to run a complete database search of any similar cases around the country. We located a 1999 Vermont verdict on remarkably similar facts on behalf of a 10 year-old girl who was severely burned when her cotton shirt burst into flames while she was standing before a wood-burning stove.

The important factor we learned from that case was the longstanding lobbying efforts by the cotton industry to stop any labeling of their product as being a fire hazard.

On the strength of that case we filed a claim against the manufacturer of the bedclothes and the retailer who sold the clothing. Our argument was not only the longstanding lobbying against informing the public, but more importantly the volumes of information generated by the cotton industry indicating just how explosive the fabric is. Not only does the fabric "explode," but it also has one of the highest burn rates and is one of the most difficult to extinguish. Further, cotton has what experts term as a "self-propagating" factor, and that is it will re-ignite suddenly even if one believes the fire has been extinguished.

Unfortunately, the retailer had filed bankruptcy subsequent to the sale of the product; therefore, the case proceeded against the manufacturer only.

After retaining fabric experts and documenting the longstanding lobbying efforts of the industry of which the manufacturer was a member of the association, the case was then mediated by court order. After a protracted mediation, the case was ultimately resolved to the client's satisfaction.

Statistics Tell the Story

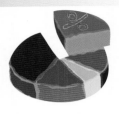

FLAMMABLE CLOTHES

According to the Consumer Products Safety Commission's June 2000 press release, there are nearly 300 emergency room treated burn injuries to children each year from garments that catch fire easily and burn rapidly.

Despite federal legislation requiring standards for flammability on children's sleepwear, there have been many reported cases of the industry ignoring important safety requirements and marketing dangerous sleepwear:

⇨In August of 2001, The Limited Inc. and its subsidiary Masc Industries agreed to pay a half-million-dollar civil penalty for violating the Federal Flammable Fabrics Act "by knowingly importing it and selling flammable children's sleepwear including pajamas and bathrobes." The pajamas were sold as a two-piece pullover or front button style, with sleeveless, short, or long-sleeved tops and bottoms in various colors and patterns sold in girls' sizes six through 14.

⇨In 2000, Kmart recalled 42,000 fleece garments, which failed to meet federal mandatory standards for fabric flammability.

⇨In 1999, Gap Inc. voluntarily recalled 231,000 children's pajamas sold at Gap and Old Navy stores.

⇨Unfortunately, as noted consistently in this book, a recall does not mean that the product is located and destroyed. A recall simply means that the manufacturer does not distribute, and the retail outlets do not sell. Those clothes which are already in consumer hands still pose an inherent danger to children.

⇨Volunteers from the Keenan's Kids Foundation on two occasions have found previously recalled children's sleepwear in Goodwill Clothing Stores and the Salvation Army Thrift Shops.

DRAWSTRINGS

From 1985 to 1999, there were 22 deaths and 48 serious injuries involving entanglement of children's clothing drawstrings, according to the Consumer Products Safety Commission. The drawstrings will entange on playground equipment, school bus doors, or almost any object, thus causing risk of suffocation.

FLAMMABLE CLOTHES

S ince 1972, the Consumer Products Safety Commission has mandated fire standards for children's pajamas. Before these standards an average of 60 children died every year from burning pajamas. After the standards were adopted, the average dropped fewer than four per year.

In 1996, the Consumer Products Safety Commission changed the standards to exempt sleepwear of infants nine months or younger and also tight fitting sleepwear in children's sizes up to 14 years old.

Beginning in June of 2000, the Consumer Products Safety Commission (CPSC) has required all manufacturers of snug fitting cotton sleepwear to attach to the clothing either hangtags or a permanent affixed label to remind consumers that the garment is NOT flame resistant and needs to fit snugly for safety.

Several prominent members of Congress were concerned when the standards that protected children for many years were suddenly watered down. Thus in 2002, Congress introduced the Children's Sleepwear Safety Act (S.2208), which was intended to revoke the 1996 Amendment that loosened the standards for the flammability of children's sleepwear and returned them back to the ones which had kept our children safe since 1972.

In addition to prominent members of Congress and consumer groups, the legislation was also backed by the National Volunteer Fire Counsel and virtually every fire prevention association in the country.

The 2002 Legislation is still pending.

DRAWSTRINGS

No federal legislative exists; however, in 1996 the Consumer Products Safety Commission issued guidelines.

Taking Action

In order to adequately protect your child please follow the checklist below to safeguard while sleeping:

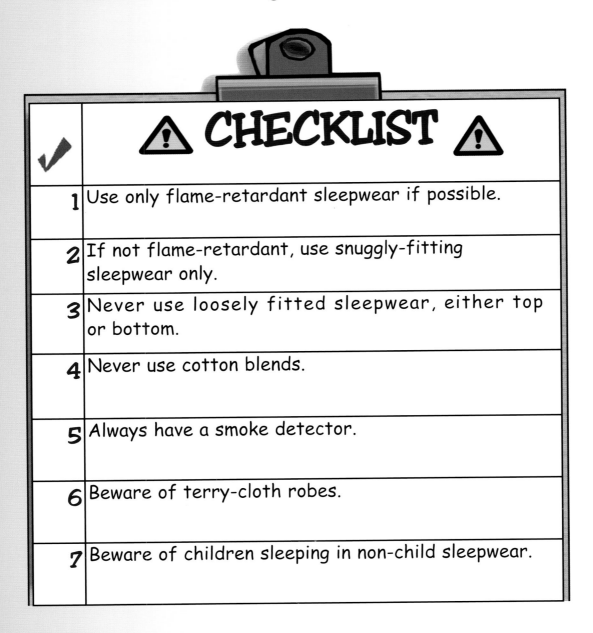

⚠ CHECKLIST ⚠

✔	
1	Use only flame-retardant sleepwear if possible.
2	If not flame-retardant, use snuggly-fitting sleepwear only.
3	Never use loosely fitted sleepwear, either top or bottom.
4	Never use cotton blends.
5	Always have a smoke detector.
6	Beware of terry-cloth robes.
7	Beware of children sleeping in non-child sleepwear.

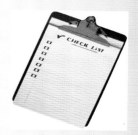

1.USE ONLY FLAME-RETARDANT SLEEPWEAR IF POSSIBLE.

All fabric which has a flame-retardant will have an applicable label. Fabrics such as polyesters are normally the best.

2. IF NOT FLAME-RETARDANT, USE SNUGGLY-FITTING SLEEPWEAR ONLY.

The author strongly believes that the CPSC was wrong in relaxing the regulations and that only flame-resistant fabric should be used in children's sleepwear. However, since the law now permits non-fire-resistant fabrics the following explanation is added:

Snug-fitting sleepwear is made of stretchy cotton or cotton blends that fit extremely close to the child's body. Snug-fitting sleepwear is less likely than loose t-shirts to come in contact with a flame and does not ignite as easily or burn as rapidly because there is little air under the garment to feed a fire.

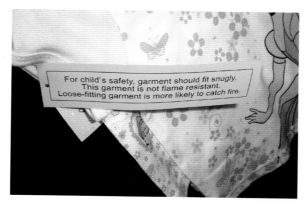

Current Warning Label

Flammable Clothes and Drawstrings 25

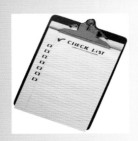

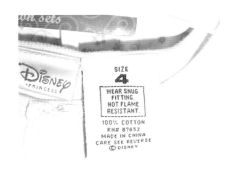

Current Warning Label

Beginning in June of 2000, the Consumer Products Safety Commission (CPSC) has required all manufacturers of snug fitting cotton sleepwear to attach to the clothing either hangtags or a permanent affixed label to remind consumers that the garment is NOT flame- resistant and needs to fit snugly for safety.

3. NEVER USE LOOSELY FITTED SLEEPWEAR, EITHER TOP OR BOTTOM.

Not only can the excess fabric become a target for an ember or a flame, but also as noted above, it provides a lot of oxygen to feed the fire once there is an ignition and becomes extremely dangerous.

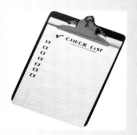

4. NEVER USE COTTON BLENDS.

As indicated from the case story in this chapter, cotton is the most susceptible fabric to quick ignition and burns faster and is harder to extinguish than any fabric. Also noted above it has the "self-propagating" that will often re-ignite after the flames has seemingly been extinguished.

5. ALWAYS HAVE A SMOKE DETECTOR.

Check its functioning and change batteries twice a year. The easiest way to remember is to change the batteries on the day you switch from Daylight Savings Time.

6. BEWARE OF TERRY-CLOTH ROBES.

Terry cloth robes are extremely flammable so don't permit the child to sleep in the robe.

7. BEWARE OF CHILDREN SLEEPING IN NON-CHILD SLEEPWEAR.

The child will desire to sleep in a t-shirt, football jersey, or ballerina suit. Just say no.

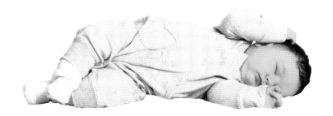

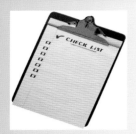

In order to help reduce deaths and serious injuries from **DRAWSTRINGS**, the following checklist should be used:

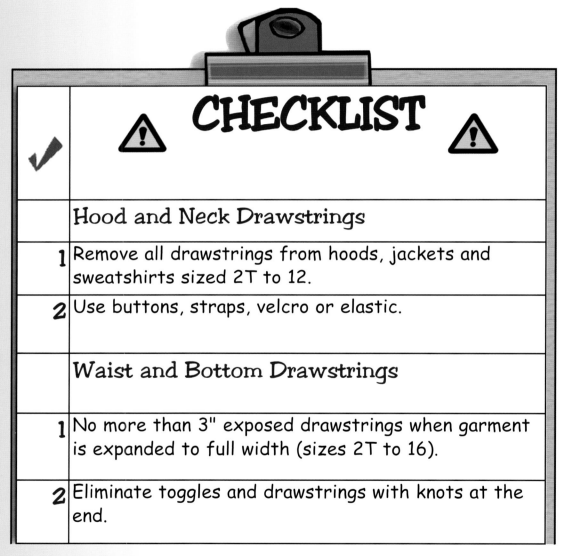

✔	⚠ CHECKLIST ⚠
	Hood and Neck Drawstrings
1	Remove all drawstrings from hoods, jackets and sweatshirts sized 2T to 12.
2	Use buttons, straps, velcro or elastic.
	Waist and Bottom Drawstrings
1	No more than 3" exposed drawstrings when garment is expanded to full width (sizes 2T to 16).
2	Eliminate toggles and drawstrings with knots at the end.

These checklists were adapted from CPSC guidelines.

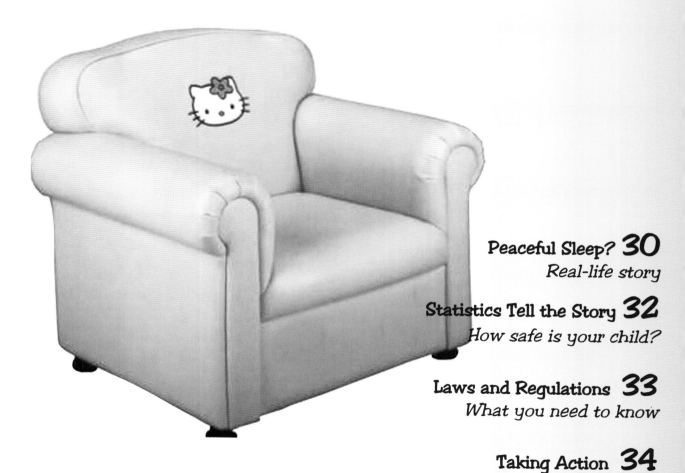

Dangerous Furniture

3

Peaceful Sleep?

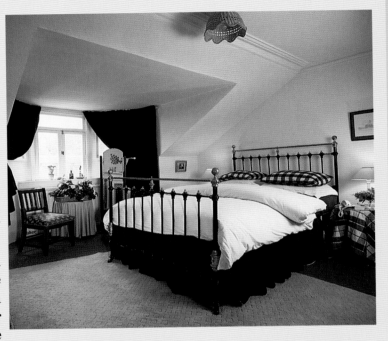

Every Sunday the Wilsons stopped at their rural drugstore to buy a newspaper from the state's capital city. Dad settled in with the sports page and business section, while Mom enjoyed the news and the lifestyle section. The two boys, six and eight years-old, shared the comics. One Sunday the insert section held some especially enticing advertisements. The boys had outgrown their bedroom furniture sometime ago and had been pleading with their parents for an updated look. There in the colorful insert was the room of their dreams. Decorated with a baseball theme, the bedroom sported beds in the shape of baseball mitts, headboards made from baseball bats and even a large circular rug in the shape of a baseball.

The following Saturday, the family made the 350-mile roundtrip to the furniture store in the capital city. Two weeks later, the bedroom set arrived at their home. The boys instantly became the envy of the town, with even the elderly neighbors stopping by for a tour of the newly furnished bedroom.

One night Mike, the older boy, put a floor lamp close to his bed so that he wouldn't disturb his sleeping brother while he read his sports magazine. Mike dozed off without noticing that the floor lamp was tipped so that it touched the foam pillows at the end of the bed. During the early morning hours, the light became hot enough to ignite the pillows. Within seconds the bedroom was engulfed in flames. The boys narrowly escaped with their lives, but their legs were severely burned, and their lungs permanently damaged from smoke inhalation.

The Keenan Law Firm was hired to investigate whether the fire was preventable and, if so, who was at fault. The first suspicion was that a short in the light fixture had caused the fire. But the arson investigators soon discovered that the origin of the fire was the foam pillow, which was made of highly flammable chemicals; chemicals that ignite upon exposure to extreme heat. In fact, all of the new upholstered furniture the family had purchased was made with non-fire-retardant materials, materials that would burn like straw in a wheat field fire.

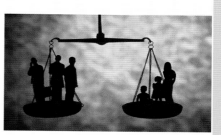

LEGAL ACTION and OUTCOME

With their bedroom purchase, the Wilsons, like millions of Americans, brought into their home a product that accounts for more deaths than any other of the 15,000 products regulated by the Consumer Products Safety Commission. *(John Hendren, "Furniture fires kill as feds debate," AP National Wire 17 April, 1999).*

Our law firm learned the shocking statistics concerning the frequency of these preventable fires. We accumulated evidence that U.S. furniture manufacturers have known for over 30 years that non-fire-retardant fabric and materials lead to a high number of deaths and serious injury. Yet, according to the CPSC 1997 report, the cost of fire retarding a sofa is a mere $24 to $30 *(see Hendren Article note five).*

Had the Wilsons lived in California or Great Britain, where only fire retardant upholstered furniture may be sold, the tragedy would not have happened to their sons.

With the overwhelming evidence of negligence, we filed a lawsuit against the furniture store and the 11 manufacturers who made portions of the bedroom furniture. Once all the incriminating documents were secured, establishing their knowledge of the danger and the low cost of making safe furniture, the case was settled and the boys' future medical bills and economic needs were secured. Unfortunately, as a condition of the settlement, we were required to return all the "smoking guns" we obtained. We had no choice: the parents were adamant that the case be settled, and the judge held the return of the documents to be a lawful request.

Statistics Tell the Story

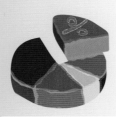

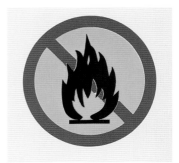

⇨ Upholstered furniture fires are the leading cause of residential fire deaths. (*Consumer Products Safety Commission*. October 1997. "Upholstered Furniture Flammability: Regulatory Options for Small Open Flame and Smoking Material Ignited Fires.")

⇨ Approximately 15 to 25 percent of all civilian fire fatalities are caused by upholstered furniture fires. (Hall, John R., Jr. 2001. "Targeting Upholstered Furniture Fires." *MFPA Journal*. March/April: 58.)

⇨ Between 1980 and 1997, an average of 920 people per year were killed as the result of such fires (Hall article).

PLASTIC BAGS

The CPSC receives an average of 25 reports a year describing a child suffocating from plastic bags. Almost 90 percent are children under one year of age.

LIGHTERS

Children under five years old playing with lighters cause more than 5,000 residential fires a year with 150 deaths and more than 1,000 injuries according to the CPSC. Although the disposable lighter industry was required to make disposable lighters "child resistant," the frequency of fires continues.

WINDOW COVERING CORDS

Between 1991 and 2000, the CPSC reported 160 strangulations involving cords on window blinds: 140 strangulations involved outer pull cords and 20 involved the inner cords that run through the blind sets. The strangulation victims ranged in age from nine months to 17 months.

Sadly, there are no federal laws to protect consumers from the danger of non-fire-retardant upholstered furniture. Well over 30 years ago, the U.S. Department of Congress issued a report titled "Upholstered Furniture Notice of Finding that Flammability Standard or Regulation May be Needed in Institution of Proceedings." In the report, the Secretary of Commerce stated the following:

> There now exists no national flammability standard for upholstered furniture affording the general public protection from an unreasonable risk of fire. Upholstered furniture, therefore, may be produced and made available for consumer purchase which through ordinary use would present a foreseeable hazard and is continuous slow-burning or smoldering and the resultant production of smoke or plastic atmospheres leading to death, injury or significant property damage. (*Report of the Secretary of Commerce* 1972.)

California is the only state that protects its citizens. There are three specific technical bulletins issued by the California Bureau of Home Furnishings and Thermal Insulation that set forth the need to test and the need to fire retard furniture.

PLASTIC BAGS

No laws exist.

LIGHTERS

Since 1994, all disposable lighters must be "child resistant."

WINDOW COVERING CORDS

A CPSC investigation began in 1999, which prompted the industry to redesign their window blinds in November of 2000. Since 1995 the CPSC has eliminated pull cords ending in loops.

Taking Action

Many of the report cards and checklists in this book suggest seven to 10 prevention points. This chapter, however, is very simple. The bottom line is:

To help prevent deaths and serious injury from **UPHOLSTERED FURNITURE**, use the following checklist:

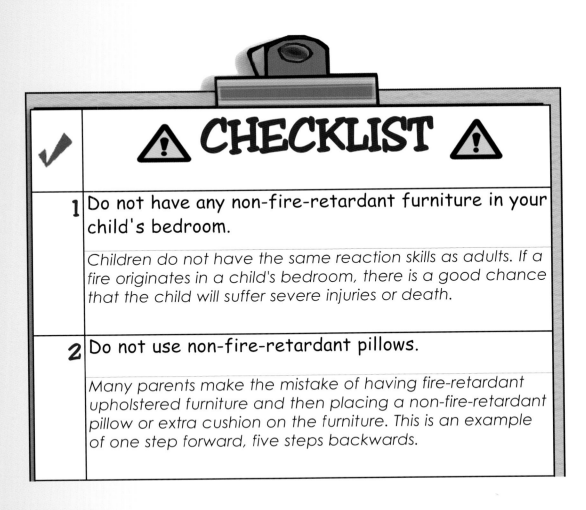

✔ ⚠ **CHECKLIST** ⚠

1 Do not have any non-fire-retardant furniture in your child's bedroom.

Children do not have the same reaction skills as adults. If a fire originates in a child's bedroom, there is a good chance that the child will suffer severe injuries or death.

2 Do not use non-fire-retardant pillows.

Many parents make the mistake of having fire-retardant upholstered furniture and then placing a non-fire-retardant pillow or extra cushion on the furniture. This is an example of one step forward, five steps backwards.

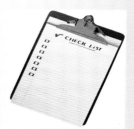

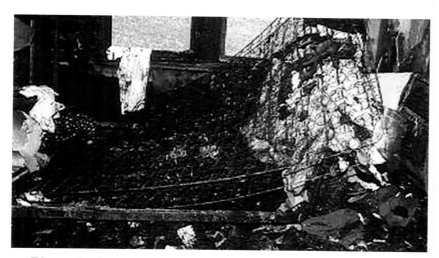

Photo is from actual case showing the fire damage.

Non-fire-retardant upholstered furniture is not the only furniture danger posed to our children. Consider the following:

➥ In the summer of 2004, the U.S. Consumer Products Safety Commission ordered a recall of 3,800 folding chairs manufactured by the Tennessee-based Meco Corporation. These folding chairs were part of a five-piece juvenile table furniture set that included a green table, blue chair, yellow chair, green chair and red chair. All of the red chairs were found to have dangerous levels of lead, posing an immediate health risk. (*Associated Press* August 19, 2004.)

➥ In a landmark Arkansas case, parents purchased a dresser made by the Bassett Furniture Manufacturing Company in anticipation of the birth of their daughter. They placed the dresser in the baby's room and brought her home. Several family members remarked on the "new" smell of the dresser. When the baby developed health problems, including rapid breathing, eye redness, and other chronic ailments, the family had an industrial hygienist run tests on the new dresser. Dangerous levels of formaldehyde had caused severe problems for the baby's undeveloped immune system. (*Lawyer's Weekly USA* November 20, 2004.)

Dangerous Furniture   **35**

To help prevent deaths and serious injury from **PLASTIC BAGS**, use the following checklist:

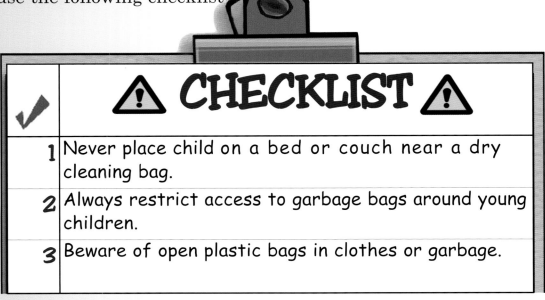

⚠ CHECKLIST ⚠

✔	
1	Never place child on a bed or couch near a dry cleaning bag.
2	Always restrict access to garbage bags around young children.
3	Beware of open plastic bags in clothes or garbage.

To help prevent deaths and serious injuries from **LIGHTERS**, use the following checklist:

⚠ CHECKLIST ⚠

✔	
1	Remember only disposable lighters are "child resistant." Children are attracted to reusable lighters and materials.
2	"Child resistant" lighters are NOT child proof.
3	BOTTOM LINE: Keep all lighters and matches out of a child's reach.

To help prevent deaths and serious injuries from **WINDOW COVERING CORDS**, use the following checklist:

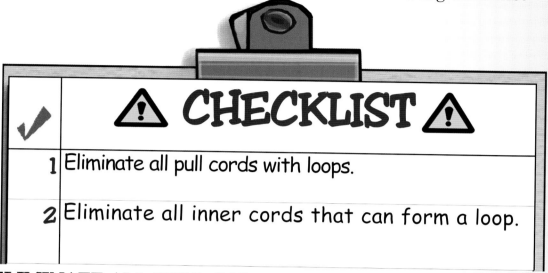

✔	⚠️ CHECKLIST ⚠️
1	Eliminate all pull cords with loops.
2	Eliminate all inner cords that can form a loop.

1. ELIMINATE ALL PULL CORDS WITH LOOPS.

As indicated in the Laws and Regulations section, all pull cords manufactured since 1995 are prohibited from having a loop by federal regulation. However there are millions of blinds in use manufactured prior to 1995. As shown from the statistics, 140 child strangulation occurred when children's neck are caught in the outer cord when a loop exists. Therefore, replace the old cords with ones that have no loop.

2. ELIMINATE ALL INNER CORDS THAT CAN FORM A LOOP.

The inner cords caused 20 strangulations. These entrapments occur when a young child pulls on an inner cord and it forms a loop that a child can hang in. All of these deaths involved children in cribs or playpens placed next to windows. In most cases, the outer pull cords were placed out of reach, but the children still strangled when they pulled on the inner cords of the blinds.

Although in 2000, the industry redesigned their blinds to prevent looping, there exist millions of loop potential blinds in use. Unlike the outer cord where disposal is the only solution, the industry has provided a free kit for consumers to make all blinds safe.

The CPSC has advised: "Consumers who have window blinds with loops should immediately visit WCSC (www.windowcoverings.org) or call (800)506-4636 to receive a free repair kit for each set of blinds. The repair kit includes small plastic attachments to prevent inner cords from being pulled loose.

Instructions for cord stop installation are easy and repair can be done in minutes without removing blinds. (www.windowcoverings.org/howtorepair.html)

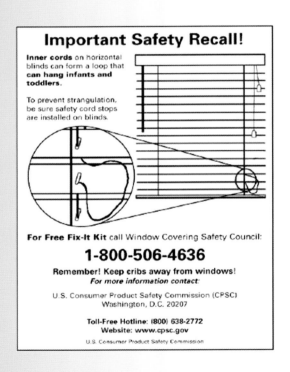

Important Safety Recall!

Inner cords on horizontal blinds can form a loop that **can hang infants and toddlers.**

To prevent strangulation, be sure safety cord stops are installed on blinds.

For Free Fix-It Kit call Window Covering Safety Council:

1-800-506-4636

Remember! Keep cribs away from windows!
For more information contact:

U.S. Consumer Product Safety Commission (CPSC)
Washington, D.C. 20207

Toll-Free Hotline: (800) 638-2772
Website: www.cpsc.gov

U.S. Consumer Product Safety Commission

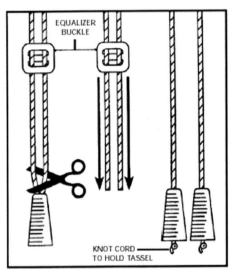

EQUALIZER BUCKLE

KNOT CORD TO HOLD TASSEL

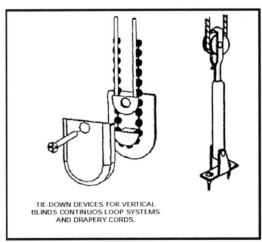

TIE-DOWN DEVICES FOR VERTICAL BLINDS CONTINUOS LOOP SYSTEMS AND DRAPERY CORDS.

These illustrations are courtesy of the Consumer Products Safety Commission (www.cpsc.gov).

4 Choking Hazards

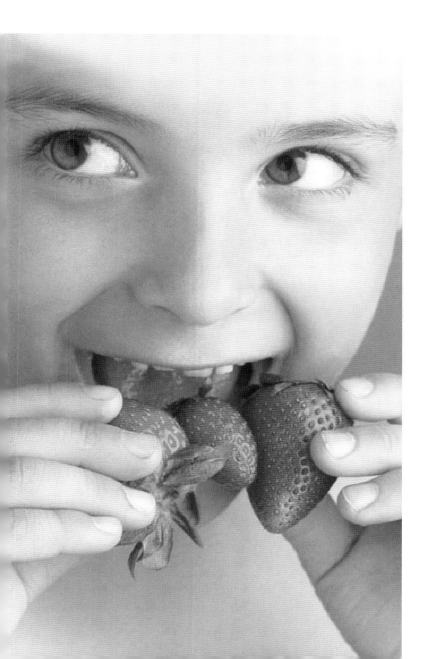

Is Danger Lurking at Your Table?

"Hot dogs and beans, please," said four year-old Jeffrey when asked what he wanted for lunch one summer day. His mother, Jennifer Allen, had fixed that meal many times before but she had always fried and cut up the hotdogs separately before adding them to the beans she'd warmed up in another pot.

But this time Jennifer had bought a can of franks and beans manufactured by a major food company. It had both the hotdogs and beans already mixed together in the same can. As she cooked the contents of the can, Jennifer noticed that the hotdog pieces were a little bigger than the way she cut them but not so large as to alarm her. After the meal, Jeffrey happily ran out and resumed play in the backyard with his friends.

Thirty minutes later Jeffrey's friends came screaming, "Come quick, Mrs. Allen, come quick!" Jennifer was shocked to discover Jeffrey's lifeless body stretched out on the ground in front of her. After calling 9-1-1, she tried to rouse her son while waiting for the ambulance, but had no success. Neither did the EMS team. At four years of age, Jeffrey choked to death in his own backyard.

The autopsy revealed a partially chewed piece of hotdog that obstructed Jeffrey's airway, which caused his death.

LEGAL ACTION and OUTCOME

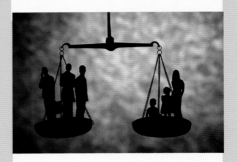

Jennifer Allen, a single parent, asked me to investigate to see if anyone was at fault and whether her son's death had been preventable. I had to inform her that, although such deaths are alarmingly common, under current case law, there was no case. My opinion is that, as public awareness increases in coming years, there will be a potential case.

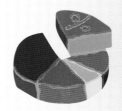

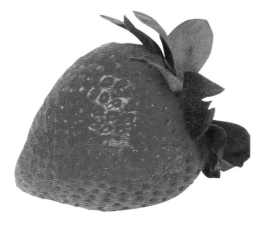

⇨ Approximately every five days a child in the United States dies from choking on food. More than 90 percent of these children are younger than age five, according to 2004 statistics from the Center for Science in the Public Interest *(CSPI)*. (<u>www.cspinet.org</u>)

⇨ In 2001, more than 10,000 children were treated in emergency departments for choking on foods, according to the Centers for Disease Control and Prevention. (<u>www.cdc.gov</u>)

⇨ Nearly 2,000 people (with 62 percent being children) unintentionally swallow "button" batteries used to power hearing aids, watches and calendars, according to the National Capital Poison Center. (<u>www.poison.org</u>)

Laws and Regulations

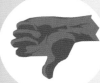

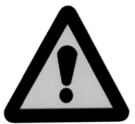

Against the backdrop of this shockingly high frequency rate of death and injury from choking, there are currently no legal protections whatsoever. No laws, no regulations.

In 1984, the Center for Injury Research and Policy at Columbus Children's Hospital issued a report that called for minimum labeling on packages of high risk foods.

In 2004, the Center's director, Dr. Gary Smith, said that "It is remarkable that almost 20 years after our study was published, more has not been done to protect children from the foods that can kill and injure them."

Ironically, I was able to give Jeffrey's mom some peace when I found the July 17, 2003 congressional testimony of Joan Stavros Adler. This bereaved mother tearfully recounted the death of her four year-old son, Eric, from, you guessed it, choking on a hotdog.

The good news is that there is now pending legislation in congress co-sponsored by Congressman Mike Honda (D-CA) and Michael Fergunson (R-NJ) that will establish an Office of Choking Hazards within the Food and Drug Administration. *(House Bill 2773, 2003)*

Also, many congratulations should be given to the perseverance and advocacy of the CSPI, most notably the leadership of Michael F. Jacobson, Ph.D., its executive director. Please note that their Nutrition Action Health Letter is available at their Web site, **www.cspinet.org**.

The proposed office would:
1. Establish a national database of food choking incidents.
2. Authorize the FDA to require informational labels for certain foods.
3. Be able to issue mandatory recalls for subsequent and unacceptable choking hazards.
4. Provide educational materials on food choking prevention to pediatricians and hospitals.

As to the "button batteries," there is no risk of mercury or heavy metal poisoning if swallowed because of a 1996 federal law prohibiting the manufacture of mercuric oxide "button batteries."

Parents and caregivers of children under five years-old should pay special attention when following the checklist below:

⚠️ CHECKLIST ⚠️

✔	
1	Be aware that children under five years old have smaller air passages and less physical ability to cough out obstructions than older children do.
2	Any food that is small, round, cylindrical or compressible poses a choking hazard for children under five years old. *This includes:*
	Hotdogs
	Sausages
	Candies, particularly hard candy
	Chewing gum
	Popcorn
	Nuts
	Seeds
	Grapes
	Peanut butter
	Raisins
	Raw carrots
	Apple chunks
3	Avoid all hard candy for children under five years of age.
4	Avoid serving hotdogs and raw carrots to children under five years old unless you take these steps:
	First, cut them into quarters
	Then, cut them lengthwise
	Finally, cut into small pieces

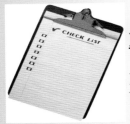

BUTTON BATTERIES

Lodgment in the esophagus is the most dangerous factor of swallowing a button battery. The battery can cause perforation of the esophagus and severe burns. As noted in the Laws and Regulations section, there is no danger in mercury or heavy metal poisoning.

IMPORTANT: When a button battery is swallowed it is impossible to predict whether it will "pass" or get hung up, causing serious damage or death.

Therefore, use the following checklist to help prevent serious injury or death from swallowing a **BUTTON BATTERY** (*guideline is adopted from the NCPC guidelines*):

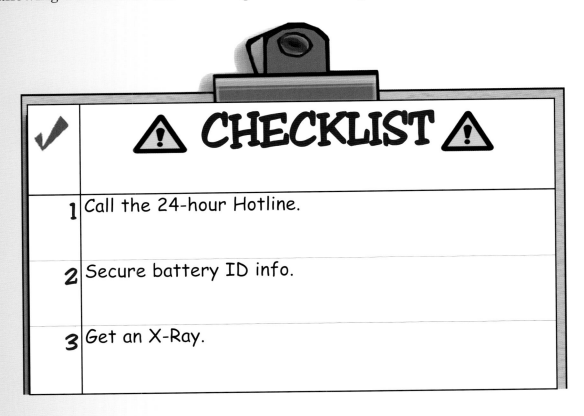

✔	⚠ CHECKLIST ⚠
1	Call the 24-hour Hotline.
2	Secure battery ID info.
3	Get an X-Ray.

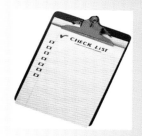

1. CALL THE 24 HOUR HOTLINE.

Call the 24-hour National Button Battery Ingestion Hotline at (202)625-3333 IMMEDIATELY (TDD (202)362-8563). Feel free to call collect. Your physician or emergency room may also call. They are on duty 24-hours a day, 7 days a week.

2. SECURE BATTERY ID INFO.

If available, provide the battery identification number (from the package or from a matching battery).

3. GET AN X-RAY.

An x-ray must be obtained immediately to be sure that the battery has gone through the esophagus into the stomach. Do not wait for symptoms to develop before getting an x-ray. If the battery remains in the esophagus, it must be removed IMMEDIATELY.

CAUTION: Batteries lodged in the esophagus can cause severe burns in JUST TWO HOURS!! Battery removal is done with an endoscope; surgery is rarely, if ever, indicated. Do NOT give ipecac.

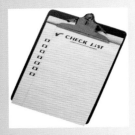

Also note the following advice and recommendations from the National Capital Poison Center (www.poison.org):

If a battery has moved beyond the esophagus, it can be expected to pass by itself. Passage may take many days, or even months. Removal is NOT indicted if the battery has passed beyond the esophagus and the patient is asymptomatic. Once you are sure the battery is not in the esophagus, the patient can be sent home to wait for the battery to pass. Watch for fever, abdominal pain, vomiting or blood in the stools. Report these symptoms immediately to your physician and to the Battery Hotline at (202)625-3333.

Watch the stools until the battery has passed. Clean the battery, tape it to a card or wrap it carefully, and mail it to:

National Capital Poison Center
3201 New Mexico Avenue, Suite 310
Washington, DC 20016

Be sure to include your name, address and telephone number. To learn more about battery ingestions, a toxicologist analyzes each battery and correlates the severity of the patient's clinical effects with the degree of corrosion noted on the battery.

Many thanks for the excellent work of the people at the National Capital Poison Center.

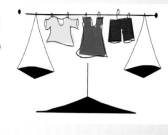

Dangerous Garage Doors

5

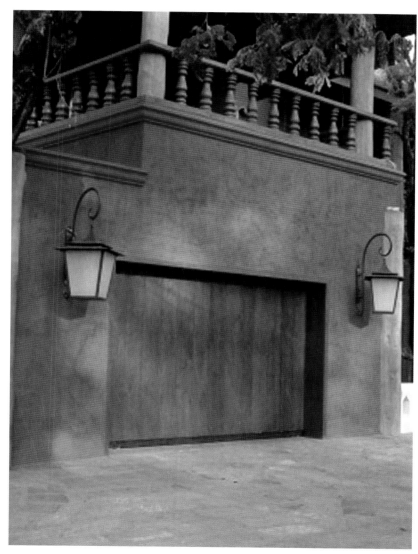

47

Not Kid's Play

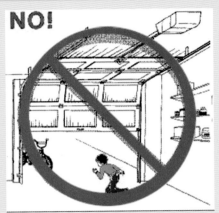

NO!

The Pentacost family loved the charm of their old house. Built in 1930, the home had a large front porch, high ceilings and spacious rooms. The garage was also charming and had a massive door with an operating system that was 15 years old but strong and secure and able to lift the door. One day, nine year-old Daniel was playing with his eight year-old friend, Jamal, at the tool desk of Daniel's father. The tools were stored in the garage. Daniel's mother was busy in the backyard.

After becoming bored with the tools, Daniel and Jamal began playing "Garage Door Chicken," a game taught to them by a neighborhood friend. The game consisted of clicking the remote, then darting in and out under the garage door while it slowly opened and closed. The object, of course, was to successfully beat the garage door.

Suddenly, Jamal knocked his head on the bottom of the garage door. He fell to the floor, dazed and semi-conscious. The advancing door came down directly on Jamal's neck.

Daniel called for his mother, Shirley, to come quickly but it was too late. They found Jamal on the floor of the garage with his neck pinned by the heavy garage door. Shirley refused to believe the boy was dead and did not face reality until the paramedics registered no pulse, heart rate or respirations.

My firm was hired to discover the facts and examine whether anyone was at fault. We learned that a substantial number of children die each year of preventable garage door malfunctions. While older houses have their charm, they also have deadly garage doors.

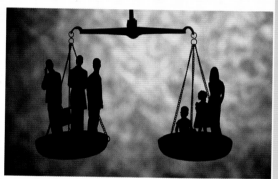

Consider that the garage door is the largest and heaviest moving object in the house. All it takes to move these spring-loaded doors is the simple touch of a button. Add the convenience of mounted key pads and remote controls, and the fact that the garage door is often the most used entrance of the home, and it becomes clear that garage doors must be treated with great caution and respect.

We determined that the manufacturer knew of the dangers their doors posed. In fact, four other children had died under similar circumstances. What's more, the Pentacost family also understood the danger because, a year earlier, the family pet was crushed under the same door that killed Jamal. Yet the family took no precautions following the pet's death.

Jamal's family filed a lawsuit. After expert depositions were taken, we were able to conclude the case to the satisfaction of Jamal's family.

Statistics Tell the Story

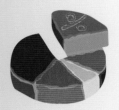

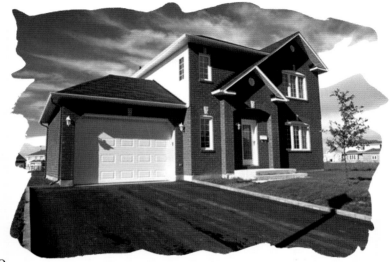

According to the Consumer Products Safety Commission, approximately 60 children between the ages of two and 14 have been trapped and killed under automatic garage doors since March 1982. This is approximately four deaths a year. Untold additional children have suffered brain damage and serious injury.

During the year 2003, there were two brain anoxic injuries from garage door malfunctions, according to the National Electronic Injury Surveillance System.

On January 1, 1993, the Consumer Products Safety Commission began requiring that all new garage doors manufactured or imported for sale in the United States be outfitted with an external entrapment protection system. This system can be an electric eye, a door edge sensor, or any other device that provides equivalent protection. The important thing is that once an object is encountered, the door will reverse. The regulations further state that if an electric eye is used, it should be installed at a height of 4 to 6 inches above the floor.

Please note: This law applies to garage doors manufactured after 1993. It requires no retrofitting of existing garage doors, nor any warnings or notices to be sent. Therefore, there are hundreds of thousands, if not millions, of dangerous garage doors manufactured before 1993 that currently pose lethal dangers to children.

Taking Action

The following is a helpful checklist to remove the hazards of **GARAGE DOORS**:

⚠ CHECKLIST ⚠

✔	
1	Take whatever steps are necessary to ensure that your children are not able to be in proximity to any garage door manufactured before 1993.
2	Test your garage door once a month as outlined. (Following)
3	Mount the keypad wall control at least five feet off the floor so that your children cannot reach it.
4	Keep remote controls out of reach of children.
5	Know how to operate the emergency release.
6	Maintain the garage door according to the manufacturer's recommendations.
7	Teach children the dangers of garage doors and never to "play chicken" or any other game involving garage doors.

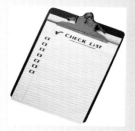

1. TAKE WHATEVER STEPS ARE NECESSARY TO ENSURE THAT YOUR CHILDREN ARE NOT ABLE TO BE IN PROXIMITY TO ANY GARAGE DOOR MANUFACTURED BEFORE 1993.

As we have seen from Jamal's death, care must be taken that your child does not come into contact with any old garage doors at the home of a friend, neighbor or relative.

2. TEST YOUR GARAGE DOOR ONCE A MONTH AS OUTLINED BELOW.

This advice applies even for doors manufactured after 1993. Despite this strong warning from the Consumer Products Safety Commission, Underwriter Laboratories and virtually every child safety group in America, virtually no one tests their door on a monthly basis.

Reverse Testing- Your door should reverse itself automatically when it comes down on a roll of paper towels. Do not use a firm object such as a block of wood for this test, because only a soft object will indicate whether a door would reverse without causing injury to a child in its path. All doors that fail the paper towel test should be disconnected until they are professionally serviced.

Balance- To check its balance, start with the door closed and trip the release mechanism so that you can maneuver the door by hand. If the door is balanced and runs freely on its tracks, you should be able to lift the door smoothly without much effort. The door should stay open three to four feet off the ground.

Force Setting- Test the force setting of the opening by holding the bottom of the door as it closes. If the door does not reverse as you apply moderate resistance, the force setting is dangerously excessive. Consult your owner's manual or the manufacturer's Web site for how to adjust this setting.

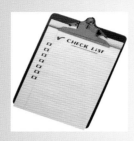

3. MOUNT THE KEYPAD WALL CONTROL AT LEAST FIVE FEET OFF THE FLOOR SO THAT YOUR CHILDREN CANNOT REACH IT.

The location should be where the user has a clear view of the door's motion.

4. KEEP REMOTE CONTROLS OUT OF REACH OF CHILDREN.

Since children are great imitators, they will quickly understand where the remotes are located. If they are within reach, children may be tempted to treat the garage door as a toy.

5. KNOW HOW TO OPERATE THE EMERGENCY RELEASE.

Since 1982, each door opener is required to have an emergency release that disconnects the motorized opening system so that the door can be lifted by hand. This is the only way to free an entrapped child. Look for a short rope hanging from the motor, usually with a red tip or cord.

6. MAINTAIN THE GARAGE DOOR ACCORDING TO THE MANUFACTURER'S RECOMMENDATIONS.

Virtually every manufacture recommends cleaning the tracks and then applying a light machine oil except on plastic parts once a month. As we have seen with the monthly performance checks, far too few households oil their garage doors monthly. This must change to safeguard our children.

7. TEACH CHILDREN THE DANGERS OF GARAGE DOORS AND NEVER TO "PLAY CHICKEN" OR ANY OTHER GAME INVOLVING GARAGE DOORS.

This precaution is listed last because it is the least effective. Statistics tell us over and over again that children who do not properly understand dangers will engage in conduct that they know is prohibited. In fact, some children will engage in the conduct simply because it is prohibited. Therefore, while it is important to instruct children in proper safety measures, wise parents know better than to rely on their children's cooperation to keep them safe.

6
Gun Locks

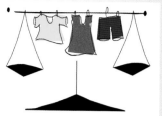

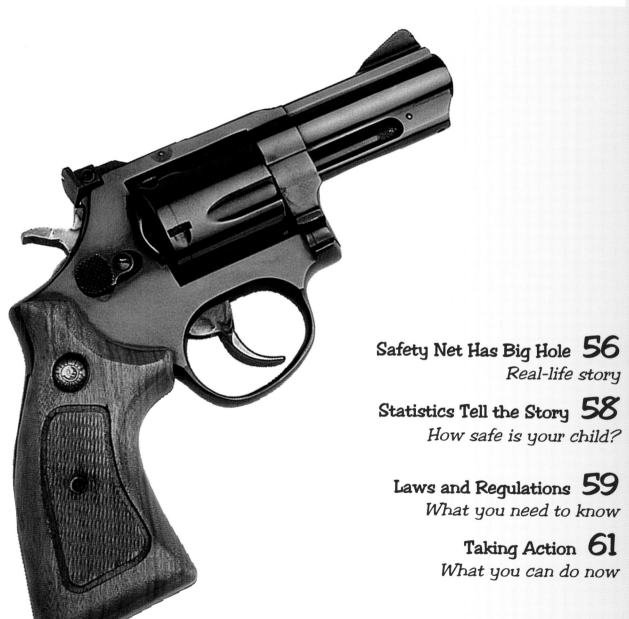

Safety Net Has Big Hole

Patrick and Mildred were frightened by the nightly news reports of home burglaries and violent crimes in nearby neighborhoods. They would never describe themselves as gun lovers, but, like many Americans, they were convinced they needed a small handgun in their home for protection. They realized that meant taking precautions to keep the gun out of the reach of their 10 year-old son, Chad.

They placed the Smith and Wesson 38 in a locked nightstand and the key in the clothes closet on a hook behind hanging ties. To guarantee Chad would never be in harms way because of the gun, they also purchased a safety trigger lock with a combination.

The parents believed that they had accomplished two things. The first was their ability to get the gun quickly in the event that they needed it. Two drills assured them that it would take only five and a half seconds to get the nightstand drawer key, unlock the drawer and spin the three numbers on the gun lock. The second accomplishment was the reassurance that Chad would never fire the gun. Not only would he not be able to find it, he would be stopped by the trigger lock, even if he had the gun in hand.

After school one Wednesday, Chad was home alone for about 30 minutes before Mildred arrived home from work. Patrick would be home another hour later. When Mildred arrived, she knew Chad was home because there was a dirty milk glass on one counter and some cookie crumbs scattered on the other counter. Mildred assumed Chad was upstairs, likely playing on the computer in his room. About 30 minutes later, just as Patrick was pulling in the driveway, a loud shot rang out. Chad's parents thought it might be a firecracker, or worse, maybe the upstairs furnace or hot water heater had blown.

Patrick and Mildred ran upstairs and discovered the unthinkable. Chad was lying on his bedroom floor, the 38 Smith and Wesson right beside him, a screwdriver not far from his hand. Chad had found the closet key, unlocked the nightstand drawer, taken the gun to his bedroom, and with the aid of a screwdriver-removed the trigger lock.

Why did this tragic death occur? Specifically, why had the lock failed? The family hired The Keenan Law Firm to investigate the facts. As described below, Keenan's Kids Foundation has much experience with gun locks; many have saved lives, but a number of poorly constructed gun locks simply do not work.

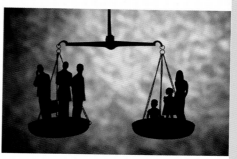

Our firm retained a gun and safety engineer who inspected the lock and gun. He reported that the lock had many breakable plastic parts: it had simply popped open when Chad wedged the screwdriver between the lock and the gun.

We also discovered, after filing the lawsuit, that the manufacturer's cost of this defective gun lock was less than $2. Patrick and Mildred had paid over $20 for the lock. We also learned through the subpoenaing of records that other owners of trigger locks reported similar failures, though fortunately no other deaths had occurred. The company, despite customer complaints and known failures of their product, took no corrective action.

All reputable manufacturers are cognizant of safety in the design of their products. They consider the potential for misuse of their products and will, at the very least, minimize the dangers of misuse. This is the case not only with gun lock manufacturers, but also with manufacturers of lawn mowers, toaster ovens and virtually every manufactured product. In the case of a gun lock, it is clearly foreseeable that a child might attempt to circumvent the lock. A reputable gun lock manufacturing firm, like the company used by our children's foundation (which distributes gun locks for free), will absolutely prevent child misuse.

The case was ultimately settled, and the company now uses all metal parts in their gun locks.

Statistics Tell the Story

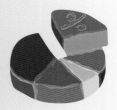

⇨Every two and a half minutes a child dies as a result of a gun discharge.
(*National Association for Gun Safety* 2003.)

⇨ All of the studies indicate that many of these deaths can be preventable.
(Kellerman AL, Somes GS, Rivara FP, et al. 1998. Injuries and Death Due to Firearms in the Home. *Journal of Trauma.* 45(2): 263-267.)

⇨Three-quarters of Americans support a requirement that trigger locks be used for all handguns.
(Smith, Tom W. 2000. *2000 National Gun Policy Survey of the National Opinion Research Center.* National Opinion Research Centers, University of Chicago.)

There are virtually no federal laws concerning mandatory gun locks, standards for gun locks, or safe firearms in general.

In 1998, and again in 1999, Congress attempted to pass the *Child Gun Violence Safety Act (House Bill 4073 and Senate Bill 2185)*. However, on both occasions the act failed to make it out of committee. Faced with the possibility of legislation, however, 20 gun manufacturers agreed to voluntarily ship gun locks with all new guns. Unfortunately, a survey by the Violence Policy Center (VPC) found that only four of these gun manufacturers followed through and included gun locks with their guns.

On the federal level, because of the concern over the safety of gun locks (discussed below), a bipartisan bill was introduced in the 2001 session calling for the Consumer Products Safety Commission to create specific safety standards for the manufacturer of gun locks. Once again, the bill never made it out of committee.

BOTTOM LINE: THERE IS NO FEDERAL LEGISLATION.

Four states-California, Massachusetts, Connecticut, and New Jersey- do require that gun locks be provided with the sale of all new handguns. In fact, the California law *(California Penal Code §1287)* is the most comprehensive of all the state laws. It requires that the California Department of Justice test and approve gun locks to comply with the law. California further requires that a DOJ -approved gun lock be provided with all gun resales.

WHAT HAPPENS WHEN THERE ARE NO MANUFACTURING STANDARDS?

Keenan's Kids Foundation began distributing free gun locks in 1995. To date, over 10,000 of these locks have been distributed through PTA groups and at kiosks at several Atlanta malls. The gun lock we distribute is manufactured by Armadillo Co. It's a model 9000, and it has a perfect safety record.

In 2000, our foundation did a focus group comprised of eight children, ages five to 12. We chose six different manufactured gun locks, and we partnered with a local TV station and the DeKalb County Sheriff's Office in Decatur, Georgia. We conducted the group at the sheriff's office, and it was monitored by the chief firearms instructor for the department.

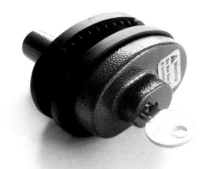

The eight children in the focus group were presented with six locked but unloaded handguns, and they were given one simple task; by whatever means they chose to use, they were to attempt to remove the gun lock from the gun. To accomplish this, the children were provided what they might find at home- a screwdriver, a hammer, pliers and a fork. It took only 20 minutes before six of the gun locks failed and the children were able to unlock the guns. Of the remaining two, one was the gun lock that we have distributed for years. It passed the test. All of the children except one abandoned the task after six were opened and two were not. The only child who continued was a pig-tailed petite little girl of five who kept working. With only one minute to spare before time ran out, she finally popped the other gun lock. The footage of the experiment was run on local TV. The focus group not only opened our eyes, but also the eyes of the public. Gun locks, we learned, are not created equal.

Additionally, consider the following: On July 24, 2000, the well-known Master Lock Company, in cooperation with the U.S. Consumer Products Safety Commission, voluntarily recalled three-quarter million gun locks from retail stores such as Walmart, Kmart and Sports Authority between June 1999 and July 2000. All of the recalled gun locks were keyed trigger locks and were sold separately or in combination with certain Smith and Wesson and Walther handguns.

In good faith, Project Home Safe distributed over 400,000 gun locks free of charge between September 1999 and October 2000. Unfortunately, these gun locks, made in China, gave children access to guns because they could be opened without the key.

BOTTOM LINE: NOT ALL TRIGGER LOCKS ARE CREATED EQUAL.

The following checklist will assist in removing the hazards posed by a gun in the home:

CHECKLIST

✔		
1	If you do not need a gun - do not have a gun around children.	
2	If you can, put the gun in a locked safe or lockbox.	
3	Buy the best trigger lock available.	
4	Not all gunlocks fit all guns.	
5	The trigger lock must have a key lock or combination.	
6	The trigger lock must come with instructions.	
7	Rules one through six apply wherever a child goes throughout the house.	

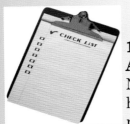

1. IF YOU DO NOT NEED A GUN - DO NOT HAVE A GUN AROUND CHILDREN.

Never assume that a child will be unable to find a gun, no matter how well you hide it. There have been countless studies in which parents have watched through one-way mirrors as their children found and used guns. Further, be aware that while you may not have children in your home, visiting children must be protected by safeguards as well.

2. IF YOU CAN, PUT THE GUN IN A LOCKED SAFE OR LOCKBOX.

If you do not need immediate access to the gun, the safest place to keep it is in a locked gun cabinet or a home safe. Lockboxes are also okay and in the opinion of Dr. Arthur Kellerman, a leading expert in handgun technology, are much better than a trigger lock.

3. BUY THE BEST TRIGGER LOCK AVAILABLE.

United Laboratories has tested and rated several that appear very good. If it looks inexpensive, do not buy it. If there is an overabundance of plastic in the gunlock, do not buy it.

4. NOT ALL GUNLOCKS FIT ALL GUNS.

There are many guns that still can be fired and access to the trigger accomplished even when the gun lock is firmly locked.

5. THE TRIGGER LOCK MUST HAVE A KEY LOCK OR COMBINATION.

Several fly-by-night manufacturers have come up with different variations, which simply do not work.

6. THE TRIGGER LOCK MUST COME WITH INSTRUCTIONS.

If the manufacturer has not taken the time to set forth easy-to-understand directions, then that should tell you what type of attention they paid to the quality of their product.

7. RULES ONE THROUGH SIX APPLY WHEREVER A CHILD GOES THROUGHTOUT THE HOUSE.

It is not enough simply to protect your home by following these guidelines: your child is equally at risk in the homes of neighbors, friends or relatives who have guns. Make sure your child is equally safe away from home.

* A trigger lock is a device which encloses the gun's trigger guard so that the trigger cannot be pulled and thus the bullet will not fire. The lock usually comes in two pieces-one piece has a metal shaft that fits through the gun's trigger guard and into a hole in the other locked piece. The inside face of each piece is made of rubber with small molded rubber cleats that then fit around the trigger guard. The locks are either key or a combination. There is also the cable gun lock, which looks like a bicycle lock with a cable that runs through the barrel of the gun and prohibits the trigger from firing.

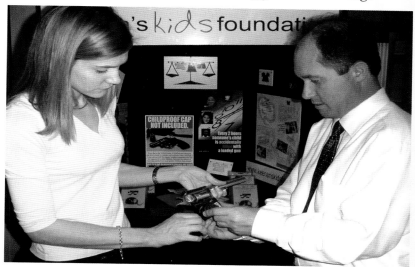

April Swanson and Ben Wilcox demonstrate the proper use of a gun lock.

IMPORTANT NOTE

There is no one thing or one action that will prevent a tragedy like Chad's. Instead, a combination of factors must be at work. One of these factors is education of the child. Dr. Kellerman's research has found that only half of kids ages eight to 12 can tell the difference between a real gun and a toy gun. The NRA, a long opponent of any restriction on firearms, has an education program for children and young adults called Eddie Eagle. To date, "Eddie" has not produced any peer reviewed studies that its education program works. Thus, the child's certificate from an "Eddie Eagle" program creates a false sense of security. Therefore we as adults must take full responsibility, because children do not have the same ability to rationalize as adults. While children may understand the "don'ts," they simply don't understand the "whys." Therefore, while child safety education may be important, no safety program should depend on it.

THE FUTURE

Child advocates agree that action must be taken to reduce dramatically the number of child deaths due to guns. The devil is clearly in the details on this issue. Some advocate complete abolition of guns, others urge strict control of handguns, while others believe that child safety education is the answer. These approaches are unfortunately unrealistic.

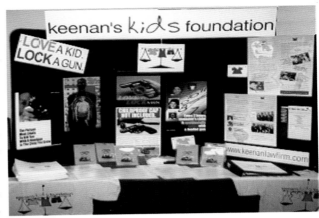

Others allege that gunlocks should be mandatory, and gunlocks must be made safe, therefore, the government must promulgate standards and play a role in the certification safety process.

Clearly, we believe that following all seven points set forth in the "Taking Action" section is the most reasonable approach today in order to bridge us to the future.

There are exciting developments on the horizon in the field of gun safety for children. Arthur Kellerman, M.D., of the Emory School of Public Health is the country's leading advocate for using modern technology to make guns safe for children. Ironically some of this technology dates back to the Civil War when the Colt Company was able to make the first inroads. Guns can be designed so that only adults can fire the weapon. These are so-called "child resistant" guns. Still another option is to make guns with electronics that only recognize the owner, so-called "smart guns."

In 2002, New Jersey passed the first "Smart Gun Law" mandating that all guns sold in New Jersey have the "smart gun" mechanism enabling only the adult owner to fire the gun. The law requires the State Attorney General to certify that the technology is available for retail sale by 2005.

Unfortunately, after a demonstration in December of 2004, state officials announced it would be another five years before technology is ready. (*Associated Press* December 10, 2004, Bayonne, New Jersey.) The smart gun is being developed by the New Jersey Institute of Technology, which just received a 1.1 million dollar federal grant. According to Donald Sebastian, NJIT vice president of research and development, the prototype works more than 90 percent of the time using 20 pressure sensors mounted inside the handle of the gun to distinguish the particular characteristics of the user's grip.

Currently, the "Smart Gun" technology is being incorporated by Metal Storm Inc. of Arlington, Virginia, and once perfected, will be easy for immediate distribution.

The NRA opposes the New Jersey "smart gun" law and advocates no change in existing firearms.

We strongly believe that the Smart Gun is the answer to help prevent the senseless and unnecessary deaths of children, and we applaud the efforts of Arthur Kellerman, M.D., and the research at NJIT.

Manufactured Homes

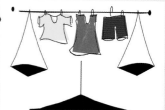

7

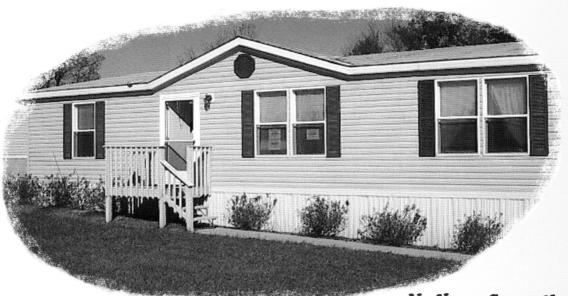

No Home Sweet Home

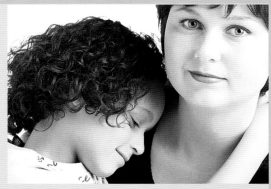

Suzanne and Billy Martin married as teenagers so that their soon-to-be-born child would be born in wedlock. Being married and caring for newborn Bobby put a strain on the fledgling family's finances, so they moved in with Suzanne's parents.

Billy promised that the family would move to a home of their own as soon as possible. Three years later, after a great deal of hard work, the couple had saved enough for a down payment on a new doublewide manufactured home.

Some would call it a mobile home. Suzanne and Billy simply called it their home. At the closing, the Martins paid an additional $957 for what the agent called "tie-downs." They didn't understand what the charge was for, so the agent explained that tie-downs are devices required by federal law to prevent the home from tipping over in high winds.

The property the couple purchased was beautiful rolling land that leveled off at the top of a small hill. The home was delivered to this flat portion on the top of the hill. During installation, Billy noticed the installers putting the home on cinder blocks and attaching a cable to the metal portion of the home to anchor it to the ground.

A fine home it was, a place to experience their first holiday season together as homeowners. Spring rolled around, bringing with it tornado season. Then one night in April, tragedy struck.

A tornado cut a path right through the young couple's property, lifting their home and sending it tumbling down the hill. Both Suzanne and Billy sustained serious injuries, including broken bones, concussions and severe blood loss.

But worst of all was what happened to Bobby, their four year-old son. The boy's tiny body was hurled 25 yards before striking a tree. He died instantly.

Billy instinctively knew this tragedy should not have happened and found his way to my law firm. We have had many experiences with cases of children suffering severe injuries and deaths at the hand of manufactured homes.

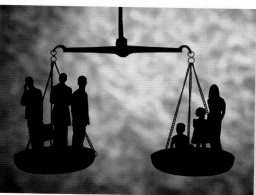

LEGAL ACTION and OUTCOME

We knew all about the federal law that the agent referred to at Billy and Suzanne's closing. This law requires all manufactured homes to be secured to the ground to "guarantee" that they can withstand wind forces up to 115 miles an hour. That wind speed is defined as an F-1 tornado.

Congress in the 1970s was concerned with the high number of tornado injuries and deaths of persons living in mobile homes. They wondered why mobile homes were the first to be destroyed while wood and brick site-built homes were left intact. What Congress decided to require is that the manufactured home industry be held to the same standards as conventional homebuilders.

The law does not specify by what means each manufactured home should be secured. Installers can use concrete bedding, welding, or the tie-down system used on Suzanne's and Billy's home. But all systems are required to withstand winds up to 115 miles an hour.

So this case centered on two issues. First, what was the wind speed at the time of impact? Second, if the wind speed was less than 115 miles an hour, why did the anchoring fail?

The wind speed calculation was easy to determine thanks to the National Weather Service's Storm Tracking Center. Even though several years had passed since Bobby's death, it was a simple matter for me to gain online access to the federal government's weather database to determine the precise wind speed within an eighth of a mile of Suzanne's and Billy's home. According to indisputable government findings, the wind speed was no greater than 87 miles per hour. Thus, the house should have been intact after the tornado.

We next had a team of engineers go to the home site to determine why the anchoring failed. The engineers quickly determined that there were several glaring installation failures. First, the type of anchors used were designed for rock surfaces and not soil. Second, the number of tie-downs needed for this particular home was 16 based on its size and weight. Sadly, the engineers' inspection revealed that the installers had used only four tie-downs. No wonder the home toppled!

The manufactured home company, one of the nation's largest, was notified of the claim, and they quickly offered to mediate the case. The mediation took place over a two-day period and was quite adversarial. I remember well how the executives who made their living from selling these manufactured homes argued that the value of a child's life who lived in a "mobile home" was not worth much. Their hypocrisy was palpable and made us only strive harder for a just resolution, which we achieved at midnight on the second day.

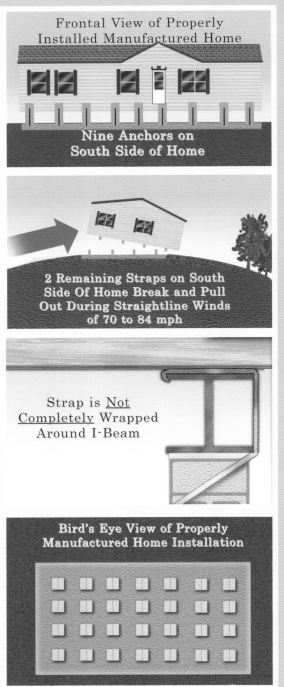

Frontal View of Properly Installed Manufactured Home

Nine Anchors on South Side of Home

2 Remaining Straps on South Side Of Home Break and Pull Out During Straightline Winds of 70 to 84 mph

Strap is Not Completely Wrapped Around I-Beam

Bird's Eye View of Properly Manufactured Home Installation

⇨   In 2001, one out of 7.5 new single-family housing starts were manufactured homes. Manufactured housing retail sales were estimated at $9.5 billion in 2001, according to the Manufactured Housing Institute.

⇨ There are "at least 100 deaths and over 1,000 injuries" from wind-force impact on the homes.

⇨ The U.S. Weather Service in 2003 estimated that over the past 20 years, more than 40 percent of wind-force-induced deaths were caused to persons residing in mobiles homes. This despite the fact that less than seven percent of people lived in mobile homes during the same time period.

⇨ *The Atlanta Journal-Constitution* reported that in 1998 in Georgia and Florida alone, there were 52 deaths in mobile homes that sustained wind-force impact. *(April 18, 2000 edition.)*

Laws and Regulations

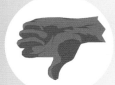

As noted before, the U.S. Congress in 1974 enacted the *Manufactured Housing and Construction Safety Standards Act* of 1974 (42 USCA 5401-5426). In so doing, Congress declared that all manufactured homes should withstand the same wind force as conventional homes, the force of an F-1 tornado.

The U.S. Department of Housing and Urban Development audited the manufactured home industry for compliance with this important law in 1987 and 1997. Sadly, they found the industry to be well out of compliance in both audits.

Congress' attempt to protect manufactured home buyers has in part failed because of lack of enforcement. Many state agencies are headed by former industry representatives.

In 2000, the *Manufactured Housing Improvement Act* was passed into law. However, the legislation creates another layer of bureaucracy - "private sector consensus committee"- that offers little protection for the consumer. The act is entirely funded by the manufactured home industry.

The following is an important checklist in assisting in removal of the hazards of a **MANUFACTURED HOME**:

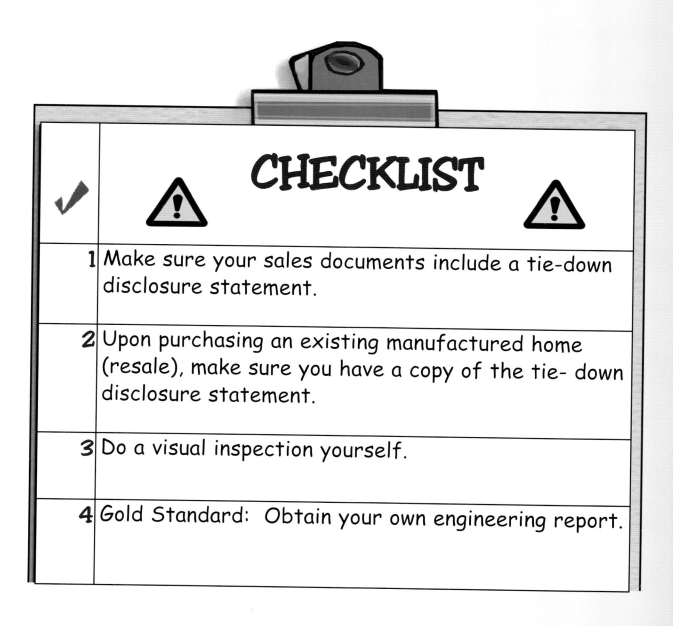

CHECKLIST

✔	⚠	⚠

1 Make sure your sales documents include a tie-down disclosure statement.

2 Upon purchasing an existing manufactured home (resale), make sure you have a copy of the tie- down disclosure statement.

3 Do a visual inspection yourself.

4 Gold Standard: Obtain your own engineering report.

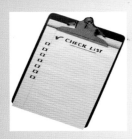

1. MAKE SURE YOUR SALES DOCUMENTS INCLUDE A TIE-DOWN DISCLOSURE STATEMENT.

If you do not receive this disclosure, assume it was not done. Many manufactured homes businesses operate for a year or two before shutting down and starting up under another name.

2.UPON PURCHASING AN EXISTING MANUFACTURED HOME (RESALE), MAKE SURE YOU HAVE A COPY OF THE TIE-DOWN DISCLOSURE STATEMENT.

3. DO A VISUAL INSPECTION YOURSELF.

Although this is not scientific, look under the home. Does it appear to be properly secured? Are the anchors tight? Do there appear to be enough tie-downs to hold the home against heavy winds?

Note: Your visual inspection should be in addition to, not instead of, the tie-down disclosure statement.

4. GOLD STANDARD: OBTAIN YOUR OWN ENGINEERING REPORT.

For an estimated $500 to $800, or even less, you can hire an engineer to perform a site inspection. He or she will perform the necessary calculations to ensure that the home's tie-downs are sufficient to withstand an F-1 tornado.

Note: About 40 percent of all U.S. tornados are F1 with wind speeds above 115 miles per hour. In such storms, manufactured homes as well as concrete, lumber and other structures will be equally devastated. Congress only intended manufactured homes to be as secure as-not more secure than- other structures.

Rule of Thumb: If, after a storm, site-built homes are intact, but manufactured homes are not, then assume the manufactured homes were not tied down properly.

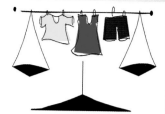

Carbon Monoxide

8

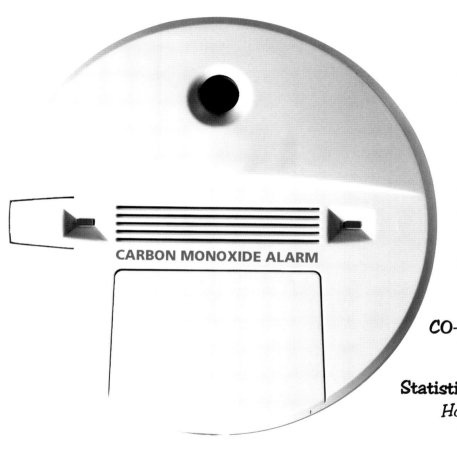

CARBON MONOXIDE ALARM

CO - The Silent Killer

The Parker family was overjoyed when William's new job afforded them an upscale new apartment. The apartment was more spacious and livable than their old one, and they obtained an extra peace of mind when the rental agent informed them that not only did the three-bedroom apartment have a smoke detector, but also a carbon monoxide detector, as well. The Parkers were aware that carbon monoxide posed a threat but, frankly, did not know from what source or how it could be prevented. All they knew was that a detector was a good idea and would tell them when things were bad.

The family, which was comprised of older daughter, Millie, and younger son, Jimmy, had a set schedule on Friday night and Saturday mornings. Friday night they would pick out a rented DVD, order pizza and have a family night. The kids would be able to stay up a little longer, which meant everyone slept in a little longer on Saturday morning.

Therefore, on Saturday morning the Parkers were not alarmed when neither of their children were up running around. However, when 10 o'clock came they decided to knock on the two bedroom doors and get the kids up and moving for a fun Saturday.

What occurred next was far from fun because they could barely arouse Millie, who was immediately groggy and complained of a bad headache and nausea. The younger Jimmy could not be aroused, and an emergency 911 call was made. Both Millie and Jimmy were transported to the emergency room, where the worst fears were realized concerning Jimmy's condition. Despite the valiant efforts of the E.R. team, Jimmy had died. Millie was admitted to the hospital, where toxicology tests indicated severe carbon monoxide poisoning.

The Parkers told the doctors that carbon monoxide poisoning could not have happened because they had a detector in their new apartment, and it never made a noise.

The medical examiner's office, while investigating the cause of Jimmy's death, visited the apartment and noted that the carbon monoxide alarm was located in the ceiling at the rear of the hallway, the furthest distance away from the children's rooms. Further, the detector was battery-operated only and did not activate when the button was pushed.

Because of the questions regarding the carbon monoxide detector, the family retained me to file suit to discover if Jimmy's death and Millie's serious injuries were preventable. The expert we retained told us that there was no local or state law requiring carbon monoxide detectors. Further, that the detector itself lacked a very important safety feature, an LCD light indicator, which would flash and activate a sound when the batteries got dangerously low. At the time of Jimmy's death and Millie's injuries, the batteries were dead, and the Parkers had no way to discover it.

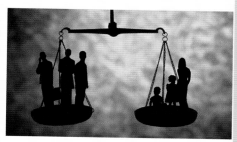

The investigation further revealed that the source of the carbon dioxide had been an older furnace located two floors below the children's bedrooms. The safety valve had become stuck permitting release of carbon monoxide to the outside air, which traveled up the heating ducts and into the children's bedrooms.

In summary, the apartment complex owners were negligent in placing only one carbon monoxide detector in the apartment, rather than having one in each of the sleeping rooms. The apartment complex owners were further negligent by either not hardwiring the detectors directly into the DC current that powers all electrical devices in the apartment or, rather than hardwiring, to instead have purchased carbon monoxide detectors with an LCD indicator that would have alerted that the batteries were not working. Finally, the apartment complex owners were responsible for the creation of the release of the deadly carbon monoxide by not detecting and correcting the defective furnace safety valve.

Remarkably, the apartment complex owners, who own properties throughout the United States, defended by stating they were under no obligation to provide carbon monoxide detectors in the first place and, therefore, their act of placing the detector was one of a good Samaritan, and therefore, they were entitled to immunity under law. The judge ruled that because the Parkers were told about the detector, and that was one of the factors that caused them to sign the lease in the beginning, the case would proceed to trial. The apartment complex owners cross-claimed, bringing an action against the furnace manufacturer, the outside maintenance company and the manufacturer of the carbon monoxide monitor. The monitor company responded to that suit by stating that the apartment complex owners knew what they were buying and simply exercised a choice in buying the cheapest product offered, the one without the LCD indicator. The furnace company responded by stating that the apartment complex owners had not notified them when they had moved the furnace from an older apartment complex into the new building, and therefore, they were not in a position to take corrective action. The maintenance company defended by alleging that it had twice notified the apartment complex owners of the need to not just fix the furnace, but replace it because of its dilapidated condition.

The one thing that was completely true is that the Parkers were pure victims and were not responsible for their son's death or their daughter's serious injuries. As the case proceeded to trial, all parties contributed to a global settlement, with the apartment complex owners paying the vast majority of the funds necessary to secure justice for the Parkers.

Statistics Tell the Story

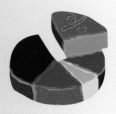

⇨ According to the Consumer Products Safety Commission, a child is far more susceptible to carbon monoxide poisoning because they require more oxygen and use it faster than adults. The CPSC also notes that the child's central nervous system (CNS) is not fully developed and, thus, susceptible to the toxic exposure of carbon monoxide poisoning.

⇨ According to the medical literature, in addition to death carbon monoxide can also cause severe learning disability, memory loss and personality changes.

⇨ Approximately 24 children a year under the age of 14 die from carbon monoxide poisoning, with an additional 3,500 emergency room reported injuries, according to the National SAFE KIDS Campaign, (www.safekids.org), who have been at the forefront for years on carbon monoxide danger and prevention in children.

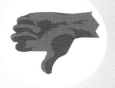

At least five states require carbon monoxide detectors in the home: Alaska, Rhode Island, West Virginia, New Jersey and New York, according to the National SAFE KIDS Campaign. The New York law, which is the most extensive, indicates that all living structures must have carbon monoxide detectors by November of 2004. The law requires a reporting function by landlords and, as well, prescribes penalties for noncompliance. The law also provides penalties for the tenants' willful destruction or removal of carbon monoxide detectors. Finally, the law requires that in all new buildings the carbon monoxide detection must be hardwired and not exclusively battery-operated.

Taking Action

The Consumer Products Safety Commission, in September 1996, in Release 189, proclaimed that carbon monoxide deaths and injuries of children can be prevented. (www.kidsource.com/cpsc/monoxide.html)

Unfortunately, most parents and caregivers are like the Parkers. They do not understand carbon monoxide, nor how it can be prevented, and naively believe that one only needs a detector and the world for children is safe.

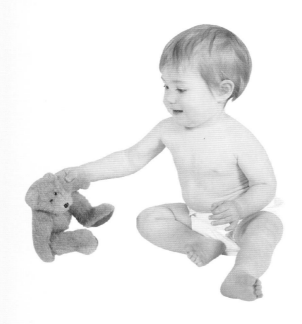

The following checklist will help detect and reduce **CARBON MONOXIDE** poisoning:

✔ CHECKLIST ⚠

✔		
1	Detectors are not a substitute for fixing unsafe conditions.
2	Use only United Laboratories (UL) approved detectors.
3	Install CO detectors in all sleeping rooms.
4	Keep detectors at least 15 feet from furnaces and heat sources.
5	Hardwire detectors if possible.
6	If batteries are used, detector must have an LCD indicating light.
7	Test batteries once a year.
8	Periodically test gas detection function.
9	Beware of recalls.
10	Beware of malfunctioning cutoff switches.
11	Beware of charcoal and gas grills.
12	Never operate a generator inside the home.

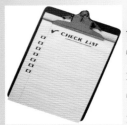

1. DETECTORS ARE NOT A SUBSTITUTE FOR FIXING UNSAFE CONDITIONS.

The best prevention is to make sure that carbon monoxide is not improperly released and, therefore, the detector will not sound.

The most common source of carbon monoxide release is defective appliances, inadequate ventilation, improper flues or vents.

In the September of 1996 CPSC release, the following are recommended to have a yearly inspection by a professional:

Furnaces, hot water heaters and stove. If they burn natural gas, heating oil, wood or other kinds of fuel, these appliances are potentials for carbon monoxide.

Chimneys, flues, vents. Have flues and chimneys inspected before each heating season for leakage or for blockage by creosote or debris. Creosote buildup or leakage could cause black stains on the outside of the chimney or flue. These stains can mean that pollutants are leaking into the house. Have all vents to furnaces, water heaters and boilers checked to make sure they are not loose or disconnected.

High temperature plastic venting (HTPV) pipes. CPSC has received reports that high temperature plastic venting pipes, which are used in mid efficiency appliances, may separate or crack. This could allow carbon monoxide from the furnace to enter the home. Homeowners with gas-fired mid efficiency furnaces or boilers installed between 1987 and 1993 should have them inspected for cracking and separating.

Improper Ventilation. Make sure that your appliances have adequate ventilation. A supply of fresh air is important to help carry pollutants up the chimney, stovepipe or flue and is necessary for the complete combustion of any fuel.

Finally, consumers should be aware that charcoal grills are also a potential source of carbon monoxide. Never use charcoal grills in enclosed spaces such as a home, garage, vehicle or tent, and never bring grills with live coals indoors after use. Never use charcoal grills as an indoor heat source.

2. USE ONLY UNITED LABORATORIES (UL) APPROVED DETECTORS.

The UL symbol is clearly marked on the outside of all smoke detectors. It is highly advisable that the independent testing company of Consumer Reports be consulted. The last ratings of carbon monoxide detectors by Consumer Reports, (www.consumerreports.org), were done in October of 2004, during which 20 different detectors were tested. These included hardwired, battery and combination smoke/carbon dioxide detectors. As with many Consumer Report tests and recommendations, the most expensive carbon monoxide detector ($110) got the lowest rating.

3. INSTALL CO DETECTORS IN ALL SLEEPING ROOMS.

It does not matter where you put it in the child's sleeping area, the detector should be somewhere in the room.

4. KEEP DETECTORS AT LEAST 15 FEET FROM FURNACES AND HEAT SOURCES.

It is very important that a detector be placed within 15 feet of fuel burning appliances because this is the most likely source of carbon monoxide release, and the detector will sound immediately upon improper release.

5. HARDWIRE DETECTORS IF POSSIBLE.

Virtually all direct current detectors also have an auxiliary battery backup so that, if there is a power outage, the batteries will act as a backup. All safety experts agree that direct current hardwire carbon monoxide detectors are the safest because the human error of not replacing batteries is evident.

6. IF BATTERIES ARE USED, DETECTOR MUST HAVE AN LCD INDICATOR LIGHT.

It is remarkable that battery-operated carbon monoxide detectors are even sold in the United States without an LCD indicator. While most consumers, if given the choice, will always opt for the LCD indicator model, unfortunately, as we saw from the tragedy case above, many penny-pinching landlords will opt for the lowest cost, often not even realizing that they have just purchased the carbon monoxide detector which does not have the LCD light. All they realize is they got the lowest price.

7. TEST BATTERIES ONCE A YEAR.

It is recommended that a particular holiday be chosen for the annual battery test. That can be the child's birthday, the Fourth of July, it does not matter what the date so long as it is done once a year on that same date.

8. PERIODICALLY TEST GAS DETECTION FUNCTION.

The only thing that the battery test does is to test whether the battery is working. This sounds like common sense, but a battery test does not indicate whether the carbon monoxide detector in fact can detect carbon monoxide. Many consumers assume that if the batteries work then the detector works. Not so. Consumer Reports (www.consumerreports.org) advises the periodic use of an artificial carbon monoxide aerosol can called Detectagas. These aerosol cans can be purchased over the Internet at www.gogeisel.com for approximately $18. Some hardware stores, in fact, carry this product. Simply spray it near the detector, and if it activates the detector, then, obviously, the detector is working.

Consumer Reports does advise, if you do not wish to go to the trouble of the gas detecting test, peace of mind can be obtained by simply installing a second detector beside the installed detector. The likelihood of both detectors failing is statistically remote.

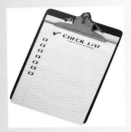

9. BEWARE OF RECALLS.

In recent history, 650,000 carbon monoxide detectors were recalled by the Nighthawk Company. They were made in 1999 and may still be on retail shelves in certain locations around the country. In 1998, 350 Life Saver detectors were recalled. As with other recalls, this does not mean the product was removed from the marketplace: It simply means they are not being sold. There was no attempt to track down the nearly million people who purchased these defective carbon monoxide detectors.

10. BEWARE OF MALFUNCTIONING CUTOFF SWITCHES.

Virtually all appliances, such as boilers and water heaters, have safety cutoff switches that will shut down the appliance or equipment if carbon monoxide is being improperly released. This is the first line of defense. Make sure that all cutoff switches are properly operating, which will probably require a professional or a trained mechanic to make such an inspection.

11. BEWARE OF CHARCOAL AND GAS GRILLS.

According to the Consumer Products Safety Commission, (www.cpsc.gov) there are 20 deaths each year and more than 300 emergency room visits from injuries from carbon monoxide poisoning from charcoal grills. Thus the CPSC recommended:

⇨ NEVER BURN CHARCOAL INSIDE HOMES, VEHICLES, TENTS OR CAMPERS.

⇨ CHARCOAL SHOULD NEVER BE USED INDOORS, EVEN IF VENTILATION IS PROVIDED.

⇨ SINCE CHARCOAL PRODUCES CO FUMES UNTIL THE CHARCOAL IS COMPLETELY EXTINGUISHED, DO NOT STORE THE GRILL INDOORS WITH FRESHLY USED COALS.

As to gas grill the CPSC advises:

⇨ Check grill hoses for cracking, brittleness, holes and leaks. Make sure there are no sharp bends in the hose or tubing.
⇨ Move gas hoses as far as possible from hot surfaces and dripping hot grease.
⇨ Always keep propane gas containers upright.
⇨ Never store or use flammable liquids, like gasoline, near the grill.
⇨ Never keep a filled container in a hot car or car trunk. Heat will cause the gas pressure to increase, which may open the relief valve and allow gas to escape.

12. NEVER OPERATE A GENERATOR INSIDE THE HOME.

In Florida, after the hurricanes many families used gas generators to power their homes which sadly resulted in death. As we will note in Chapter 20 Houseboats, a gas generator near a living space is very dangerous and should always be placed outside with proper venting of the carbon monoxide fumes.

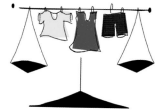

9
Lead Hazards

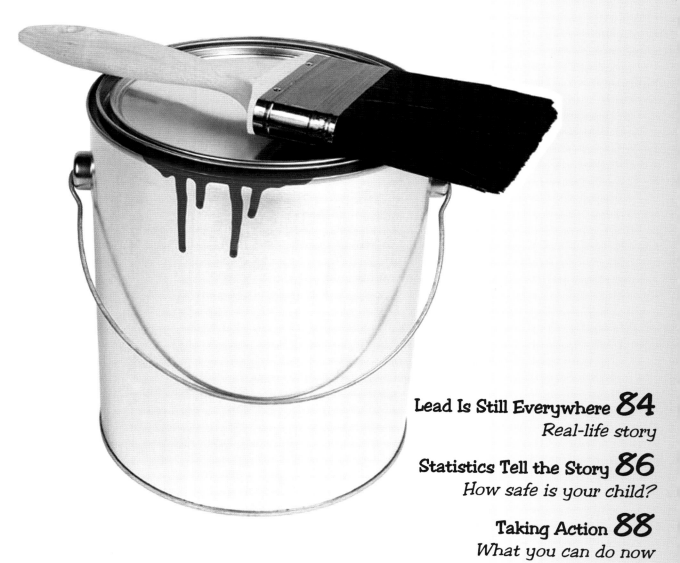

Lead Is Still Everywhere

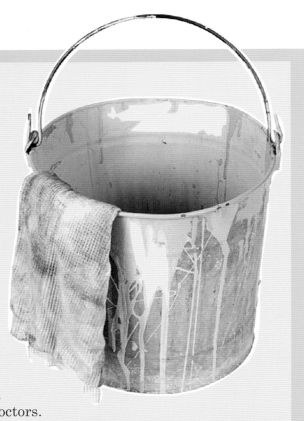

Marlene was a single mom with two small children, Josie and De De. The family had been on a waiting list for a year to get accepted into public housing in their major metropolitan city. Although they moved into the oldest project in the city system, they were nonetheless thankful to have a roof over their heads. Marlene worked every day, and her extended family came by the apartment to take care of the children.

After a short time in their new living space, Marlene began to notice subtle changes in Josie: things just weren't right with her daughter. Marlene took time off from work to take Josie to three different doctors. Despite long waits in the doctors' offices, each doctor, without conducting any tests, told Marlene that she was being an overprotective Mom and that nothing was wrong with Josie.

Almost a month later, though, Josie developed troubling neurological symptoms and was rushed to the emergency room. Initial toxicology screens indicated large levels of lead in the child's blood. Marlene wondered where her daughter could have come in contact with lead and contacted my office for advice.

LEGAL ACTION and OUTCOME

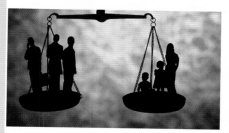

All of the Public Housing Commission meetings are public record, so it did not take long to discover that the Commission knew for several years of the high levels of lead in Marlene's housing project. In fact, the U.S. Department of Housing and Urban Development (HUD) had cited the housing development for not taking action in protecting families from potential lead poisoning. After a lawsuit was filed, the Commission offered the defense that they were in the process of finding land for new housing projects, and they simply had no choice but to offer the existing housing unit, as is, to Marlene and her children.

After reviewing the housing project, our experts developed some simple lead removal procedures that the Housing Authority could have employed at little or no cost to remove the danger. The primary source of lead in the complex was lead paint. Areas that were painted were in such dilapidated condition that the lead paint was chipping onto the ground. Children could receive the highest dosage of lead poisoning possible simply by picking up those chips and placing them in their mouths.

Stripping the old paint off the walls and repainting them with a non-lead paint could easily have removed this danger. (In fact, lead has been removed from paint-by federal law-since the late 1970s.) There is no reason that the housing unit could not have been made safe for this family.

After depositions and expert testimony, the case was ultimately settled to the satisfaction of the family. Josie has been provided with the medical care and treatment she will need for the rest of her life. The specific developmental delays and the reduction in her IQ that she will suffer are not clear at this point, but funds have been set aside in trust to help take care of the damages as needed.

Statistics Tell the Story

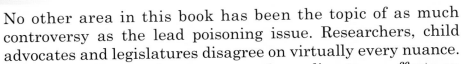

No other area in this book has been the topic of as much controversy as the lead poisoning issue. Researchers, child advocates and legislatures disagree on virtually every nuance. Yet one fact is indisputable: lead exposure can have disastrous effects on a developing young child and even on babies before they are born. In fact, even children who appear healthy, with no symptoms, can exhibit dangerous levels of lead in their bodies. Let us now turn to what constitutes a dangerous level.

CONTROVERSY OVER WHAT LEVELS OF LEAD ARE DANGEROUS

The Centers for Disease Control (CDC) (**www.cdc.gov**) has determined that 10 micrograms per deciliter is a dangerous level of lead in the blood. As late as October of 2004, the CDC issued a bulletin titled "Why Not Change the Blood Lead Level of Concern at this Time?" and in their two-page disposition statement held fast to the 10 micrograms per deciliter cutoff. However, the leading private sector researcher and child advocate in blood level dangers, Bruce Lanphear, M.D., MPH, strongly disagrees. Dr. Lanphear, who is the director of environmental health at the prestigious Cincinnati Children's Hospital Medical Center, challenges the 10 microgram per deciliter cutoff. In a five-year study with Cornell University and the University of Rochester School of Medicine, Dr.Lanphear determined that children experiencing lead exposure levels less than 10 micrograms per deciliter showed pronounced impairment on a number of tests.

Because we must always err on the side of safety with children, most child advocates are urging the adoption of five micrograms per deciliter cutoff and rejecting the higher level embraced by the CDC.

WHAT PERCENTAGE OF CHILDREN HAVE DANGEROUS LEVELS OF LEAD?

The CDC in September of 2004 estimated that 2.2 percent of America's children have lead levels above their 10 micrograms per deciliter limit.

Other researchers have to put the figure of children with elevated lead blood levels at one in 11.

WHAT ARE THE SOURCES OF LEAD INGESTION IN CHILDREN?

According to the EPA, specifically the National Lead Information Center (NLIC) (www.epa.gov/lead/leadinfo.htm), the leading source of lead poisoning comes from homes. Four million homes today have lead paint, and 12 million children live in older housing. It is noted that any home manufactured or built before 1978 has some form of lead-based paint. The CDC estimates that 10 percent of all lead poisoning in children comes from home remodeling.

Dr. Lanphear points out that 10 years ago, 90 percent of his pediatric patients with lead exposure were lower income or poor. Today, over half of his pediatric patients with high levels of lead come from moderate to middle-income families. The remodeling of older homes is thought to be responsible for much of the lead poisoning in middle to upper-middle-class children.

Soil around the home, household dust, drinking water, old painted toys and furniture also constitute primary sources of lead poisoning in children, according to the National Lead Information Center.

Drinking water has also been implicated, but this is yet another area of controversy.

The annual cost of childhood lead poisoning is estimated at $40 billion (*Environmental Health Perspective*. 2002. 110: 721-728.)

Taking Action

Regardless of whether you embrace the 10 microgram per deciliter or the five-microgram per deciliter figure, it is necessary that you take preventative steps as set forth in the following checklist:

✔	⚠ CHECKLIST ⚠
1	Screen your child regularly.
2	Be aware of the house paint danger.
3	Be aware of the dirt danger.
4	Be aware of the water danger.
5	Be aware of the wallpaper danger.
6	Be aware of the vinyl mini-blind danger.
7	Be aware of the playground equipment danger.

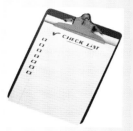

1. SCREEN YOUR CHILD REGULARLY.

A routine lead level test costs approximately $25, and it is noninvasive. Although many states have mandatory testing for all children participating in Medicaid programs, many doctors unfortunately do not routinely test children for lead levels. It is recommended that the test be done every year for the first three years of a child's life and then every five years thereafter.

2. BE AWARE OF THE HOUSE PAINT DANGER.

As noted above, house paint is the primary source of lead poisoning. A home lead test is the only way to determine the exact levels. DO NOT home test yourself. Although there are some kits available, they are extremely unreliable. Instead, call an EPA-certified examiner. Testers in your area can be located by calling the National Lead Information Center and Clearinghouse (NLICC) at 1-800-424-LEAD. Your local HUD office will also have a list.

3. BE AWARE OF THE DIRT DANGER.

Soil can contain lead, particularly if the soil is located near high-traffic roads or around old buildings. Children playing in the soil can track it into the home, where it can be particularly dangerous over long periods of time. If you believe there may be lead in your backyard or neighborhood soil, the EPA-certified tester who tests home paint for lead can also test the soil.

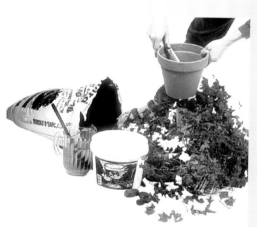

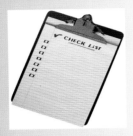

4. BE AWARE OF THE WATER DANGER.

There is much controversy about the danger of lead in drinking water. Once again, the CDC is at the forefront in calming public concern by issuing a number of question and answer documents. These can be found at **www.cdc.gov/lead/quanda.htm**.

In Washington D.C., in 2004, the CDC issued a warning titled "MMWR Concerning High Levels of Lead in Their Drinking Water." Two-thirds of the tested homes had water exceeding the EPA lead limits, some by as many as 36 times, as the result of additives that corroded the lead pipes. Nonetheless, the CDC issued no corrective advice and simply said, "The elevated lead level in D.C. water is under review."

The EPA does advise that you use a NSF International water filter, which has been proven to be effective in removing lead. The NSF International nonprofit testing group has been certifying water filters for a number of years.

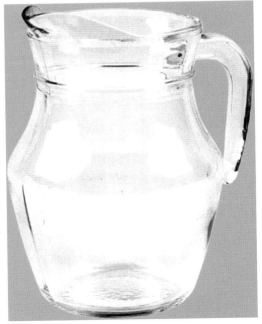

Finally, there are several cities that add substances to the water supply in order to reduce the presence of lead. Check with your local water authority.

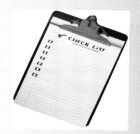

5. BE AWARE OF THE WALLPAPER DANGER.

The NLICC has indicated that some wallpaper is made with lead materials, and wallpaper made prior to 1978 most likely contains lead.

6. BE AWARE OF THE VINYL MINI-BLIND DANGER.

The NLICC and several advocacy groups have noted that several vinyl mini-blinds, particularly those manufactured in the far East, contain high levels of lead and should not be used.

In 2000, Ace Hardware voluntary recalled 87,000 vinyl window blinds that contained lead. Over time, vinyl deteriorates from exposure to sunlight and heat, forms lead dust on the surface of the blinds.

7. BE AWARE OF THE PLAYGROUND EQUIPMENT DANGER.

In Chapter 14 on Playground Hazards, we discuss how the Keenan's Kids Foundation has been conducting playground report cards for a number of years. One of the things participants check for is the presence of lead paint, which can be found on metal equipment in public playgrounds. Our volunteers have found a shocking number of playgrounds with chipped lead paint. In fact, to our surprise, a playground located in one of the affluent areas of Atlanta- circled by multi-million-dollar homes–had three pieces of equipment with chipped lead paint fragments that could easily be ingested by children.

Part Two

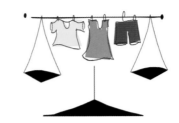

The Neighborhood

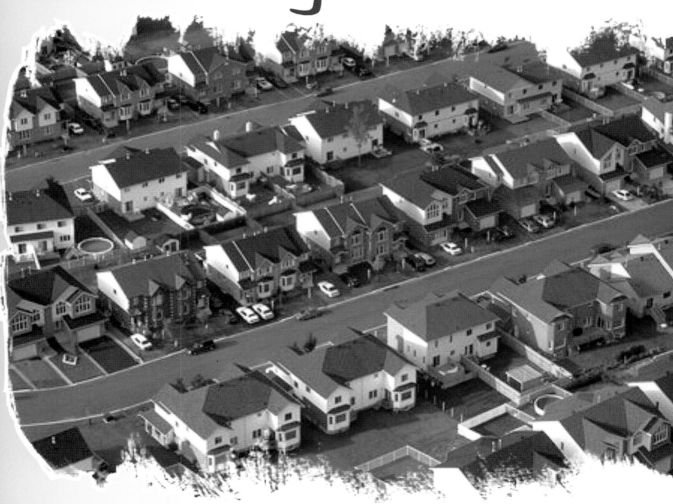

10
Hazards in Outside Play Areas

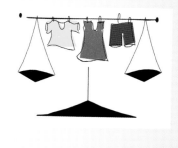

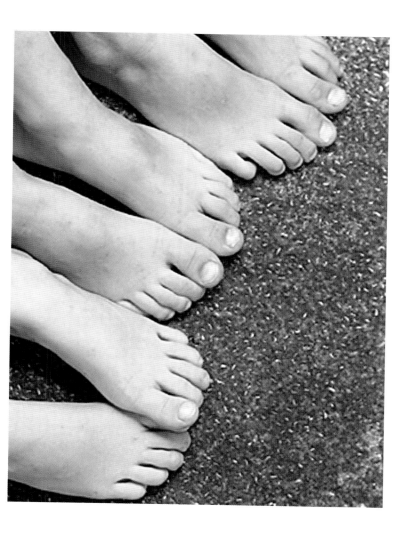

Tarzan at the Wrong Place and Time

Montel was an energetic eight year-old boy living in a typical suburban neighborhood surrounded by his friends. Together they claimed the entire neighborhood to be their play area, and "Tarzan" was one of their favorite games.

Virtually every neighborhood has a telephone pole that is secured in the ground with a GY wire on either side of the pole. These metal GY wires attach to the top of the pole and descend at a roughly 45-degree angle into the ground where they are anchored. These telephone or power poles often contain near the top of the pole a powerful electric transformer; telephone wires as well as cable television wiring are often also attached.

The transformer is the most dangerous element of the telephone/power pole. It emits a strong electrical current, fatal to anyone who touches it. To prevent children from climbing the pole, utility steps are located far above the ground so the children cannot reach them. And whenever anyone is working around the pole, power to the transformer is often turned off in order to prevent any electrocution.

These GY wires, which are fixed to the ground, are very enticing to children who will jump and grab it, swing on it, even make tepees or tents on it by draping blankets over the wire. These GY wires used for play are limited only to the imagination of the child. In Montel and his friend's world, it was the "vine" that helped them play Tarzan. Each of his friends would grab the GY wire and swing as far out as they could, pretending that they were reaching out to another "vine," much like the movie character. The best GY wire for Tarzan play was located two blocks away from Montel's house.

Unfortunately for Montel, the GY wires on that pole were present before a new transformer was affixed to the top of the pole by the power company. Installers, limited in placement by telephone and cable lines, placed the transformer dangerously close to the GY wires. So as the children would swing back and forth on the GY wire, it would reach dangerously close to the transformer at the top of the pole.

Then one day as Montel was swinging back and forth on the GY wire, an ark jumped from the transformer over to the metal GY wire, sending a huge electrical current down the GY wire and through Montel's hands that clutched the wire. The electricity traveled through his entire body as if he had been hit by lightning.

The electricity was so strong that it literally melted Montel's sneaker bottoms onto the grass. According to the neighbors who arrived immediately, Montel hung to life but died moments later on the neighborhood grass before the emergency medical team arrived. The cause of death was electrocution.

A parent's worse nightmare was realized when the mother came running down the sidewalk because she was alarmed at the appearance in the neighborhood of the EMTs. She fainted into the arms of the neighbors. On arriving home within the hour, Montel's father learned the fate of his son.

LEGAL ACTION and OUTCOME

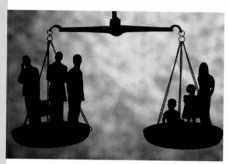

The parents hired me to get the answers and to hold the wrongdoers accountable. Shamefully, when we notified the power company, their first response was that Montel had committed a "criminal trespass." He did not have their permission to use the GY wire, said the company. Such a tactic only enraged the parents further to hold the power company accountable. We hired a former power company safety executive, who found in addition to the improper placement of the transformer (in relationship to the GY wire) the GY wire also lacked an important $30 shield that should have been affixed to the top of the pole connected to the GY wire. This $30 sheath would have prohibited the transfer of electricity down the wire and would have shorted and thus shut off the transformer. We also were able to secure the testimony of construction workers who indicated that they were placed on tight work quotas that made proper installation almost impossible because of the extra time it would take to make the conditions safe. After all of the facts were proven against the power company, they wanted mediation. After two days of heated mediation, the case was settled to the satisfaction of the parents.

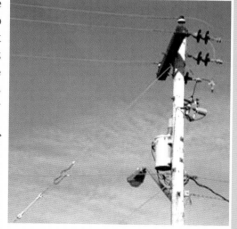

However, as a condition of the settlement the parents demanded that the power company perform a widespread audit of nearly 1,000 power lines located in or near neighborhoods. As a result of this audit, many similar dangerous power lines were retro-fitted, made safe, so that even if children in the future did play "Tarzan" or any other game involving the GY wire, their lives would not be in harm's way.

One final note, parents should be discouraged from permitting their children to play on GY wires or near power lines of any type. However, in the case of Montel's parents, they did not know of their child's activity several blocks away from their home.

Statistics Tell the Story

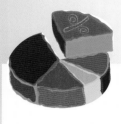

There are a multitude of outside hazards which are found in many neighborhoods that pose serious dangers to children. The following is just a sample:

PESTICIDES

⇨　In 2002, there were an estimated 69,000 children involved in pesticide exposure in and around the home, according to the American Association of Poison Control Centers.

⇨　Nationwide, 85 percent of households store at least one pesticide, and 47 percent of households with children under the age of five were found to store at least one pesticide within reach of children.

⇨　From the 2004 Natural Resources Defense Council database, Note: Just because your home is properly secured from pesticide exposure be aware of your neighbor's homes and your neighborhood.

⇨　Unfortunately science does not know the full effects of pesticide exposure to children. The EPA has tested only nine of 750 registered pesticides for their effects on the developing nervous system (**www.epa.gov**).

LAWNMOWERS

⇨　Power mowers were responsible for over 100,000 injuries each year with 8,000 of the victims being children. Fifteen children died on riding mowers alone.

⇨　In 2001, 9,400 children younger than 18 received emergency treatment for lawnmower related injuries according to the American Academy of Pediatrics (**www.aap.org**). It should be noted that males accounted for approximately three-quarters of the injuries.

TREES

⇨　Although there are no national statistics, in Atlanta, Georgia between January 1, 1999 and August 31, 2004, the medical examiner investigated 65 deaths resulting from falling tree limbs or involving trees in some manner. No specific children's statistics were available. (*Fulton County Medical Examiner* September 2004.)

TRAMPOLINES

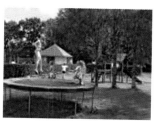

⇨ While many parents recognize the inherent danger of trampolines and thus do not have one in their household, there are many neighborhoods containing one or more trampolines for access by neighborhood children. During the year 2003, there were 80,703 injuries to children ages one month to 14 years reported by the Consumer Product Safety Council (www.cpsc.gov).

⇨ In addition to the high number of injuries from normal use of a trampoline, in 2005 the Consumer Product Safety Commission (www.cpsc.gov) ordered the recall of 1.296 million trampoline manufactured by the JumpKing Corporation due to faulty parts.

ATTRACTIVE NUISANCES

A term used to describe objects which draw children's attention that pose potential dangers such as abandoned appliances, most notably refrigerators, empty buildings and construction sites.

There are no national statistics available; however, the following news reports are noteworthy:

⇨ The most famous incident involved 18-month-old Jessie McClure who was rescued from a well 20 feet deep and eight inches wide in Midland, Texas where she had been trapped for two and a half days.

⇨ In October of 2004, a 22-month-old baby fell 14 feet into an abandoned hole in Frisco City, Alabama where she stayed trapped for 13 hours.

⇨ In May of 2004, a 17-month-old in Mulvane, Kansas fell into a 15 foot well and it took 50 emergency workers to extract her.

FIREWORKS

According to the National Center for Injury Prevention and Control, a division of the Centers for Disease Control (www.cdc.gov) :

⇨ In 2003, four persons died and an estimated 9,300 were treated in emergency departments for fireworks-related injuries in the United States.

⇨ An estimated five percent of fireworks-related injuries treated in emergency departments required hospitalization.

⇨ About 45% of persons injured from fireworks are children ages 14 years and younger.

⇨ Males represent 72% of injuries.

⇨ Children ages five to nine years have the highest injury rate for fireworks-related injuries.

Laws and Regulations

As to pesticides, there are volumes of regulations regarding proper containers, storage requirements and warning label content. Unfortunately adults violate these safety rules everyday and the warning labels are ineffective for children. In fact, one study conducted by the Center for Injury Control at Emory University found that the classic poison symbol of the skull and cross-bones in fact attracted children's curiosity to the container rather than the intended effect of the warning itself.

As to lawnmowers, trees and trampolines, there are virtually no state regulations and not one federal regulation. Also, although the CPSC estimates there are 80 million gas cans across the nation, there is a glaring loophole in the law...these gas cans are not required to be "child resistant."

As to the general topic of attractive nuisances, there does exist state law concerning a landowner's responsibility to cover sink holes and shafts. However, once again adults routinely ignore these regulations. As for abandoned appliances, most cities and counties have laws requiring complete removal or at least removal of the door. These regulations are frequently ignored.

Fireworks: In spite of federal regulations and varying state prohibitions, "class C" and "class B" fireworks are often accessible by the public. It is not uncommon to find fireworks distributors near state borders, where residents of states with strict fireworks regulations can take advantage of more lenient state laws.

Among "class C" fireworks, which are sold legally in some states, bottle rockets can fly into one's face and cause eye injuries; sparklers can ignite one's clothing (sparklers burn at more than 1,000°F); and firecrackers can injure one's hands and face if they explode at close range (*U.S. CPSC 1996*).

Under the *Federal Hazardous Substances Act*, the federal government prohibits the sale of the most dangerous types of fireworks to consumers. These banned fireworks include large reloadable shells, cherry bombs, aerial bombs, M-80 salutes and larger firecrackers that contain more than two grains of powder. Under this same Act, mail-order kits to build these fireworks are also prohibited (*Banned Hazardous Substances* 2001.), information from www.cdc.gov/ncipc/factsheets/fworks.htm.

The following check list should assist you in making the neighborhood and surrounding areas of your child's play safe.

⚠️ CHECKLIST ⚠️

✔	
1	Survey often your child's play area.
2	Know basic lawnmower safety.
3	Trees: know the 3-D's.
4	Eliminate all neighborhood nuisances.
5	Beware of construction sites.
6	Prohibit the use of trampolines.
7	Examine local power line poles.
8	Push ownership of empty lots.
9	Beware of fireworks.
10	BB guns are not toys.
11	Remove five-gallon buckets.
12	Guard halogen torchiere floor lamps.
13	Laundromat stores are not play areas.

1. SURVEY OFTEN YOUR CHILD'S PLAY AREA.

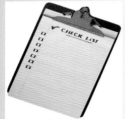

Dangers lurking in a child's world are not always apparent to the parent or care-giver. We do not often get on our hands and knees and go underneath porches or crawl up into storage spaces, but the inquisitive mind of a child takes them often to such places. It is not enough to make your home safe because your child will play in other person's homes and public buildings as well. Therefore, often survey for open chemical cans, gasoline containers, sharp tools, and some of the more obvious dangers such as sink holes, abandoned appliances and dangerous ladders.

2. KNOW BASIC LAWNMOWER SAFETY.

There are three basic rules for lawnmower safety;

Rule 1: Never let a child less than 12 years of age be anywhere near a power mower while in operation.

Rule 2: Make sure your lawnmower and/or your neighbor's mower has a "dead man" control handle that turns the power off when it is let go.

Rule 3: Never let a child younger than 14 years of age operate a ride-on mower.

According to a July 2004 article in *Medical News Today,* (www.medicalnewstoday.com), "despite common belief, lawnmower injuries do not always occur in children operating the mower. Twenty-four percent of pediatric mower-related injuries occur in children younger than the age of five. Children must not be allowed to ride as passengers on mowers or be towed behind mowers in trailers or carts. Young children should not be allowed to play near areas where lawn-mowers are being used."

3. TREES: KNOW THE 3- D'S.

Tree limbs except on rare occasions do not suddenly drop out of the sky. Arborists, professionals dealing with tree maintenance, ask lay people to adopt the 3-D approach: know there are three stages. There is first the disease, followed by the dying process, and then the dead tree limb will fall to the ground. There is usually ample time to realize that a tree limb is vulnerable to falling from the sky. Therefore, with tree limbs that are in the diseased or dying stage, immediate removal should be done.

We will learn in Chapter 14 Playgrounds about the sad death of two-and-a-half-year-old Rachel Johanson from a falling dead tree limb that claimed her life-a dead tree limb that twice had been scheduled to be removed.

4. ELIMINATE ALL NEIGHBORHOOD NUISANCES.

In order to safeguard your child's well-being, you must be proactive on removing the neighborhood nuisances. Require the landowner to haul the appliances away, fill the sink holes and make sure that all construction material is removed after a building project is complete. If a gentle request does not bring about removal, then be insistent in calling city or governmental officials to enforce the law. If possible, if gentle persuasion and contacting the authorities does not work, offer yourself or yourself and others to remove the appliances, fill the sink holes and clean up the construction site. Whatever needs to be done to make the neighborhood safe, do it.

5. BEWARE OF CONSTRUCTION SITES.

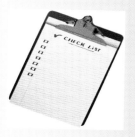

Construction sites are known to attract children. They like the construction site to be their play area. Sitting on the heavy equipment, climbing the ladders, pounding the lumber, the child's imagination has no limit. Beware that often a child would rather play on a construction area than on a ball field. Therefore, careful attention to making sure that dangerous equipment and conditions are properly secured away from the harm of the child.

6. PROHIBIT THE USE OF TRAMPOLINES.

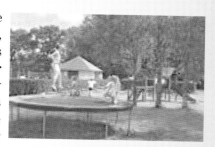

The American Academy of Pediatricians, which comprises the largest group of physicians whose role is to treat injuries of children, has for many years been on record as demanding that trampolines not be used with children under any circumstances. Their May 1999 policy statement reads as follows: "The injury data support the American Academy of Pediatrics reaffirmation of its recommendation that trampolines should NEVER be used in the home environment, in routine physical education classes, or in outdoor playgrounds." The statement could not be clearer.

7. EXAMINE LOCAL POWER LINE POLES.

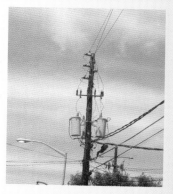

As we saw from the case story of Montel that opened this chapter, there are deadly dangers of closely configured power lines. The transformer is usually easily identifiable and should not have a GY wire anywhere close to it. Further, there should not be any other wires close to the transformer that come to the ground in close proximity of the child's play. As we saw from the case story, the GY lines or any wires within the reach of the child attract child's play. If you do view a circumstance which your gut tells you is dangerous, contact the local authorities and be persistent until you get the proper answers.

8. PUSH OWNERSHIP OF EMPTY LOTS.

According to the EPA (www.epa.gov), empty lots pose a significant risk to children in urban areas because they can contain dangerous chemicals as well as act as a dumping site for appliances, sharp objects and other items which could hurt or kill children. The EPA has worked with local cities to urge transfer of vacant lots to local residents. Their most notable project was in Providence, RI where there were over 4,000 vacant and abandoned lots. The EPA, together with local officials and community groups, transferred ownership of these lots to local residents for the cost of $1 in exchange for the new owners promise to clean and make safe the empty lots.

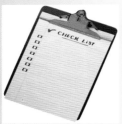

9. BEWARE OF FIREWORKS.

Unsupervised children have a 11 times greater chance of injury according to a 1996 study by the Consumer Product Safety Commission (www.cpsc.gov). Being a child carries inherent risks. First, their curiosity often supersedes their sense of safety. Second, they lack the hand/eye coordination of adults. Therefore, children often get too close, don't know the proper procedure to ignite and disaster occurs.

IMPORTANT: Many children are injured when playing at their friend's home where the supervision is lacking. Also, children often find fireworks that adults thought were safely hidden away from children. If you use fireworks, use all you have; do not store.

10. BB GUNS ARE NOT TOYS.

Four deaths a year occur with BB guns, according to Consumer Products Safety Commission (CPSC) (www.cpsc.gov). Some BB guns have muzzle velocities higher than 350 feet a second. Therefore the CPSC recommends that only those over of 16 years of age should use.

11. REMOVE FIVE-GALLON BUCKETS.

In less than 20 years, the CPSC (www.cpsc.gov) has reported 275 child deaths by drowning and 30 serious hospitalizations from five-gallon buckets containing liquids, some with only small amounts of liquids. Children are curious and are attracted to water. Most five-gallon buckets are 14 inches high, which is about half the height of a young child. Therefore, top heavy infants and toddlers are unable to free themselves when they fall and thus can drown in a small amount of water.

Don't leave any water or liquid in the five-gallon buckets around children under any circumstance.

12. GUARD HALOGEN TORCHIERE FLOOR LAMPS.

Since 1992, the CPSC (www.cpsc.gov) has reported 189 fires and 12 deaths, of which 10 were children, from halogen torchiere lamps. Since 1997, most HT lamps have been manufactured with a wire guard; however, the CPSC warns the guard is only effective with bulbs 300 watts or below. CPSC also recommends:

⇨ Never place the lamp near curtains or other cloth window treatments.
⇨ Never drape clothes over the lamp.
⇨ Keep the lamp away from bedding.
⇨ Never leave the lamp on when you leave a room or are not at home.
⇨ To reduce the likelihood of tipover, keep children and pets away from the lamp.
⇨ Only use a halogen bulb of 300 watts or less in the lamp.

13. LAUNDROMAT STORES ARE NOT PLAY AREAS.

Children love to climb into coin-operated washers. There have been many reported deaths where the machine started before the coins were inserted.
(*Associated Press* August 5, 2005. Reports 6 deaths since 1986.)

Neighborhood Animals

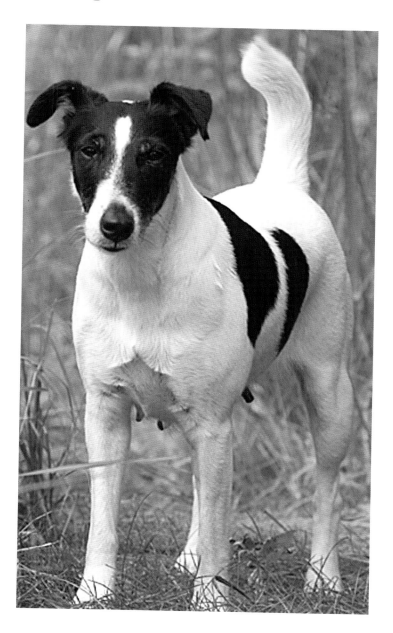

Man's Best Friend is Little Girl's Enemy

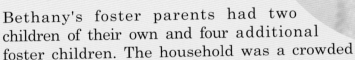

Bethany did not have a happy start in life. Her father was an alcoholic who regularly beat her mother. Bethany's mother became addicted to painkillers and admitted herself to a rehabilitation program. The State Child Protective Agency stepped in and placed seven year-old Bethany in foster care, where she would be safe until her parents could provide a stable home for her.

Bethany's foster parents had two children of their own and four additional foster children. The household was a crowded one, but Bethany was happy to be out of harm's way. Besides, Bethany found peace and quiet in the backyard, where she would sit under the elm tree and read or daydream. One day, while Bethany sat in the yard, a neighbor's four-year-old Rottweiler meandered slowly across the yard. Bethany, who had never seen a dog that large, was petrified and began to cry. Her crying attracted the dog, which came closer. Bethany then began screaming, further agitating the dog. Disaster fully struck when the child began to run, overcome with the need for flight.

The dog gave chase. Bethany stumbled. The dog began to tear and maul her legs, then her buttocks, her face, and her skull. The actions of a resourceful neighbor finally caused the dog to retreat, but not before it inflicted bites and tears that required over 110 stitches.

During her hospitalization, Bethany received transfusions to replace 50 percent of her body's blood volume. She has a permanent limp and lifelong scars.

Because of her disabilities and medical expenses, Bethany's newly appointed guardian hired The Keenan Law Firm to bring a claim on her behalf. Our investigation revealed that the dog had previously bitten two other children. The neighborhood newspaper boy had even abandoned his bike delivery because of the danger of this dog. His mother now drives him on his paper route when he is in the vicinity of the dog.

LEGAL ACTION and OUTCOME

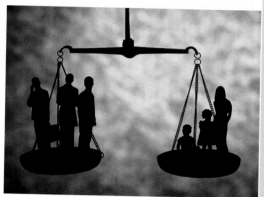

The dog owner claimed not to know anything about the past violent history of the dog, even though the children who had been bitten and their parents testified that they notified the owner of the assaults. One parent had even sent a letter, and one had called the police. The owner took no responsibility.

Ultimately, on the eve of the scheduled trial, the insurance company for the dog owner- over the owner's objections- paid the policy limits of his homeowner's policy, thus ending the lawsuit. Bethany's life is forever changed, but she now has funds to help take care of her, including her medical needs and her college education.

Statistics Tell the Story

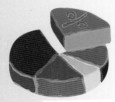

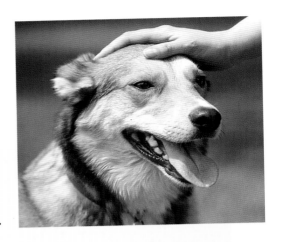

Unfortunately, Bethany's experience isn't unique. News stories tell of infants taken from their cradles by dogs and children being bitten in the face, mauled, or killed.

⇨ Dogs bite 4.7 million Americans every year. (*CDC, National Center for Injury Prevention and Control.*)

⇨ In 2001, 368,245 people were treated for dog bite-related injuries. (*CDC.*)

⇨ About 42 percent of dog bites occur among children less than 14 years of age. (*CDC.*)

⇨ The majority of injuries to children under four years of age are to the head and neck area. (*CDC.*)

⇨ Dog bites account for about a dozen deaths each year. (*CDC, Morbidity and Mortality Weekly Report (MMWR).*)

⇨ Children are the victims of the most serious dog attacks. (*CDC, National Center for Health Statistics.*)

⇨ The highest rate of dog bites is among children ages five to nine, and boys are bitten more often than girls. (*MMWR.*)

⇨ Insurance companies paid $250 million for dog bite liability claims in 1996 alone. (*Insurance Information Institute.*)

Laws pertaining to dogs and other pets vary locally. Some states have statues related to pets and dog bites, but some don't. Check your state laws (often available online) and your county and municipal codes. (Ask your city clerk and county clerk, or check online or at the library).

Some communities outline regulations pertaining to vicious or dangerous dogs, in particular. Most have some kind of ordinance to deal with pets in the community (regulations regarding allowing pets to run free, for example). Often these regulations outline what will happen if a dog is violent in terms of removal of the dog and/or punishment of the owners. Of course, when these regulations come into play, the damage has already been done. Become involved in your local government in order to make your community safe from dangerous animals.

Taking Action

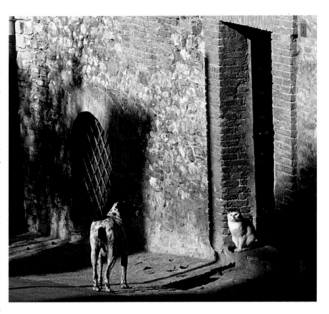

There will always be irresponsible dog owners who fail to protect their families and neighbors from a dog with a dangerous propensity. Therefore, we must take an assertive approach to protect our children. Become proactive.

In my opinion, the best approach has been set forth by Kelly Voight, a young teenager in Palatine, Ill. In 1999, at the age of seven, a neighbor's dog attacked Kelly. Like Bethany, Kelly required over 100 stitches as a result of the attack. During her rehabilitation and subsequent therapy, Kelly decided to do something positive-she decided to spread the word on dog-bite prevention. Her message, "Kid to Kid," is quite powerful. Her non-profit organization, "Prevent the Bite," has a wonderful Web site, **www.preventthebite.com**, full of excellent information. The checklist below is adapted in part from Kelly's good work.

There are several other good sources, including: **www.safekidssafedogs.com**, and a site run by State Farm Insurance (insurance companies also want to reduce dog-bite injuries), **www.statefarm.com/consumer/dogbite.htm**

Here are some guidelines for removing the hazards
of **NEIGHBORHOOD DOGS:**

CHECKLIST

For Non-Threatening Situations

Kelly has developed an acronym-WASP-to instruct children how to approach leashed dogs accompanied by their owners. (Of course, these are the only dogs that should be approached.)

W — **Wait and watch** the dog's body language.
(Kelly teaches children to recognize angry, afraid, and happy dogs.)

A — **Ask** the owner for permission to pet the animal.

S — Let the pet **sniff** you.

P — **Pet** the dog in the direction of the fur.

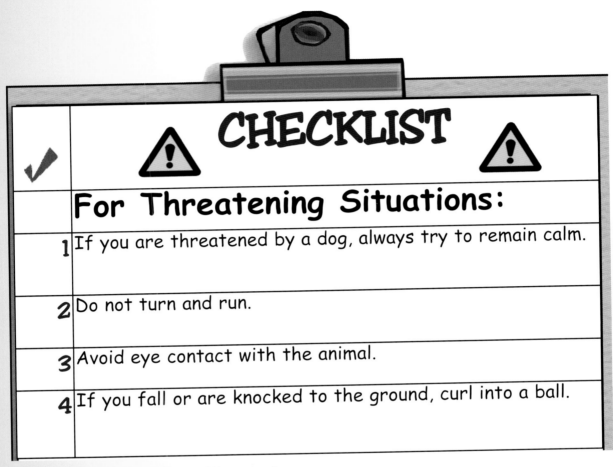

CHECKLIST

For Threatening Situations:

✔		
	1	If you are threatened by a dog, always try to remain calm.
	2	Do not turn and run.
	3	Avoid eye contact with the animal.
	4	If you fall or are knocked to the ground, curl into a ball.

For Threatening Situations:

1. IF YOUR ARE THREATENED BY A DOG, ALWAYS TRY TO REMAIN CALM.

Do not scream. If you say anything, speak calmly and firmly. Try to stay still until the dog leaves, or back away slowly until the dog is out of sight.

2. DO NOT TURN AND RUN.

Such action only aggravates the dog and will invite an attack.

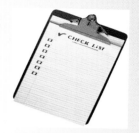

3. AVOID EYE CONTACT WITH THE ANIMAL.

The dog will see eye-to-eye contact as a precursor to a fight. Watch the Discovery channel sometime and see animals make eye contact before battle commences.

4. IF YOU FALL OR ARE KNOCKED TO THE GROUND, CURL INTO A BALL.

Immediately put your hands over your head and neck, and remember always to protect your face.

If you would like to see a complete review of the statistics, prevention, and community approaches to prevention, please review the fine article in the *Journal of the American Veterinary Medical Association, JVMA,* volume 218, no. 11, June 1, 2001, pages 1732 through 1749.

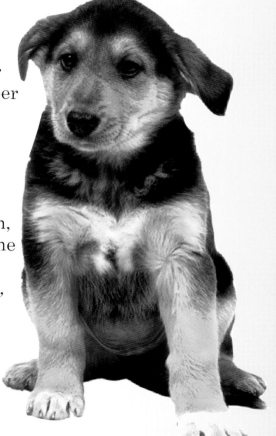

Dangerous Animals

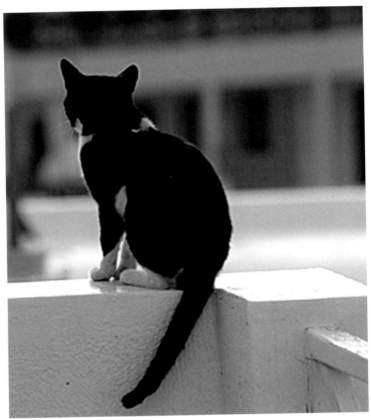

Dogs aren't the only animals that pose a danger. Tigers and other exotic animals that people keep as pets are killing children. In Texas, for example, a 10 year-old girl was killed by a tiger she was grooming with her stepfather when the tiger clamped her head in its jaws. "Wild animals, even if they are raised by hand from infancy, grow up to be unpredictable and dangerous," says Richard Farinato, director of captive wildlife protection for the Humane Society of the United States. Yet people can buy these animals for as little as $300. Owners don't often consider before their purchase what it will take to properly care for an animal that's built to run 100 miles a day, swim rivers, and bring down prey for dinner. Tigers and other big cats are programmed to attack and kill, and even the tamest of them can revert to their hard wiring at any given moment.

➯In the United States, 15,000 big cats are currently being kept as pets or in roadside zoos. *(Humane Society of the United States.)*

➯There have been ten fatalities due to exotic pets in the past five years. *(Humane Society of the United States.)*

The U.S. Department of Agriculture, the American Veterinary Medical Association, and animal shelters across the country oppose the ownership of dangerous exotic animals. The Captive Wildlife Safety Act currently bans the interstate shipment of lions, tigers, and other exotic animal for pet sale. Of course, this doesn't prevent in-state breeding or sales. The Humane Society of the United States is working to increase the number of states that ban the keeping of dangerous wild animals as pets. Contact your legislator to tell him or her that you support such legislation.

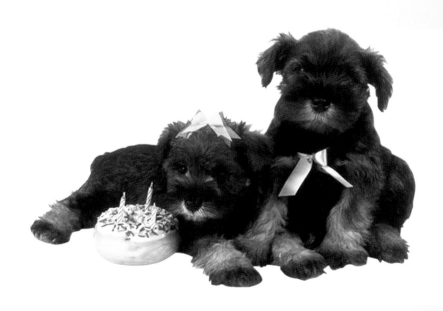

Neighborhood Animals

Petting Zoos

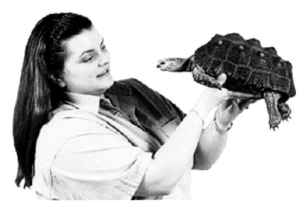

In 2000, Philadelphia reported the first cases of E. coli from a petting zoo; 16 children were ultimately diagnosed. In 2005, 22 children in central Florida were hospitalized with E. coli. The state health department confirmed the source was the petting zoo. At present there are few regulations and many petting zoos don't even posses a business license. Unfortunately eight percent of people infected by E. coli are later stricken with a potentially fatal kidney disease know as Hemolytic Uremic Syndrome (HUS). Because of the evolving immune system of a child, all children are at greater risk.

There has been calls for widespread testing of all animals in the zoos. However, experts contend the testing would need to be done daily because the E. coli bug can appear within hours. The most common sense solution is provided by Dr. Jeff Bender at the University of Minnesota School of Veterinary and Public Health. Dr. Bender advises that parents should wash the hands of their children immediately after the animal petting with soap and water or sanitizing gel. The State of Florida recently added a number of washing stations at the state fair and has commenced a public awareness campaign.

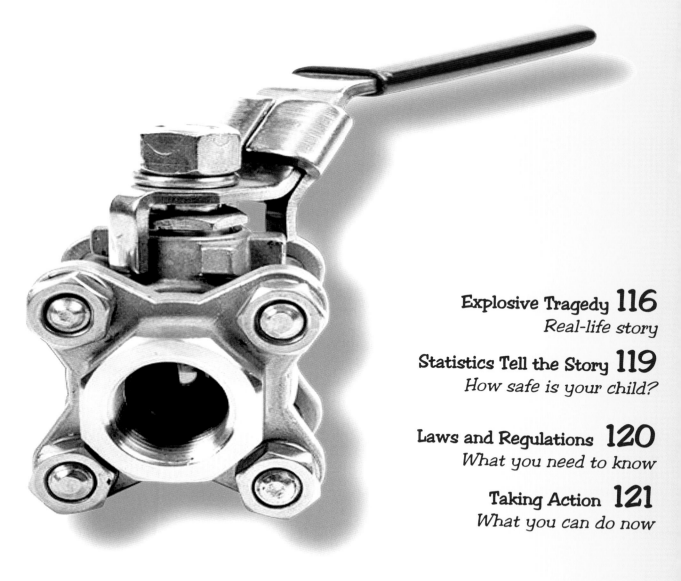

12

Natural Gas

Explosive Tragedy

Charles and Peggy Walker were high school sweethearts. They married shortly after graduation and looked forward to beginning their family. First came a son, Glenn, followed two years later by little Molly. Charles, who worked the graveyard shift at the local factory, came home early in the mornings and slept until one or two o'clock each afternoon.

One Saturday morning, Charles was sleeping in the downstairs bedroom while Peg and the children were upstairs on the main level. Glenn, age seven, played on his XBox in the living room, and Molly, age five, played on the back deck.

Shortly before noon, an explosion rocked the Walker home. The neighbors later likened it to "a bomb being dropped on the house." The first floor, where Charles slept, was immediately engulfed in flames. Moments later, the main floor, where Peg and the children were located, was also engulfed. Fortunately, Peg was able to rescue Molly from the deck. Glenn barely escaped, receiving severe burns as he exited the house. Charles, however, was charred from head to toe and was life-flighted to the local burn unit, along with his son. Glenn's hospitalization lasted three weeks, and he received multiple surgeries to repair skin damage. Charles, on the other hand, was in and out 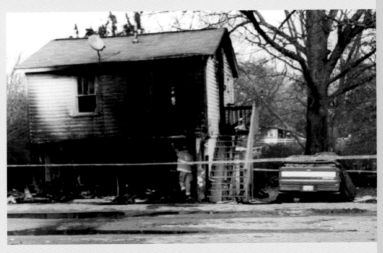 of a coma for almost 30 days. In an effort to save his life, doctors performed several debridement surgical procedures to remove the dead, burned skin. In the end, fluid filled Charles' lungs, and he died of adult respiratory distress syndrome (ARDS).

How did this horrible tragedy occur? The local fire inspector determined that the flame from the gas hot water heater ignited natural gas fumes, causing the explosion. The question remaining, however, was what caused natural gas fumes to accumulate near the water heater in the first place?

LEGAL ACTION and OUTCOME

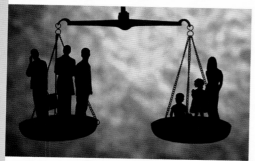

The Walker family retained me to obtain reimbursement for Glenn's medical expenses as well as justice for the family for the loss of their father and husband. What unfolded in our investigation revealed a great deal about corporate monopolies and greed.

Our expert examined the gas water heater, noting that there were no defects or malfunctions in the appliance. Instead, something else caused the natural gas to accumulate around the flame. The investigation revealed that a pipe running under the street delivered natural gas to the homes in the neighborhood. Each house had a connecting pipe that would draw the gas from the pipe under the street into the home. The pipe in the street was old and decayed and had developed an underground leak. As a result, the escaping underground gas followed the erosion under the soil into an underground highway of crevices and small tunnels. It was via this network that the escaping gas found its way under the Walker's home, into their ground floor, where it made contact with the hot water heater pilot light, resulting in the explosion.

After we determined how the explosion happened, we then turned to the question of whether or not it was preventable. The natural gas industry has known for years that underground pipes corrode and cause leakage over time. To prevent accidents, they have developed a procedure called a "leak survey." To conduct the survey, they run a gas-detecting machine directly over the underground pipe. If the machine detects a leak, repairs can be made. Safety experts recommend that an annual "leak survey" (rather than a random spot check) be conducted on all pipes in an older gas line system. In fact, the gas company performed annual leak

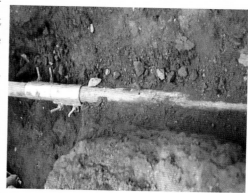

surveys in the Walker neighborhood for the first 10 years they controlled the monopoly.

The subpoenaed records show that during this time, a multitude of leaks were located and repaired. Each of these leaks had the potential for death and serious injury from unintended explosions. Remarkably, the gas company suspended the leak surveys, contending that they were costing too much money. They then petitioned the State Public Service Commission for a rate increase, using re-implementation of the leak surveys as partial justification for the increase.

Our review of the public documents shockingly revealed that while the Public Service Commission granted the rate increase, and the gas company collected the

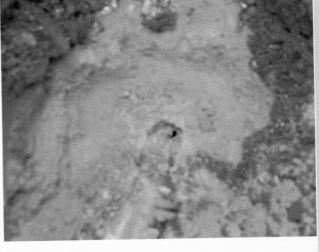

higher fees, the company did not re-institute the leak surveys. In fact, there had been no leak surveys for the three years prior to the explosion at the Walker home. If there had there been, the leak would have been noted and Charles' death and Glenn's catastrophic burns would have been prevented.

The Public Service Commission did its independent investigation of the explosion. They found that the gas company violated its leak survey promise and that its conduct had caused the death and injury. Despite this clear governmental fault finding, the gas company refused any settlement discussions until the case had been fully prepared and all experts had been deposed and the case was ready for trial. The case was ultimately settled to the satisfaction of the family. However, we learned during the prosecution of this case that what had occurred to the Walkers was not an isolated incident.

Statistics Tell the Story

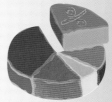

Unfortunately, no national statistics exist on the injuries and deaths resulting from gas leaks for the mail gas line. However, there are a number of news reports.

⇨ In Steamboat Springs, Colorado on February 3, 1994, there was a massive explosion as depicted in the photograph (below) in which there was severe personal injuries and massive property damage.

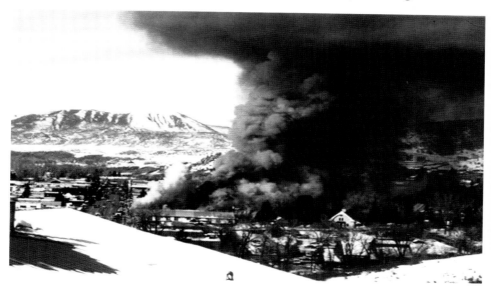

⇨ In Amarillo, Texas on September 13, 1999 a gas leak occurred similar to the Walker's tragedy outlined in the Real Life Story from this chapter. In this explosion, Forestt Harvey Miller was consumed by the fire that resulted from the preventable gas leak. Mr. Miller suffered extensive burns which later resulted in his death.

Laws and Regulations

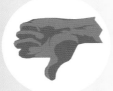

$\mathbf{E}$ach state has its own specific safety protocol for natural gas companies. Some require leak surveys; others do not. It is clear from all available evidence that annual leak surveys should be required, given the age of America's natural gas pipes.

With each passing day, the pipes become more corroded and susceptible to leaks. With the growing population, the gas companies are not keeping up with the necessary replacement of the old and decaying pipelines.

The following safeguards should be taken to prevent gas explosions:

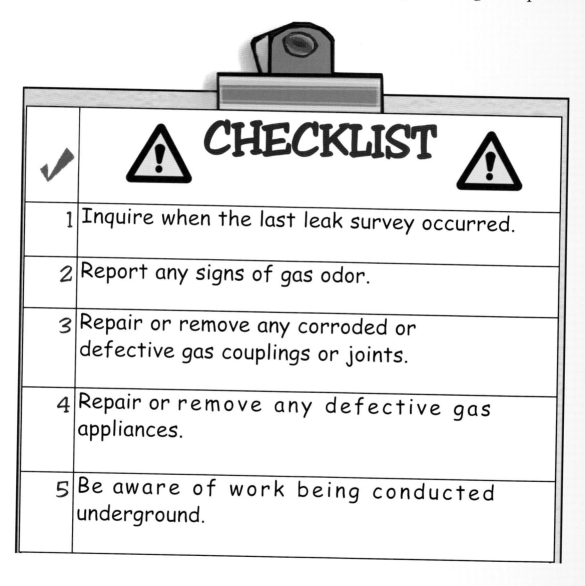

CHECKLIST

✔		
1	Inquire when the last leak survey occurred.
2	Report any signs of gas odor.
3	Repair or remove any corroded or defective gas couplings or joints.
4	Repair or remove any defective gas appliances.
5	Be aware of work being conducted underground.

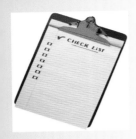

1. INQUIRE WHEN THE LAST LEAK SURVEY OCCURRED.

Call your Public Service Commission consumer advocate office. The number can be obtained via the Internet, or by calling 411. Each state has a different audit and tracking system, but the consumer advocate's office should be able to direct you to the person who can best answer your questions.

2. REPORT ANY SIGNS OF GAS ODOR.

In our reported tragedy, there was no detectable odor at any time prior to the explosion. Other victims of gas explosions also report an absence of odor. So absence of odor should not give you peace of mind. But if there is gas odor present, then be aware that it is a significant and very dangerous sign. Take action immediately. Leave the premises and call your gas company's emergency notification number.

3. REPAIR OR REMOVE ANY CORRODED OR DEFECTIVE GAS COUPLINGS OR JOINTS.

While a defective coupling did not cause the case tragedy in this chapter, there have been many reported ignition points due to corroded gas couplings. Any leakage, no matter the cause, constitutes an immediate danger and must be fixed.

4. REPAIR OR REMOVE ANY DEFECTIVE GAS APPLIANCES.

Statistics indicate that a high number of explosion injuries and deaths result from defective hot water heaters, stoves and furnaces. Carbon dioxide poisoning is a danger as well. Therefore, it is important to immediately replace any defective gas appliance.

5. BE AWARE OF WORK BEING CONDUCTED UNDERGROUND.

Gas pipes are not the only utilities below the ground. Water pipes, some electrical lines and telephone lines are often underground as well. Gas leaks can occur when the water company digs up the ground to fix a water leak, for example, or when anybody digs in the area of a gas line. Therefore, be aware of any work being done in and around the gas lines to your home and be on heightened alert for any potential leaks.

13

Neighborhood Vehicles

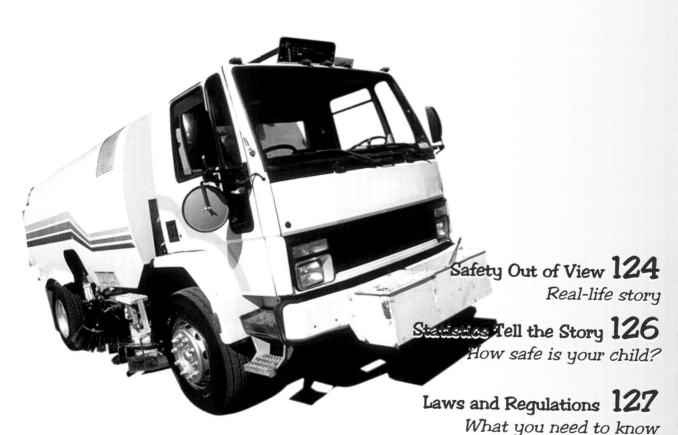

Safety Out of View

Mikey was the first member of the Lopez family to be born in America. His Puerto Rican parents dreamt of coming to America and raising a family. Five years after their marriage, they were able to save enough to make the move. Once here, both worked two jobs in order to support their family. Mikey was born and was the apple of his father's eye. Because of increases in his pay, Mikey's mother, Maria, could now stay home with the children most of the time, working just her weekend job.

The Lopez home was in a large housing project, with 10 units per building. In front of each building were reserved parking spaces, and at the corner of every four parking areas sat a large waste management bin. Once a week the big garbage truck would come through the neighborhood, its driver moving quickly to get his job done. He would connect the truck to the garbage bin, mechanically lift the bin over the front hood of the truck, deposit its contents in the back of the garbage truck, then return the bin to the ground below.

For years the garbage truck company had provided a "spotter", someone who would sit in the passenger seat and assist the driver in looking out the side mirrors in order to protect the safety of those around the truck. The extra worker also provided help in picking up the spare trash. But the multi-million dollar corporation decided to save money and eliminate the spotter. Instead, they mounted a video camera on the back of the garbage truck, with a monitor on the dashboard that would hopefully enable the driver to see persons to the rear of the truck.

A speedster on his tricycle, four and-a-half year-old Mikey pedaled furiously, his head down as he covered great distances in front of his building. While Mikey's mother was attending to his one and-a-half year-old sister, Mikey jumped on his trike and headed into the parking lot. At that moment the garbage truck connected with the trash bin. As the truck backed up, it emitted the "beep, beep,

beep" sound that alerts adults to the danger of a large moving vehicle. The problem was the sound enticed Mikey, who proceeded to pedal closer to see what was going on. Mikey moved to the rear of the truck, out of camera view and the vision of the driver. Once the preschooler perceived that he was in a dangerous situation, it was too late. The mud flap passed over Mikey's tricycle, followed by the crushing force of the back wheels. The driver, unaware that he had killed Mikey, preceded on the rest of his route.

In the split second it took Maria to realize her son's absence, she came running out of the home. She was met by a nightmare, the only recognizable item her son's New York Yankee baseball cap.

LEGAL ACTION and OUTCOME

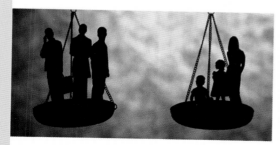

I was hired to investigate whether the company was at fault. After the suit was filed, subpoenaed documents showed that the company considered the large amounts of money it would save by eliminating the spotter position. There was even a recommendation for a second camera that could be placed to view the full range at the back of the garbage truck, rather than the limited range that the driver in our case viewed. The range of the second camera would have permitted viewing of a child.

Shockingly, evidence showed that the limited field of vision of the camera had caused numerous injuries and the death of at least one other child in the Midwest. As the case proceeded to trial, the company requested mediation. Two days into the mediation, the case was settled to the satisfaction of the family, upon the condition that the company would in the future use either spotters or a full-range vision camera.

Statistics Tell the Story

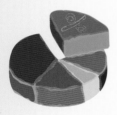

Amazingly, the National Highway Traffic Safety Administration, or NHTSA, does not collect data on non-crash, non-traffic fatalities. So a 50 year-old mother of two has stepped in and taken on the role. "Not a single surveillance system in the U.S today captures this data," Janette Fennell says.

She is the founder of *Kids 'N Cars,* a children's safety non-profit organization that works to prevent injuries and deaths to children in and around cars. *Kids 'N Cars* is the only group collecting statistics on back-over incidents from public records. Her group is at the forefront of power window safety, as well (Chapter 29).

⇨ In the United States, at least 91 children were backed over and killed in 2003-more than one child per week-often by a relative in their own driveway, and often by a larger vehicle such as van, SUV or pickup truck.(**www.kidsandcars.org**)

⇨ Most of the children killed were four years old or younger. At least 60 percent of the cars were light trucks, SUVs, minivans or pickup trucks. These are the vehicles that critics charge have poor rear visibility or "blind spots."

Consumer Reports has begun measuring the blind spots for both short and average drivers for each vehicle it tests and posting that information on its Web site at: **www.consumerreports.org/co/vehicleblindspots** or at **www.kidsandcars.org**.

⇨ 42% of non-traffic, non-crash fatalities between 1999-2003 were back-over deaths involving children under the age of 14.

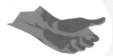

*C*urrently, there are no federal laws pertaining to this area. Garbage trucks, delivery trucks and other vehicles, both private and governmental, are regulated by the normal vehicle laws that apply to the city or town in which they operate.

Likewise, off-road use of ATVs and go-carts in neighborhoods is also governed by a variety of different local laws.

The *Safe Kids, Safe Cars Act* of 2004 was introduced in the U.S. House of Representatives and Senate, but no action was taken. The title of a press release announcing the introduction of the bill stated: "Legislation Announced as Nation Logs its 61st Child Back-over Death This Year " (2003).

Taking Action

A parent or caregiver who performs all of the hazard prevention measures outlined in the chapters of Part 1, The Home and this section, The Neighborhood (including the backyard hazard removal steps found in chapter 10), has taken great strides in providing for children's safety. But they may also have a false sense of security at home. As the statistics show, many children are seriously injured and killed in driveways, cul de sacs, neighborhood sidewalks and streets. Therefore, awareness of hazards in the neighborhood is equally important. The following checklist will help:

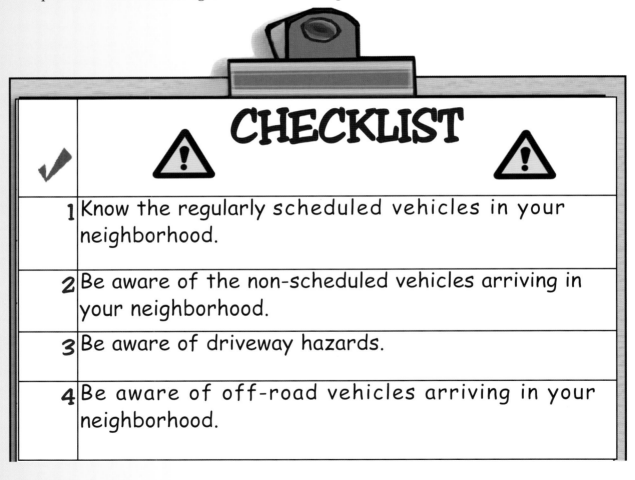

⚠ CHECKLIST ⚠

✔	
1	Know the regularly scheduled vehicles in your neighborhood.
2	Be aware of the non-scheduled vehicles arriving in your neighborhood.
3	Be aware of driveway hazards.
4	Be aware of off-road vehicles arriving in your neighborhood.

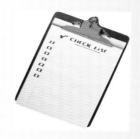

1. KNOW THE REGULARLY SCHEDULED VEHICLES IN YOUR NEIGHBORHOOD.

As noted in the tragedy above, garbage trucks have regularly scheduled routes. So do U.S. Postal Service trucks, mass transportation buses and many other vehicles. Danger is created when these vehicles enter a neighborhood, so be aware of the times and the driving habits of the operators. If the mass transit bus driver drives too fast, call in a report. If the mail truck driver stops abruptly and drives erratically, call in a complaint. Likewise, if the garbage truck driver maneuvers in a reckless manner, does not take time in backing, and is otherwise unsafe, report it. Also advise your child of the dangers and be on guard at the scheduled times.

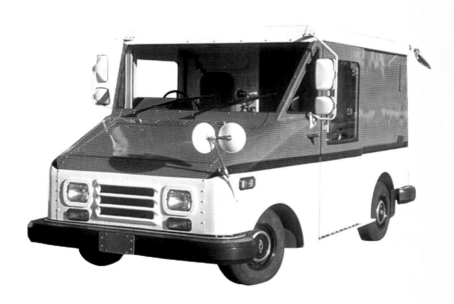

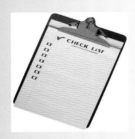

2. BE AWARE OF NON-SCHEDULED VEHICLES ARRIVING IN YOUR NEIGHBORHOOD.

Be aware of the arrival of non-scheduled vehicles, such as overnight mail delivery vehicles, florist trucks, furniture deliverers and maintenance and landscape people. All of these vehicles can present danger to your child. Report any hazardous driving that you witness by any drivers of these vehicles. Advise your child of the danger of vehicles and take preventative steps.

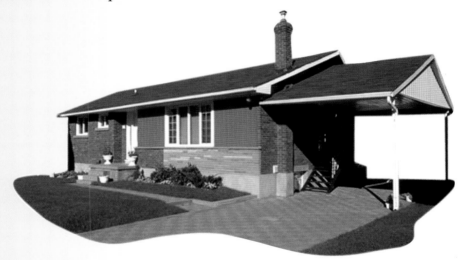

3. BE AWARE OF DRIVEWAY HAZARDS.

Since the driveway is an extension of the home, many parents and caregivers have an unrealistic sense of safety when their children play in this area. But there are many instances in which visiting family members, friends, and neighbors have tragically backed over children playing in driveways. Any vehicle in a driveway should be recognized as a hazard, and the "stop, look, and listen" guide should prevail.

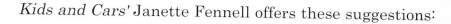

Kids and Cars' Janette Fennell offers these suggestions:

⇨ Don't let children play in the driveway.

⇨ If they are in the driveway or in an adjacent yard, Fennell's rule is that all the children must stand on the front steps-or some place visible and away from the driveway, before she moves the vehicle.If she can see everyone on the steps, she knows it's safe to pull into or out of the driveway.

⇨ Make sure that the people supervising children, particularly toddlers, know exactly when drivers are leaving so the children don't venture out to the driveway.

⇨ Install rear sensors or video cameras that mount on vehicle bumpers and provide images that span all the way to the ground.

4. BE AWARE OF OFF-ROAD VEHICLES ARRIVING IN YOUR NEIGHBORHOOD.

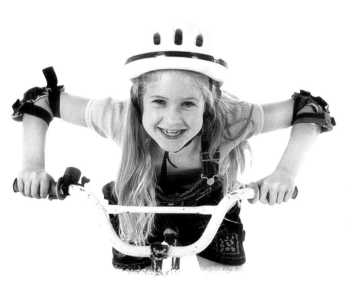

Under-age drivers who are too young to have driver's licenses and may not be mature enough to drive in a responsible manner, often operate go-carts and ATVs. Be aware of all vehicles in your neighborhood, as well as the driving habits of children who operate them. Then take appropriate preventative steps.

Neighborhood Vehicles **131**

Part Three

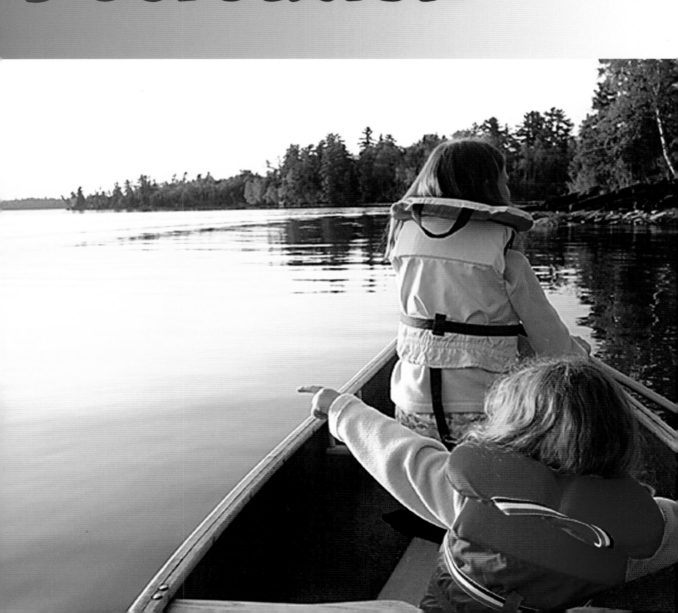

Recreation

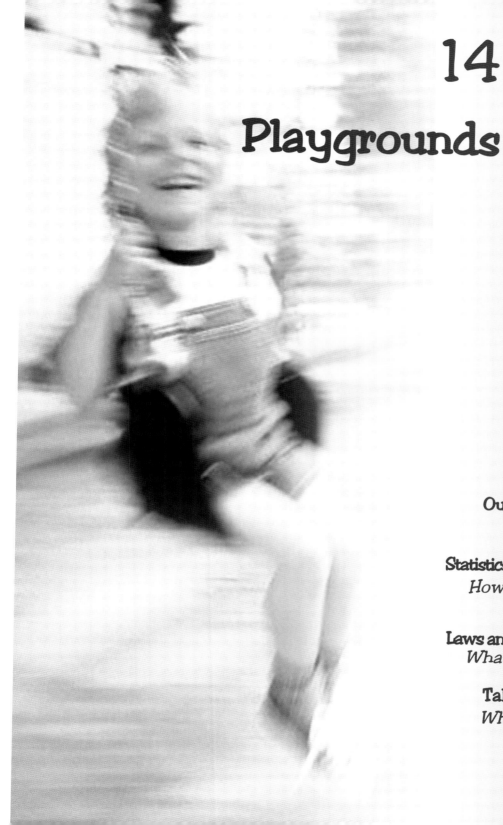

14

Playgrounds

Suzanne Johanson crouched at the bottom of the slide, coaxing her toddler. It was a sunny day in April, and Suzanne brought her children, two-year-old Rachel and five-year-old Patrick, to Pine Log Park for some healthy fresh air and exercise. The county park was just a half-mile from home and was equipped with swing sets, slides, a sandbox and jungle gym. Beautiful trees silhouetted against the blue sky and surrounded the play area. It should have been an idyllic afternoon. But Rachel never reached Suzanne's outstretched arms.

She had no way of knowing that the lovely trees had a disease that cuts off circulation to some limbs, causing sudden collapse. This had occurred so often that the park's maintenance crew set aside space at the corner of the park and dubbed it the "tree limb graveyard." Supervisors typically instructed workers to simply wait until the tree limbs fell on their own, then move them to the "graveyard."

However, there was one tree limb that had been scheduled for cutting twice. The limb was hanging high above the slide. Without warning or reason to suspect danger, the limb crashed towards the ground. It landed on Rachel's head, crushing her skull and pinning Suzanne to the ground. The helpless mother could only cry for help.

Rachel was flown 30 miles to a children's trauma center where doctors diagnosed "multiple skull fractures, severe subdural hematoma with exposed brain tissue." Rachel fought valiantly for five days, lapsing in and out of a coma, until she died with her family at her bedside.

LEGAL ACTION and OUTCOME

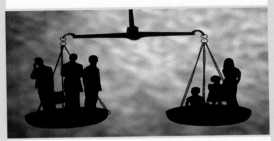

Rachel's death was completely preventable. My law firm's investigation after her death found that falling tree limbs in playgrounds are common nationwide. Safety experts even have a term for it: the "three D's"-diseased, dying and dead trees. These limbs are widely understood to require immediate removal to protect the public.

Pine Log Park had no maintenance manual and no policy regarding the inspection or removal of tree limbs. Ironically, taxpayers had paid twice for a park supervisor to attend safety seminars that specified the need for maintenance manuals and attention to the three D's.

In Rachel's case, the wrongdoers were held accountable for her death. Suzanne and her husband, Niles, filed a successful lawsuit against the county. Sadly, it was their daughter's death that forced the park's department to implement a strict maintenance schedule.

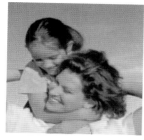

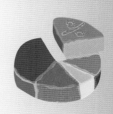

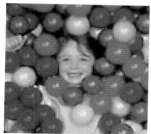

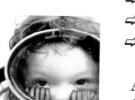

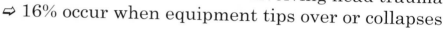

Part of a normal childhood includes accidents. But no playground should harbor serious threats of injury because adults neglected the safety of children. A child dies from a preventable injury on our nation's playgrounds every month.

What are the causes of death?
⇨ 56 % occur when a child is accidentally hanged
⇨ 21% are the result of falls involving head trauma
⇨ 16% occur when equipment tips over or collapses

A child is rushed to an emergency room with a playground injury every two and a half minutes, according to the U.S. Consumer Products Safety Commission. That is more than 200,000 preschool and elementary children a year in the U.S.
How are they hurt?

⇨ 79% involve falls
⇨ 10% involve cuts from sharp edges and pinch points
⇨ 8% involve impact with equipment

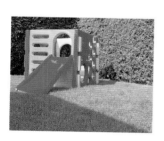

Laws and Regulations

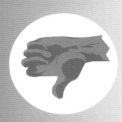

When it comes to playground safety, don't assume your child is protected. Playground safety laws and regulations are as varied as a toddler's mood swings. For example, many cities will have safety codes, but counties will not, even though the city and county playgrounds are close together.

On the state level, the patchwork is even greater. Few states specify standards based on the U.S. Consumer Products Safety Commission(CPSC) Handbook for Public Playground Safety. Most, however, rely on "working groups" or other well meaning, but toothless groups to present "educational programs" on playground safety.

At the lowest end of the rankings are states that provide no laws except those that protect manufacturers and operators of playground equipment from lawsuits. There is some hope at the federal level. A bill pending in the U. S. House of Representatives would provide $1 million grants to states that pass laws or already have laws that follow CPSC safety guidelines.

Taking Action

"Playground safety is not rocket science," says Dr. Frances Wallach, past president of the National Playground Safety Institute, part of the National Parks and Recreation Association. Inspired by Dr. Wallach and other experts, the Keenan's Kids Foundation decided to take action with a public advocacy program. According to Dr. Wallach, even an eight-year-old should be capable of recognizing unsafe conditions with some simple guidance.

The advocacy program became the Safety Report Card project of the Keenan's Kids Foundation. The grading system is simple and strict: Pass/Fail. A playground fails with one safety violation. Volunteer teams of one child over the age of eight and one retired adult used the Report Card to evaluate 30 Atlanta playgrounds during the summer of 2003. Shockingly, 29 of these failed. Virtually the same results occurred in 2004 and 2005.

Half the parks had dead tree limbs. Nearly all, 90 percent, had unsafe fall zones and sharp surfaces. Two playgrounds had deadly exposed electrical wires.

The Report Card project attracted the *Today Show* and Atlanta media. An Atlanta TV crew filmed city workers in one park hauling off dangerous playground equipment. The Report Card works! It worked in Atlanta, and it can work in your community.

Use Keenan's Kids Foundation Playground Safety Handbook 10-point Report Card to evaluate every park where your child plays. Report any defects to park, city, or county officials and keep track of results. Send a copy of your completed Report Card to your local newspaper, too. Your neighbors will thank you. If you aren't sure what to say to the newspaper, we have form letters in the Playground Safety Project Volunteer Handbook. Maybe you'll even be inspired to do what we did and investigate all the playgrounds and parks in your area.

Other information on playground safety is available on our Web site, www.keenanskidsplaygroundsafety.com

We also wish to acknowledge the good works of the Kaboom organization (www.kaboom.org) in keeping playgrounds safer. Kaboom is a dedicated and well-organized national organization. Through it's capable leadership, liaisons with local businesses and caring volunteers, many unsafe playgrounds have been greatly improved and new playgrounds have been built.

The Report Card

The following report card is used by volunteers of the Keenan's Kids Foundation. We purposely designed the report card to be used by children eight years old and above.

REPORT CARD		
	SUBJECT	GRADE
1	Condition of equipment	
2	Surfaces must be smooth	
3	Trip hazards eliminated	
4	Tipping of equipment prevented	
5	Fall zones adequate	
6	Gaps or spaces absent	
7	Electrical wires secured	
8	Dangerous tree limbs removed	
9	Surface areas safe and uniform	
10	Hazards removed	

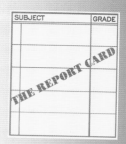

Each category receives either Pass or Fail.
To make your decision, answer the following questions:

1. CONDITION OF EQUIPMENT

⇨Are there broken or missing components, or any damaged structures?

⇨Is the paint chipping or peeling? Small children could put pieces of paint in their mouths.

⇨Are swing seats made of heavy or rigid material, such as wood or metal?
They can seriously injure a child, and the seats should be made of rubber or canvas.

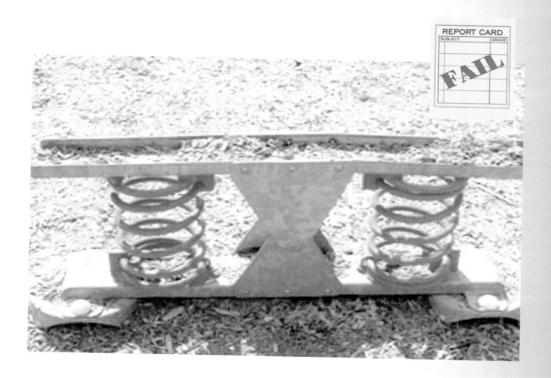

Playgrounds **139**

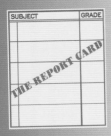

2. SURFACES MUST BE SMOOTH

⇨Are any surfaces rough or ragged?

⇨Are there sharp points or corners, edges, nails or splinters?

⇨Are there protruding nuts or hooks?

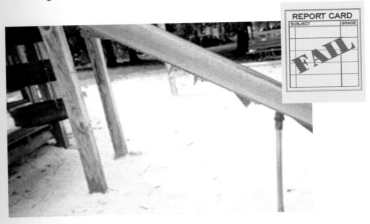

3. TRIP HAZARDS ELIMINATED

⇨Are there any objects children might trip over?

⇨Are there exposed footings, anchoring devices or environmental obstacles, such as tree roots?

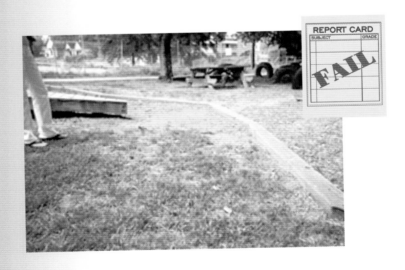

4. TIPPING OF EQUIPMENT PREVENTED

➪Is any equipment not properly secured and might be tipped?
➪Are the foundations of slides, monkey bars and swings loose and movable?

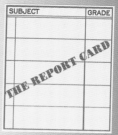

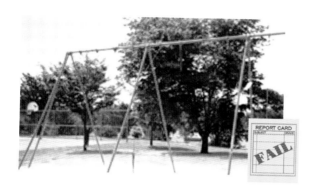

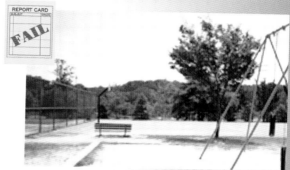

5. FALL ZONES ADEQUATE

➪A fall zone is the softened area around the equipment where a child could fall.
➪Are there buried foundations in the fall zone?
➪Does surface material extend at least six feet from the equipment in each direction?
    For slides, surface must extend the height of the slide, plus four feet.
    For swings, surface must extend twice the height in front and behind the swing.

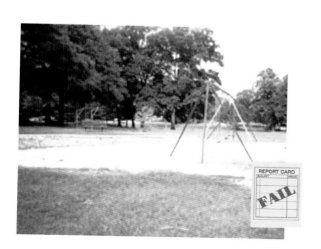

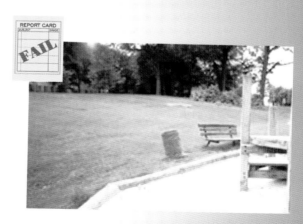

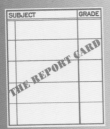

6. GAPS OR SPACES ABSENT

⇨Are there any gaps or spaces in equipment in which a child could get caught or that could catch his clothing?

⇨Are there any open spaces in S hooks? You should not be able to insert even a dime or credit card into the space.

⇨Are there gaps or protrusions in slide areas, elevated walks etc. that could snag clothing or allow a child's limbs to be caught while playing?

⇨Could a child get caught in between ladder rungs? This space should be smaller than 3 ½ inches or larger than 9 inches.

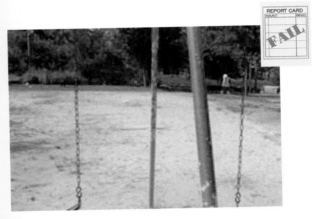

7. ELECTRICAL WIRES

⇨Are there exposed electrical wires in or around the playground?

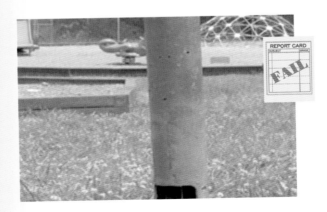

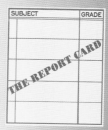
8. DANGEROUS TREE LIMBS

⇨Is there evidence of diseased or dying branches overhanging or surrounding the play area?

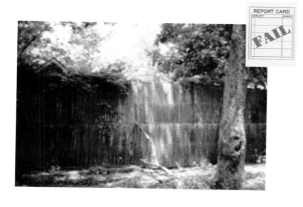

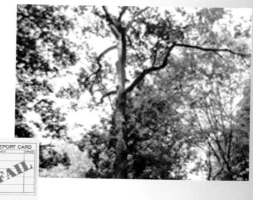

9. SURFACE AREAS SAFE AND UNIFORM

⇨What is the surface around the play equipment?
(Circle the answer) wood chips, sand, grass, cement/pavement, other substance

⇨Does the surface cover the play area uniformly? Check for erosion in high-traffic areas or exposed grass and dirt.

⇨Is the surface covering at least 12 inches deep of wood chips, mulch, sand, shredded rubber, pea gravel or safety-tested rubber mats?

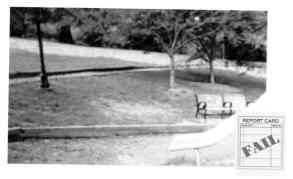

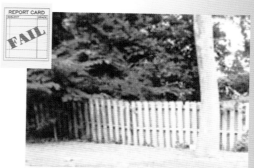

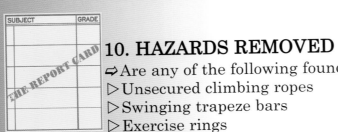

10. HAZARDS REMOVED

⇨ Are any of the following found on the playground?

▷ Unsecured climbing ropes

▷ Swinging trapeze bars

▷ Exercise rings

▷ Trampoline

▷ Old-fashioned monkey bars with interior bars with which a child may fall from a height greater than 18 inches are unsafe.

▷ Chromated copper arsenate (CCA) treated wood. CCA contains arsenic, chromium and copper. According to the Consumer Products Safety Commission (www.cpsc.gov), the wood industry stopped using CCA treated wood in the late 1970's to early 1980's, but the old playgrounds still have CCA treated wood.

▷ Solid metal animals or objects mounted on heavy duty springs, as seen in the photograph below are very hard, and children can easily injure themselves when falling off.

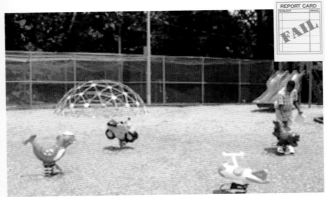

Keeping playgrounds safe for children takes diligence. Fill out a Report Card on your playground regularly. And take whatever steps to reach a perfect 10.

Long overlooked is the community of children with deficits. The vast majority of public playgrounds sadly are not friendly to children with disabilities, 5.0 million according to the U.S. Department of Education. We applaud the efforts of www.boundlessplaygrounds.org, an organization begun because of the courage of Matthew Cavedon, a 15-year-old from Bloomfield, Connecticut, who uses a wheelchair.

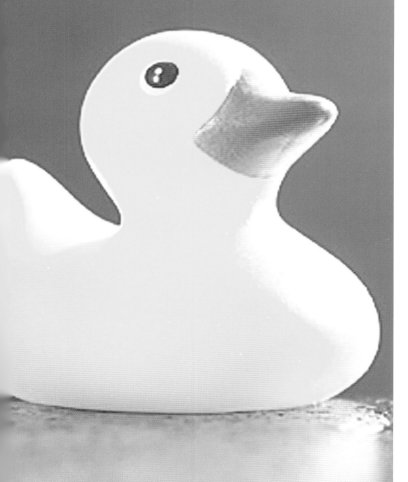

15
Toys

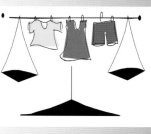

The Clock Stops

Mooki, a little girl of three, was cared for every day by her maternal grandmother, Celeste. Mooki's mother, Rosa, had recently bought her daughter a new toy, a happy face clock with large numbers and a movable hand protected by a thin sheet of Plexiglas. The manufacturer's instructions plainly stated that the toy was appropriate for children ages three to six years, so neither Mooki's mother nor her grandmother had any fear of her being hurt by it. Shockingly, this "age appropriate" toy killed Mooki.

While Mooki's grandmother was washing dishes after the nighttime meal, she turned around to check on Mooki, who was playing on the floor with her new toy clock. To Celeste's horror, the toddler had cracked the thin Plexiglas cover of the clock with the palm of her hands and placed sharp-edged pieces of the glass in her mouth. Mooki bled profusely around the lips and tongue as she smiled back at her grandmother.

Celeste quickly bundled Mooki up and rushed her to the nearby emergency room. The trauma team worked earnestly, but found that they were unable to quickly enough close the internal wound caused by a very sharp piece of the glass that Mooki had swallowed. The toddler's esophagus was severely torn, and on autopsy a piece of the Plexiglas was found in her lung.

Sadly, many inquisitive children have proven that breakable glass and Plexiglas have no place in toys that are rated safe for children three to six years of age. In addition to breaking the pieces, young children often swallow whatever it is possible to swallow. Safe, unbreakable toys can be made for them.

LEGAL ACTION and OUTCOME

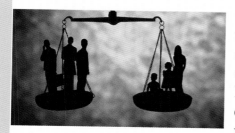

Mooki's mother wanted answers. How could this happen? A toy that was intended to bring joy killed a child. My law firm was hired and quickly discovered that this toy-manufacturer had a long history of injuries and deaths. We retained a toy safety expert who told us the toy was defective and used unsafe materials. The Plexiglas is known to easily break and cause an immediate swallowing hazard to young children.

When we took the sworn testimony of the so-called Safety Quality Assurance person at the manufacturer, we learned he had no safety background and had managed car washes before being hired as the company safety expert. We asked why the company did not use Plexiglas. He responded that any material would break and that Plexiglas was as good as the next material. Of course the company blamed the mother and the child for the death.

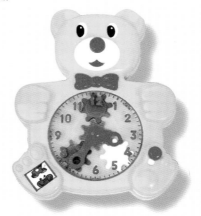

*Not the toy involved in the case.

Ultimately, after nearing two years of litigation, Mooki's parents' lawsuit against the toy manufacturer was successful.

Statistics Tell the Story

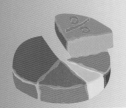

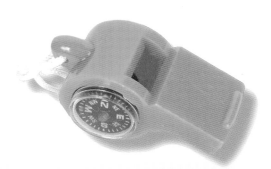

⇨ Toys accounted for 38 child deaths in 2001 and 2002, 25 in 2001, and 13 in 2002, according to the Consumer Products Safety Commission (*CPSC*). Eleven deaths occurred in 2003.

⇨ There were 155,440 emergency room visits in 2003, and 212,400 in 2002 for toy injuries according to the Consumer Products Safety Commission.

⇨ Fifty four percent of deaths in 2002 were due to choking according to the National SAFE KIDS Campaign, www.safe kids.org.

⇨ Seventy eight percent of the 165,000 toy-related emergency room visits in 2002 were with children under the age of 15 years old and 34 percent or 72,400 were children under the age of five.

In 2002, the following were the categories of death;
- ⇨ Riding toys: four deaths
- ⇨ Balloons (choking/asphyxia): three deaths
- ⇨ Toy balls (choking/airway obstruction): two deaths
- ⇨ Toy dart and dart tip (choking/asphyxia): two deaths

Laws and Regulations

The most meaningful legislation concerning toy safety is the *1994 Child Safety Protection Act,* which went into effect in 1995 and completely changed the way consumers purchased toys at their point of purchase. The Consumer Products Safety Commission came up with industry standards, such as age appropriateness and noise levels, all aimed at toy safety. There is a specific section dealing with choking hazards specifying marbles and balloons. Among the laws passed are:

The Child Safety Protection Act bans toys intended for children under age three if the toys pose a choking hazard. The act also requires warning labels on packaging for small balls, balloons, marbles and other toys and games containing small parts, when the games and toys are intended for use by children ages three to six.

The Federal Hazardous Substances Act bans toys that contain any hazardous substance, such as lead. It also bans toys that present an electrical, mechanical, or thermal hazard to children.

The Labeling of Hazardous Art Materials Act requires the labeling of art materials that contain hazardous substances as inappropriate for use by children.

The Standard Consumer Safety Specification on Toy Safety has been voluntarily set by the toy industry. The goal of these standards is to minimize the risk of injury from toys "during normal use and reasonable foreseeable abuse."

The Marking of Toy Look-alike and Imitation Firearms Regulation, set by the U.S. Department of Commerce, requires toy guns be marked in order to distinguish them from real guns.

These Regulations have helped reduce the number of children injured and killed while playing with toys. However, not all toys are tested, and even those that meet some standards may not meet others. Unsafe toys can still be found on the shelves of stores and especially online, where stringent requirements and recommendations are often overlooked.

Unfortunately these laws apply only to retail stores and currently do not apply to toys sold on the Internet. The Consumer Products Safety Commission several years ago banned the very dangerous lawn darts having caused several deaths. However, in August of 2004, for a short period of time lawn darts were being marketed via eBay by a European company which coincidentally had their product warehouse in the United States. eBay did the responsible action and banned the product.

Also, there was a significant recall of Pokemon toys distributed free at Burger King restaurants throughout the United States. The toy caused the death of a 13-month-old girl and the Consumer Products Safety Commission openly criticized Burger King's recall efforts. According to Burger King, nearly 70 million of the balls were manufactured.

Since 1994, the volunteers of the Keenan's Kids Foundation have produced a list of the "10 Most Dangerous Toys," and the list photos and descriptions are located on the Web site www.keenanskidsfoundation.com. The list is not intended to be an exclusive list but rather a representative list of the types of dangers on the market. As you will see below, we've used some of the toys on our past lists to demonstrate the dangers on our REPORT CARD.

Do not assume that the government has safety tested your child's toys. Further, do not assume the retailer has done any form of safety testing. More often than not, a product does not get recalled until several deaths or serious injuries occur. Therefore, each parent and caregiver must be vigilant in using common sense to keep dangerous toys from their child. The following report card will assist in making sure dangerous toys are not put in the hands of innocent children.

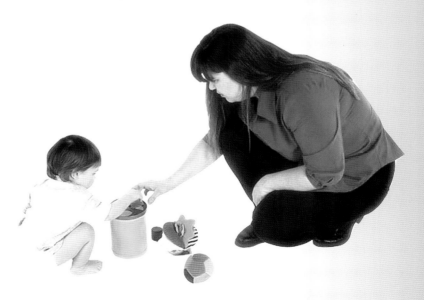

The Report Card

The following Report Card should be used when buying toys and accepting toy gifts:

REPORT CARD		
	SUBJECT	GRADE
1	No choking hazard	
2	No strangling hazard	
3	No sharp points or edges	
4	No loud noises	
5	No long cords or strings	
6	No dangerous chemicals	
7	Instructions on the package are the same as instructions inside	
8	No extreme heat	
9	No outrageous violence	
10	No obvious danger	

Each category receives either Pass or Fail.
To make your decision, please consider the following:

1. NO CHOKING HAZARD

As noted in the statistics, choking hazards account for more deaths than any other danger. There were eight deaths alone in 2002, according to the Consumer Products Safety Commission.

➪ *Never give latex balloons to children under the age of eight.*
Latex balloons were included in the 2003 Keenan's Kids Foundation's "10 Most Dangerous Toys of 2003"; the photo below is the assorted water balloon toys which are in the form of balloons and water bombs manufactured by Imperial, and we purchased them at Walgreen's Drug Store for less than $3.

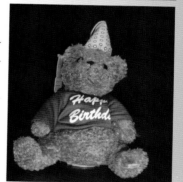

➪ *Look out for detachable parts.*
On our 2004 dangerous toy list, we included the "Happy Birthday Bear," Model 3006, manufactured by Gummy Industries and we purchased the toy at KB Toys for $11. The "ball" hands are easily detachable and swallowed by children.

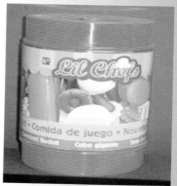

➪ *Often you must inspect the inside of the package before purchasing.*
Here is a photograph of the "Lil Chefs Play Food Bucket" which we purchased in 2003 from Toys "R" Us for less than $10. Approximately a third of the food objects inside were easily swallowed.

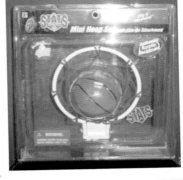

2. NO STRANGLING HAZARD

An example of this would be the "Mini Hoop Basketball Set," sold for less than $7 and listed on the 2003 dangerous toys list. The set is age appropriate for children over three, yet a child's head could easily get caught in the net.

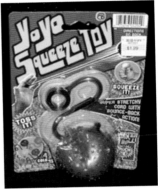

⇨ Because of its danger, we listed the "Yo Yo Ball" on both our 2003 and 2004 list. The toy has been banned in Europe and carries a risk disclaimer by the Consumer Products Safety Commission, and it is not sold by Toys "R" Us or other major toy retail establishments. Yet the "Yo Yo Ball" is easily purchased at convenience stores in most parts of the country. The toy has caused strangulations, head and eye injuries, nearly 400 according to the CPSC.

After our 2004 dangerous toy press conference, I received the following email from Linda Coleman, a mother and nurse;

Dear Mr. Keenan,

This toy should be removed from the market immediately. My son witnessed first hand what this toy can do to a child. A friend had come to visit him with his two little girls, ages 5 and 6. The adults were talking and one noticed that the five-year-old was lying on the ground. When they got to her the "Yo Yo Ball" was wrapped around her neck. She was without air. They immediately got it off and fortunately the child was okay. It was just God's will that she was found in time. There should be more strict guidelines in toy manufacturing. Thanks for your efforts.

Sincerely,
Linda Coleman, RN (Mother)

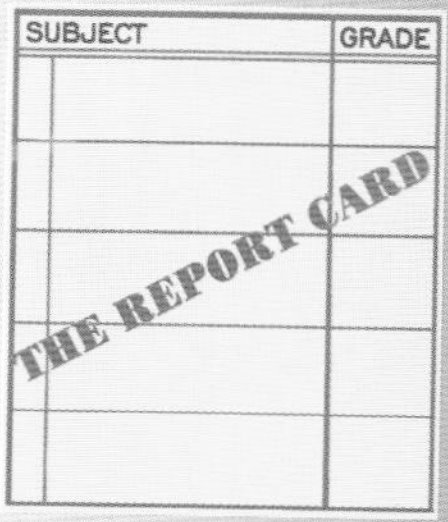

3. NO SHARP POINTS OR EDGES

For two years in a row, Ninja products were chosen as one of the 10 dangerous toys on our list. First, the "Bruce Lee Deluxe Action Set" was chosen in 2003, which had a number of sharp points.

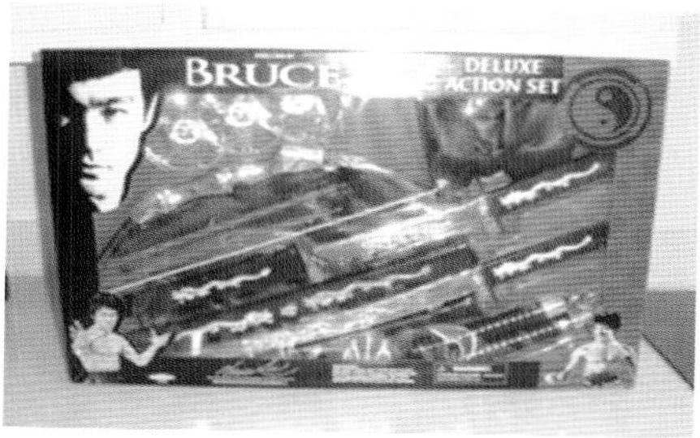

Further, in 2004, the "Ninja Force Set," Model No. 22369C, was included because of the sharp sword and knife.

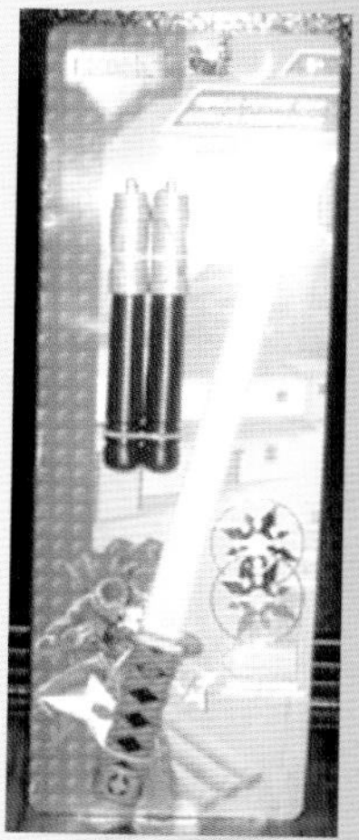

4. NO LOUD NOISES

According to the standards, the noise level on a child's toy should not exceed 90 decibels from 25 cm. A child's inner ear is still developing and is far more sensitive to harm than an adult's. The following two toys were included on our most dangerous list:

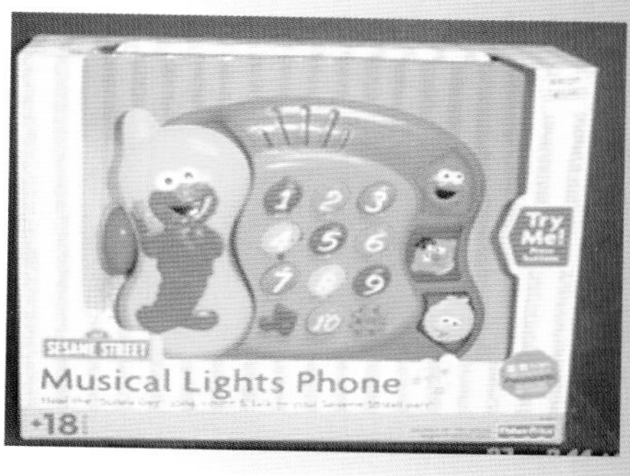

➪ In 2003, the "Sesame Street Musical Lights Phone" had noise levels far greater than permissible.

➪ In 2004, the "Learn Through Music," manufactured by Fischer Price, was found to have a decibel rating of 92 from 25cm. However, the child is more likely to play closer to the toy according to the experts, about 5 to 10 cm where the decibel reading is a whopping 110, enough to hurt an adults ear with extended use.

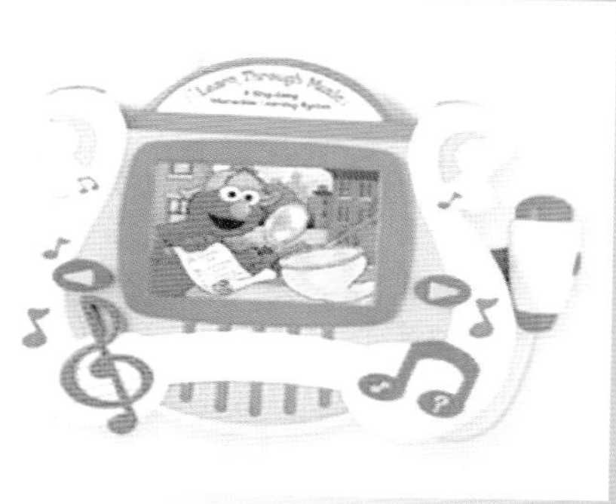

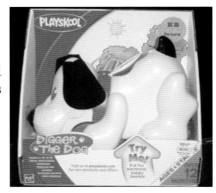

5. NO LONG CORDS OR STRINGS

⇨ In 2004, we included "Digger the Dog" because the pull string for an age appropriate of 12 months or older was longer than permissible.

6. NO DANGEROUS CHEMICALS

⇨ Remarkably, the "Hillary Duff Twinkle Toes Pedicure Set" was included in our 2004 list for containing the toxic chemical Xylene. According to the Toxic Hazards Textbook, Xylene can cause memory loss, dizziness and vomiting.

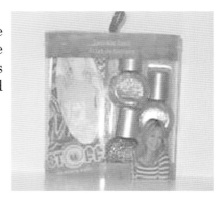

7. INSTRUCTIONS ON THE PACKAGE ARE THE SAME AS INSTRUCTIONS INSIDE

Shockingly, a high number of toys have contradictory statements on the outside package versus what you will find inside.

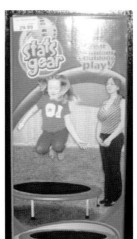

⇨ The 2004 38" "Playtime Trampoline," pictured here, clearly has a picture of a child playing on the trampoline in the backyard. In fact the photograph is in four places on the outside package, yet when the parent buys the toy and takes it home and reads the instructions they will find a whole page of WARNINGS, and they will be surprised to read "for indoor use only."

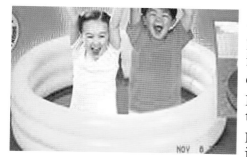

⇨ Usage is not the only contradictory piece of information. In 2003, we included the inflatable swimming pool called the "Jump Around." The outside of the package proclaimed its use for any children over the age of three. But when the parent got the product home and looked at the instructions inside, they were surprised to find that only children six years old and above would be age appropriate to play in the swimming pool.

8. NO EXTREME HEAT

⇨ In 2003, we included the "Creepy Crawlers Bug Maker," which had an oven which had the potential for both electric shock and burn injuries.

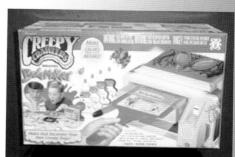

9. NO OUTRAGEOUS VIOLENCE

⇨ The Internet poses many dangers for children in toys and amusement. First, many banned toys will be distributed on the Internet. But perhaps the worst danger, given the technology skills of children, is that many times children can access dangerous and outrageous amusement and toys without the parents even being aware. In 2004 we named the outrageous "JFK Reloaded" to the list. Any child could easily go on the Internet to www.jfk-reloaded.com and play the role of the assassin of our nation's President.

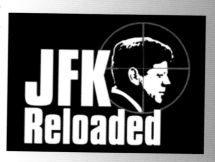

The child would be able to visualize holding the rifle and aiming at the head of President Kennedy, firing the shot and seeing his brain explode from the impact of the bullet. The producer of the Web site ironically gives the user the option between the "bloody" or the "non-bloody" re-enactment. With children now having debit bank cards, and some even their own credit cards, it is very easy for children to bypass the scrutiny of their parents and be directly exposed to outrageous violence.

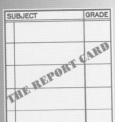

10. NO OBVIOUS DANGER

➯ Each year, there is always a toy which does not easily fall into the preceding categories but is clearly dangerous in the hands of children. In 2004, we chose the "Rocket Pocket Miniature Electric Motorcycle." This toy, according to the experts, was the fastest selling toy of the 2004 holiday season. At an expense of a $200 plus price tag, it sits low to the ground and can travel up to 18 miles an hour. The toy can easily be driven on the streets and parking lots. Because of its speed and being built low to the ground, it can and will cause serious injury and death.

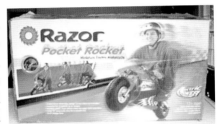

IMPORTANT NOTES:

In addition to the Keenans Kids Foundation, www.keenanskidsfoundation.com , two other notable groups release list of dangerous toys, usually in late November:

➯ www.toysafety.net, operated by the National PRIG, Public Interest Research Group.

➯ www.toysafety.org, operated by notable lawyer Edward Swartz and his equally notable lawyer son James.

To make a decision on the safety of a toy, do not rely solely on what toys have been recalled. Remember a recall does not occur normally unless/until a child dies or many are injured. Don't permit your child's death or serious injury to be the one who causes a recall. However, we still advise you to check via the Internet the list of recalled toys at www.usgovinfo.about.com/od/consumerawareness/a/toyrecalls2004.htm

For a great source of safe toys go to www.backtobasictoys.com . All of the company's toys are hazard-free.

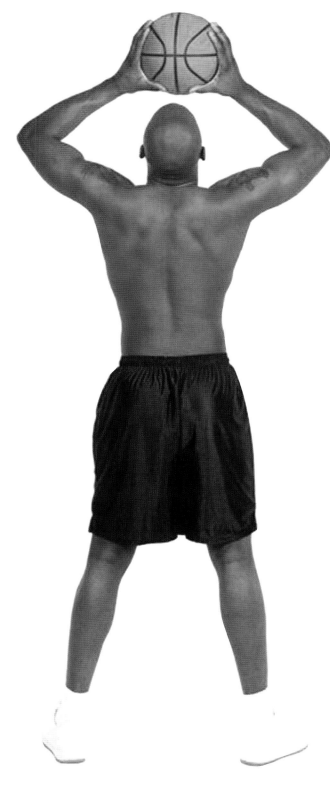

16

Sports

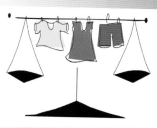

In the Heat of the Moment

*C*hip, a star teenage athlete and straight-A student, was looking forward to seeing his father, Nick, after finishing his high school basketball game. Chip's mother, Susan, was in the stands at the high school gymnasium early in the game, cheering her son on until it came time to pick up Chip's dad, who had been away on a business trip, from the airport.

The gym was unreasonably hot that night, about 82 degrees. There were no classes that spring Friday, because of a "teacher work day," so the air conditioning to the gym had been turned off since the night before. The janitor had forgotten to turn on the air conditioner to the gym six hours before Friday's night's game, as was the protocol. Both coaches decided to have their teams play the game anyway, hoping the gym would cool once the air conditioning kicked in.

Instead, as the game progressed, the body heat of the audience and the energy level of the players unfortunately increased the temperature inside the gymnasium.

Chip, the team captain, played the entire first quarter, then rested only two minutes in the second quarter. The coach later explained that Chip wanted to stay in the game to make sure his team won, and the coach admitted that he encouraged Chip and admired his spirit. No other teammates played as long or as hard as Chip that night.

Suddenly, midpoint in the third quarter, Chip collapsed on the hardwood floor. Witnesses describe him as having a seizure, "like a fish out of water." Frantically, everyone looked for the first aid kit, which was no where to be found. Sadly, neither the coach nor anyone on his staff knew first aid, nor was there a team athletic trainer in attendance. While the ambulance was called, a bystander used his hands to establish an airway and breathed life into Chip's body. No one attempted to cool Chip's body with ice or water. Chip was sped to the local hospital, where they declared that he had suffered a heat stroke.

Chip's parents arrived home from the airport, expecting to meet Chip at home. Instead, they found an empty house and a disturbing message on their voice mail, "Come to the hospital as quickly as possible."

On arrival, the doctor explained to Nick and Susan that from the onset of Chip's heat stroke there was a 20-minute window in which to administer aid, including cooling down his body. Unfortunately, because the coach and other school personnel knew nothing about saving Chip, that 20 minutes passed without help. That lack of help, combined with the decision to play rather than cancel the game or safely rotate players in the game, proved disastrous for Chip.

Chip is now mentally retarded. His scholarships, both athletic and scholastic, were cancelled. While he was once a star basketball player, he now cannot walk without assistance, and he has difficulty controlling his bowels. Chip will need a lifetime of supervised care.

LEGAL ACTION and OUTCOME

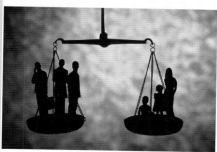

Chip's parents hired my law firm, and a claim was filed. We discovered numerous violations that caused Chip's devastating injuries. A national high school safety expert who worked on the legal case stated that the coach should not have permitted play that night, or should have limited each boy's play to five minutes at a time. A first aid kit, as well as someone who could administer CPR, should have been available. The coach in charge clearly should have insured that there was a safety plan in place to protect the boys. Severe dehydration and heat stroke are not uncommon during sporting events, either outdoors or indoors.

After a series of emotional and intense negotiations, the case was settled for a confidential sum.

Statistics Tell The Story

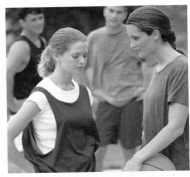

*C*hildren, who often have slower reaction times, less coordination and less accuracy in sports than adults, are at greater risk for injuries. They are also less able to assess the risks involved.

⇨ Overuse injury, the result of repeated motion over time, is responsible for nearly half of all sports injuries to middle and high-school students. Insufficient rest after an injury, poor training or conditioning, and immature bones contribute to overuse injuries among children.

⇨ Twenty-one percent of all traumatic brain injuries among children in the United States are the result of sports and recreational activities.

⇨ Higher rates of injury are associated with collision and contact sports than non-contact or individual sports. But injuries from individual sports tend to be more severe.

⇨ Approximately 55 percent of nonfatal sports injuries occur at school.

⇨ Thirty-seven percent of parents report that their child has been injured while playing a team sport. Half of these parents say the child has been injured more than once. Nearly a quarter of them report that the injury was serious.

⇨ Most organized sports-related injuries (62 percent) occur during practices rather than games.

⇨ Among athletes ages five to 14, 15 percent of basketball players, 28 percent of football players, 25 percent of baseball players, 22 percent of soccer players, and 12 percent of softball players have been injured while playing their sport.

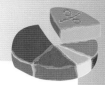

⇨ In 2002, the rate of emergency room treatment for children ages five to 14 was about:

- o 207,400 for basketball-related injuries
- o 187,800 for football-related injuries
- o 116,900 for baseball or softball-related injuries
- o 76,200 for soccer-related injuries
- o 21,200 for gymnastic-related injuries

⇨ Baseball has the highest fatality rate among all sports for children ages five to 14. Each year, three to four children die from baseball injuries.

⇨ The rate and severity of sports-related injuries increase with a child's age. Nearly 40 percent of all sports-related injuries treated in emergency rooms involve children ages five to 14.

⇨ Among children ages five to nine, sports-related injuries occur more frequently with girls than boys. However, during puberty (ages 10 to 14), boys are injured more often and more severely than girls. Boys ages 10 to 14 are two times more likely to be treated in a hospital emergency room for a sports-related injury than girls of the same age. And boys are more likely than girls to suffer multiple injuries.

⇨ Children who do not wear or use protective equipment (or who wear or use it improperly) are at greater risk of sustaining sports-related injuries. Sometimes equipment is not available because of lack of money, or because of lack of awareness regarding potential injury.

⇨ A child's stage of development is more of a factor in sports injury risk than age or body size. A less-developed child competing against a more mature child of the same age and weight is at a disadvantage and may be at greater risk for injury.

*National SAFE KIDS Campaign Sports Injury Fact Sheet 2004

Laws and Regulations

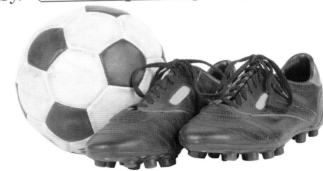

While there are some laws mandating the safety of sports equipment, there are no laws or government regulations directly pertaining to organized sports for children. The team on which your child plays may have its own set of guidelines; if so, read them and see if you agree with what's been outlined. It's up to parents and other concerned adults to see that children are safe when they participate in sports. Use the Report Card that follows to evaluate your child's sports program.

Recently, there has been a reemergence of the sport of dodgeball; a movie staring Ben Stiller is credited in part for the new found popularity. However, the National Association for Sports & Physical Education, a non-profit organization of 20,000 coaches, PE teachers, trainers and athletic directors, issued the following declaration: "Dodgeball is not an appropriate activity for K-12 school physical education programs." Some school districts in Maine, Maryland, New York, Massachuetts, Texas, Virginia and Utah have banned dodgeball, according to an AP story of November 20, 2004. Noted recreation expert, Steve Bernheim, also advises against playing the sport of dodgeball. Although no statistics are available, there are many reports of serious injury. (www.aahperd.org/naspe)

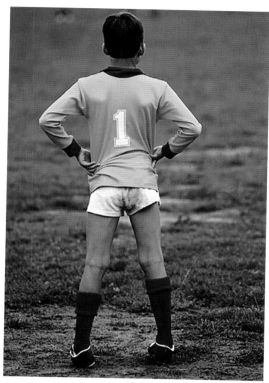

Most parents believe that there is nothing they could have done to prevent their child's sports-related injury, yet the National SAFE KIDS Campaign reports that half of all sports-related injuries ARE preventable.

In their 2003 study, the National SAFE KIDS Campaign found that more than half the parents (53 percent) surveyed expressed little concern about the possibility of their child getting hurt, despite the fact that one out of every three children is injured during team sports. Shockingly, four out of five parents surveyed whose child suffered a sports injury believe that it was part of the game and would have happened regardless of precautions. A third of the parents said they do not often take the same safety precautions during the child's practice as in the game, even though statistically most sports injuries occur during practice.

Parents need to take control and intervene when necessary in this injury-prone activity. They need to approach sports with the following REPORT CARD, designed to grade the coach and school with either a "pass" or "fail."

The Report Card

Use this report card to evaluate your child's sports activities for safety:

REPORT CARD		
	SUBJECT	GRADE
1	The coach has a clear track record of good judgement	
2	First aid equipment is available	
3	A certified trainer is available	
4	Concussion protocol is established	
5	Hydration protocol is established	
6	Lightning protocol is established for outdoor events	
7	Proper protective gear is up-to-date and in use	
8	The coach has complete knowledge of players' health conditions	
9	The coach has specific knowledge of the child's current medications	
10	Specific ambulance choice and local hospital choice are stated	

Each category receives either "Pass" or "Fail". To make your decision, please consider the following:

1. THE COACH HAS A CLEAR TRACK RECORD OF GOOD JUDGEMENT

Decisions such as whether or not to play a game and conditions of the game are often left to the sole judgment of the coach. The expert in Chip's case testified that the coach is the ultimate person in charge, the "captain of the ship." Therefore, it is important to know whether your child's coach has a proven track record of safety and whether he or she will always err on the side of safety.

2. FIRST AID EQUIPMENT IS AVAILABLE

It is essential that basic first aid equipment be within arm's reach of all sporting activities. Many schools now even have defibrillator machines. Neck stabilizers, windpipe openers, tourniquets, and surface antibiotic creams are mandatory. Access to ice and cold water is essential during the warmer months of the year. A third of parents surveyed by the National SAFE KIDS Campaign in 2000 stated that their child's team did not keep a first aid kit on hand during play.

3. A CERTIFIED TRAINER IS AVAILABLE

Only one of four organized sports activities surveyed in the 2000 National SAFE KIDS Campaign always had a certified athletic trainer on site. The study also found that more than a third (41 percent) of children's coaches are not certified in CPR. There is a recognized certifying body of athletic trainers- the National Athletic Trainers' Association (www.nata.org). This group maintains protocols regarding certain high-risk injuries, and they have a certification process to test competency.

4. CONCUSSION PROTOCOL IS ESTABLISHED

A concussion protocol should specifically outline how to access a concussion, when to refer a child to a physician, and what signs should disqualify a child from further play. In the fall of 2004, NATA issued a new position statement, "Management of Sports-Related Concussions." This protocol is quite reasonable and very attainable in the right hands (www.nata.org).

5. HYDRATION PROTOCOL IS ESTABLISHED

The CDC in 2002 found that 300 people die each year from heat-related illnesses, and that dehydration can increase the risk of heat illness. Yet the American College of Sports Medicine (ACSM) reported at its annual meeting in 2004 that two thirds of children arrived at sports practice significantly dehydrated. In the summer of 2004, Dan Marino, former quarterback of the Miami Dolphins, was the spokesperson for the "Defeat the Heat" campaign, which stressed that the ABCs will help prevent heat stroke and dehydration:

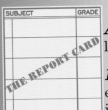

A - Always drink before, during and after activity to replace what the body has lost through sweat.

B - Bring the right fluids. For exercise lasting less than one hour, the ACSM found little evidence of performance differences between consuming water or sports drinks. For intense exercise lasting more than one hour, they recommend sports drinks plus the inclusion of sodium.

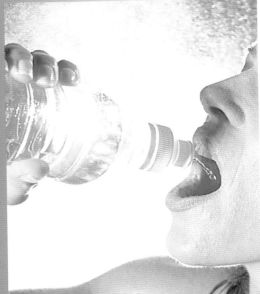

C - Consider fluids as a part of essential safety equipment for sports. Hydration of children is not rocket science-make sure the coach and school have a stated hydration policy. Children should also be given frequent rest periods during hot or humid weather.

6. LIGHTNING PROTOCOL IS ESTABLISHED FOR OUTDOOR EVENTS

Every year, millions of lightning flashes strike the ground, causing nearly 100 deaths and 400 injuries, according to the National Athletic Trainers' Association (*NATA Bulletin* September 2004.) The NATA issued a lightning protocol, which has been endorsed by the American Academy of Pediatrics (AAP). Primary to this protocol is a "flash-to-bang" ratio to avoid lightning danger. Katie Walsh, Ed.D., ATC, made the following statement: Count seconds between seeing a flash (lightning) and hearing the bang (thunder), then divide by five to determine how far away in miles the lightning is occurring. Be inside a safe structure by the time the count reaches six seconds.

The lightning protocol that has been adopted nationwide by many schools provides a specific action and recognizes that three-quarters of all lightning injuries occur between May and September, and nearly four-fifths of lightning casualties occur between 10a.m. and 7p.m. There is a higher rate of thunderstorm activity and thus higher lightning casualty rates in the seaboard, southwest, southern Rocky Mountains, and southern plain states.

7. PROPER PROTECTIVE GEAR IS UP-TO-DATE AND IN USE

See Chapter 24, "Helmets and Restraint Devices," for the specifics regarding proper gear. There should be a standard audit procedure to make sure all protective gear is up-to-date and some sanction process for repeated player violations.

8. THE COACH HAS COMPLETE KNOWLEDGE OF PLAYERS' HEALTH CONDITIONS

Most organized sports play requires a clearance letter from a physician, which simply says that the child can engage in physical activity. Often, however, these clearance letters contain specific statements about conditions like asthma, sickle cell anemia, bleeding disorders and former debilitating childhood conditions. Many times this specific knowledge is simply filed and never communicated to the coach. There must be a process in which the pertinent information travels from the doctor to the coach.

9. THE COACH HAS SPECIFIC KNOWLEDGE OF THE CHILD"S CURRENT MEDICATIONS

Unless a physician prohibits play, a coach often assumes there are no other health considerations. This is simply not true. The coach must be knowledgeable of any drugs that the child is taking. Why is this so important? It is well documented that Ritalin, for example, can drastically impact a child's hydration levels. Clearly, children taking such drugs must be hydrated properly. Ritalin is only one example of a drug that can impact a child's condition, particularly when playing full blast on the sports field.

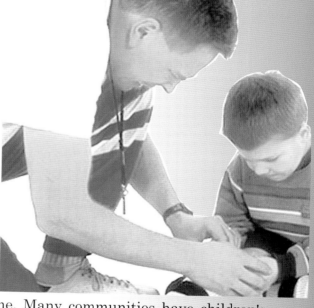

10. SPECIFIC AMBULANCE CHOICE AND LOCAL HOSPITAL CHOICE ARE STATED

The school needs to have a designated ambulance transport company and school personnel should dictate that company when calling 911, unless that company is not available at the time. Many communities have children's trauma centers located in close proximity. Oftentimes when 911 dispatches a hospital-based ambulance, that ambulance is directed to bring all patients to that specific hospital. There have been a number of cases where, due to the severity of the child's injury, the child should have been taken directly to the children's hospital trauma center rather than the local hospital. So the coach and school should know the distance and location of the nearest children's trauma center and be prepared to dictate that course of action in the face of a severe injury.

NOTE: Many coaches and schools will receive passing grades for all of the above points during actual competitive games. However, during practice, they fail on one or more account. More time is spent in practice than in games, so be certain that these guidelines apply during both.

Special thanks goes to the National Association for Sports & Physical Education (www.aahperd.org/naspe) for many years of advancing safety in sports.

SPECIAL NOTE ON MOVEABLE SOCCER GOALS

Between 1979 and 2002, the Consumer Products Safety Commission (www.cpsc.gov) documented 27 deaths and 120 serious injuries resulting from soccer goals falling over.

The majority of the deaths and injuries are from school-made or homemade soccer goals which are unstable and often heavy.

The CPSC and the Coalition To Promote Soccer Goal Safety (800-527-7510) have worked together to improve safety with the following recommendations:

⇨ Securely anchor or counter-weight moveable goals at all times.
⇨ Never climb on the net or goal framework.
⇨ Remove nets when goals are not in use.
⇨ Anchor or chain goals to nearby fence posts, dugouts, or other similar sturdy fixtures when not in use.
⇨ Check all connecting hardware before every use. Replace damaged or missing fasteners immediately.
⇨ Ensure safety labels are clearly visable.
⇨ Fully disassemble goals for seasonal storage.
⇨ Always use extreme caution when moving goals.
⇨ Always instruct players on the safe handling of and potential dangers associated with moveable soccer goals.
⇨ Use moveable soccer goals only on level (flat) fields.

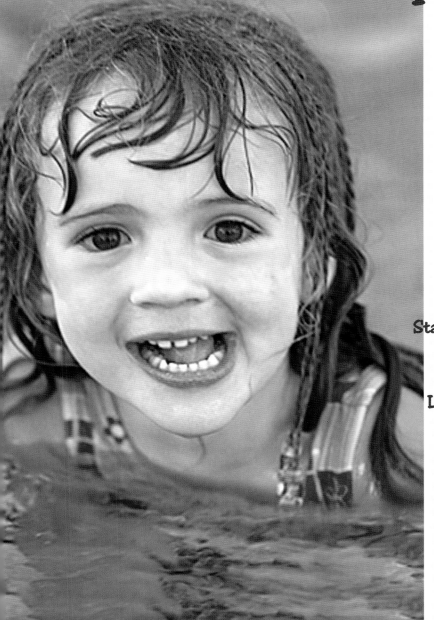

17

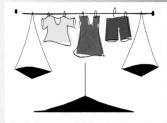

Swimming Pools, Hot Tubs and Spas

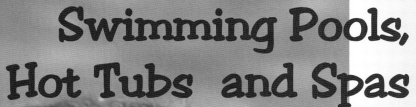

Deadly Dive

Ten-year-old Patrick looked forward to Sunday mornings throughout the summer. That's when he and his friends had the swimming pool in their apartment complex all to themselves.

Saturday, on the other hand, was singles time at the pool, when the bachelors and bachelorettes gathered around - not to swim, but to flirt and party. The couples mingled into happy hour and the Saturday pool party, where the alcohol flowed freely. Often drunk and rowdy, the last thing the singles wanted was a bunch of kids running around them and diving and splashing in the pool. The scene wasn't too enticing to the boys anyway, so they stayed away on Saturdays.

Once Sunday morning arrived, though, Patrick and his friends, Johnny and Brett, gathered to put the pool to good use. On this particular Sunday morning, the pool water was a little cloudy. The boys didn't mind; in fact, it made their play all the more exciting because they could sneak up on one another underwater in their game of "submarine." That murkiness, though, proved to be a life-threatening hazard.

After a round of "submarine," the boys took turns jumping off the diving board. Johnny and Brett each jumped, feet-first, their hands slowing their descent into the water. Without reaching the depths of the pool, each boy surfaced, and climbed out. Patrick's turn was next. Headfirst, Patrick dove expertly. The boys considered whether Patrick's dive deserved a perfect score of 10. "It's a 10," they hollered, but Patrick didn't come to the surface to receive his accolades.

At first the boys thought Patrick was playing with them, staying under in a new version of "submarine." But they soon realized that something was wrong and they ran for help. When the boys returned with their mothers, they found Patrick's lifeless body floating, facedown, in the pool. The mothers frantically tried CPR, and the ambulance team that arrived shortly did the same, but Patrick was dead.

A fresh, open gash on Patrick's head held the answer to his death. The night before, during the singles party, a drunken young man- trying to impress the girls with his strength- threw a large, heavy, chaise lounge into the deepest part of the pool. The lounge rested in the bottom of the diving area, with its back in the erect upright position. The murky water- caused by a long-standing chemical system malfunction- prevented Patrick and his buddies from seeing the chair. As Patrick dove, unsuspectingly, the impact of his head on the metal of the chair knocked him unconscious and caused him to drown.

LEGAL ACTION and OUTCOME

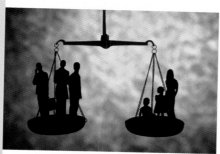

Patrick's mother hired The Keenan Law Firm to investigate the incident.

There were two culprits in this tragedy. One was the use of alcohol in the swimming pool area and the other was the lack of proper pool maintenance. The pool safety expert in the case testified that pool parties involving alcohol lead to dangerous circumstances- where an innocent bystander or party participant is hurt on a regular basis. Judgment is impaired, people do careless things, and harm frequently ensues, he explained. The expert also testified that if the longstanding problem with the pool chemicals had been remedied, Patrick and the boys would have seen the danger in the water. Proper chemical balance in a swimming pool is intended to prevent skin irritation, eye burning and exposure to bacteria. But the proper balance of chemicals can also prevent serious harm from completely unexpected hazards.

The resulting lawsuit was quickly settled, as the apartment complex management realized the overwhelming negligence that led to Patrick's death. As a result of the suit, they banned alcohol use in the pool area. This was later adopted as a municipal law. The complex management also mandated weekly maintenance checks on the swimming pool.

Statistics Tell the Story

There are 6.7 million homes in the U.S. with backyard swimming pools. Twenty percent of these households have children between the ages of one and five, the highest-risk group for drowning. **

⇨ Over 400 children drown in backyard swimming pools nationwide each year. About 250 of them are under the age of five. Half of drownings occur at children's homes or apartment complexes.

⇨ Drowning is the second-leading cause of death in children (behind motor vehicle accidents).

⇨ In 2002, 2,700 children were treated in emergency rooms for pool-related injuries. Of these, 1,600 were under the age of five. In 2003, 1,600 children were treated in emergency rooms for "submersion injuries." Children who experience near-drowning often experience serious consequences. If they require cardiopulmonary resuscitation (CPR), it is likely that they will die or be left with severe brain injury. In fact, about 2,000 children suffer neurological injury in near-drowning incidents annually.

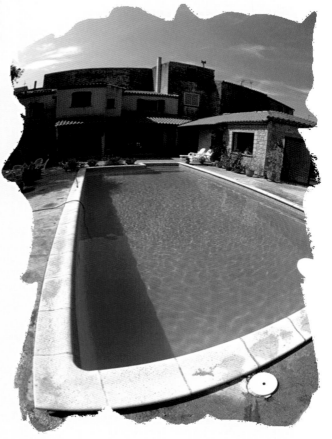

⇨ Nineteen percent of drowning deaths of children occur in public pools, with certified lifeguards present. *(The Drowning Prevention Foundation.)*

⇨ Male children have a drowning rate two to four times that of female children. And black males, ages five to nine, have swimming-pool related

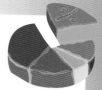

drowning rates four times that of Caucasian children. Black males ages 10 to 14 have swimming-pool related drowning rates 15 times greater than Caucasian children.

⇨ Out of all the preschoolers who drown, 70 percent are in the care of one or both parents at the time, and 75 percent are missing from sight for five minutes or less. Seven percent of the time, a sibling is supervising the victim. Drowning is called "the silent killer," because once a child slips under the water, you cannot hear that he or she is in trouble.

⇨ Between January 1990 and October 2003, there were 73 cases of body entrapment in water, including 12 deaths. Thirty-one of these incidents occurred in swimming pools and three occurred in wading pools. Seventy-seven percent of the incidents involved children under the age of 15 years.

Logically, the rate of drowning is particularly worrisome in the states of Florida, Arizona, and California, where pools are plentiful.
For example:
⇨ In Florida, where drowning deaths of children under age five are more than twice the national average, more than two-thirds of these occur in backyard swimming pools.
⇨ In Arizona, there are seven deaths for every 100,000 preschoolers, the highest rate in the nation.
⇨ In Los Angeles, where two children each week drown during peak season, 51 percent of drowning fatalities happen in backyard swimming pools.
(California State Department of Health.)

In dollars and cents:
⇨ The annual cost of drownings among children ages 14 and under is about $6.8 billion. Nearly half of these costs involve children ages four and under.

⇨ Medical costs for a near-drowning victim's family can range from $75,000 for emergency room treatment to $180,000 per year for long-term care.

⇨ The cost of a single near-drowning incident that results in brain damage can exceed $4.5 million. (National SAFE KIDS Campaign.)

**Pool and Spa Living

Laws and Regulations

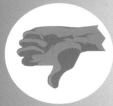

No national laws or regulations mandate the safekeeping of children in and around swimming pools. State and local regulations regarding safety equipment, pool design, water quality and record keeping do exist, but enforcement is spotty at best. At Patrick's apartment complex, for example, the pool would have been closed because of the cloudy water, had the proper authorities been alerted.

In order to minimize pool drownings of young children, the U.S. Consumer Products Safety Commission developed swimming pool guidelines. These guidelines, which are incorporated into our Taking Action section, are not mandatory. They are voluntary guidelines and recommendations.

Only four states- Arizona, California, Florida and Oregon- have enacted safety laws requiring some type of fencing around residential swimming pools.(*National SAFE KIDS* 2004.)

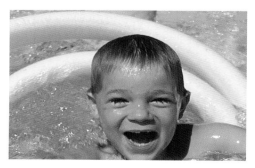

Taking Action

Children under the age of five have a far greater risk of pool injuries than older children, so at the end of our first list we've provided special guidelines for preventing swimming pool injuries for children under age five.

✔ ⚠ CHECKLIST ⚠

1	Do not permit alcohol.
2	No diving boards unless lifeguard on duty.
3	Install pool alarms.
4	No body entrapment/ entanglement potential.
5	Maintenance checks and surveillance before each use.
6	Maintain proper chemical mixture.
7	Stock first aid equipment.
8	Provide constant supervision to all children.
9	Learn CPR and rescue techniques.

1. DO NOT PERMIT ALCOHOL.

No alcohol consumption of any type should be permitted around pools where children are present or might be present at a later time. As Patrick's death showed, unintentional actions of adults can ultimately cause serious harm to children.

2. NO DIVING BOARDS UNLESS LIFEGUARDS ARE ON DUTY.

Thirty years ago, virtually every swimming pool had a diving board, but because of the avalanche of deaths and serious injuries, the vast majority of non-life guarded pools now do not have diving boards. Without a lifeguard present to administer immediate aid, the multitude of injuries and harm that can result from diving is unguarded. The bottom line is that if there is a diving board, there must be a lifeguard.

3. INSTALL POOL ALARMS.

If there is not a lifeguard with a cell phone, then there should be some other form of phone or alarm system, so that a witness can quickly call for help if needed. Floating pool alarms are also available, to alert you that something- or someone- is in the water.

4. NO BODY ENTRAPMENT/ENTANGLEMENT POTENTIAL.

Former vice-presidential candidate John Edwards once represented an eight-year-old girl whose toe got caught in a swimming pool suctioning device. The suction kept her body submerged until brain damage occurred. As a result, the May 2004 *Consumer Products Safety Hazard Release* contained the following statement:

To prevent body entrapment and hair entrapment/entanglement, have a qualified pool professional inspect the drain suction fittings and covers on your pool and spa to be sure they are proper size, properly attached, and meet current safety standards. If your pool or spa has a single drain outlet, consider installing a safety vacuum release system that breaks the vacuum to avoid potential entrapment conditions.

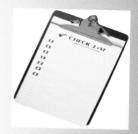

5. MAINTENANCE CHECKS AND SURVEILLANCE BEFORE EACH USE.

If there had been a maintenance or surveillance check early Sunday morning, before Patrick and his friends arrived, the pool in our sample case would have been closed until the murky water was removed. The chaise lounge would have been discovered, and Patrick's life would have been spared. Surveillance should occur before a pool is opened– every time.

6. MAINTAIN PROPER CHEMICAL MIXTURE.

At first glance, ensuring the correct chemical mixture in a swimming pool appears only to be a skin irritant safety issue. But Patrick's case proves otherwise. All safety maintenance must be done on a timely basis in order to prevent unintended dangers.

7. STOCK FIRST AID EQUIPMENT.

Because of the great potential for injury, basic first aid items must be within close proximity of the pool.

8. PROVIDE CONSTANT SUPERVISION TO ALL CHILDREN.

Constant supervision of children in and around pools is extremely important. Do not allow children to swim without a lifeguard or responsible adult on duty. If there is a pool in the vicinity, do not assume that the child will not find his or her way to it. One CPSC study showed that almost 70 percent of the young victims were not expected to be in or even around the pool. In less time than it takes to run inside for a glass of water or answer a phone call, a child can drown.

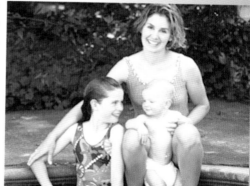

9. LEARN CPR AND RESCUE TECHNIQUES.

In the event of an incident, knowing how to administer the proper first aid might save a child's life.

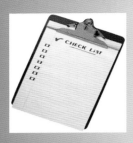

	CHECKLIST
	SPECIAL ADDITIONAL CHECKLIST FOR CHILDREN UNDER THE AGE OF FIVE: *Note: the following is adopted verbatim from the 25 May 2004 Consumer Products Safety Commission's Warning About Pool Hazards.**
1	Fences must be tall with four sides and an auto gate lock (child proof).
2	Alarms, if necessary
3	No attractive nuisances
4	Secured and locked pool steps and ladders
5	Power safety cover

SPECIAL ADDITIONAL CHECKLIST FOR CHILDREN UNDER THE AGE OF FIVE:

Note: the following is adopted verbatim from the 25 May 2004 Consumer Products Safety Commission's Warning About Pool Hazards.

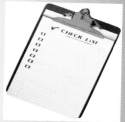

1. FENCES MUST BE TALL WITH FOUR SIDES AND AN AUTO GATE LOCK (CHILD PROOF).

Fences and walls should be at least four feet high and installed completely around the pool. Fence gates should be self-closing and self-latching. The latch should be out of a child's reach. Keep furniture that could be used for climbing into the pool area away from the fences.

2. ALARMS, IF NECESSARY

If your house forms one side of the barrier to the pool, then doors leading from the house to the pool should be protected with alarms that produce a sound when a door is unexpectedly opened.

3. NO ATTRACTIVE NUISANCES

Do not leave pool toys or floats in the pool or pool area that may attract the young children to water.

4. SECURED AND LOCKED POOL STEPS AND LADDERS

For aboveground pools, steps and ladders to the pool should be secured and locked or removed when the pool is not in use.

5. POWER SAFETY COVER

Although not mandatory, the CPSC did recommend a power safety cover, which is a motorized power barrier that can be placed above the water area and be used when the pool is not in use.

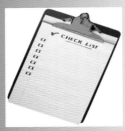

Hot Tubs and Spas

According to the CPSC, over 200 children under the age of five have died in hot tubs and spas in the last 10 years. Burns also frequently occur in small children because their skin is very sensitive to the hot water.

Follow these simple rules:
1. No child less than eight should be in a hot tub, even with an adult.
2. Always place a hard cover over the hot tub/spa and make sure it's locked.

Drain Covers

The sucking action of a drain is very dangerous to a child. Hair and or clothing can be sucked into the drain and force the child to stay submerged. Also, in small children, the child's head can be suctioned into the drain keeping the child submerged. There exist safe drain covers which prevent these dangers but they are not mandatory.
Follow these simple safety pointers.
1. If possible, buy a hot tub/spa with a safety proof drain.
2. At the least, replace the current cover with one that will prevent hair and clothed from being sucked.
3. Do not permit children to go under the water.

More information about drowning hazards and prevention can be found at the CPSC Web site: www.cpsc.gov.

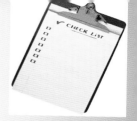

Above-Ground Pools

About one in five above-ground pools sold in the United States each year may pose a safety hazard, according to www.consumerreports.org. There exists no law or regulation requiring fences, alarms, covers and gear required of larger pools.

The extent of the deaths and serious injuries are not known because the Consumer Products Safety Commission (www.cpsc.gov) does not break down the annual 250 pool deaths and 1,800 submersion injuries into above-ground versus in-ground pools.

According to industry estimates, 30,000 to 40,000 above-ground pools are sold each year ranging from $50 to $750, standing 18 inches to four feet and having less than 200 to more than 5,000 gallons of water.

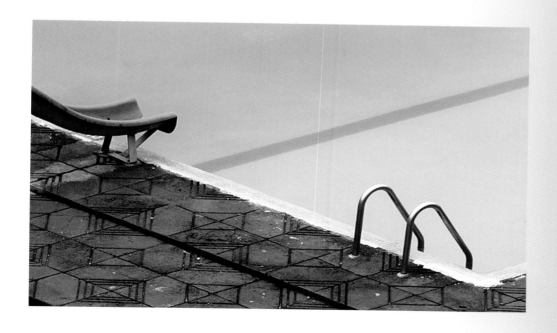

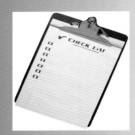

Use the following checklist to help prevent **ABOVE-GROUND POOLS** deaths and injuries:

✔	⚠ **CHECKLIST** ⚠
1	**Always supervise.** There is no substitute for visualizing and supervising. A split second can make a difference.
2	**Always fence.** Fencing is required. According to Gary Smith, M.D., of the American Academy of Pediatrics, **www.aap.org**, "the fence is the only proven safety intervention to prevent drowning."
3	**Check with CPSC.** The CPSC has some excellent recommendations in publications 359 and 362 which can be obtained online at **www.cpsc.gov**.

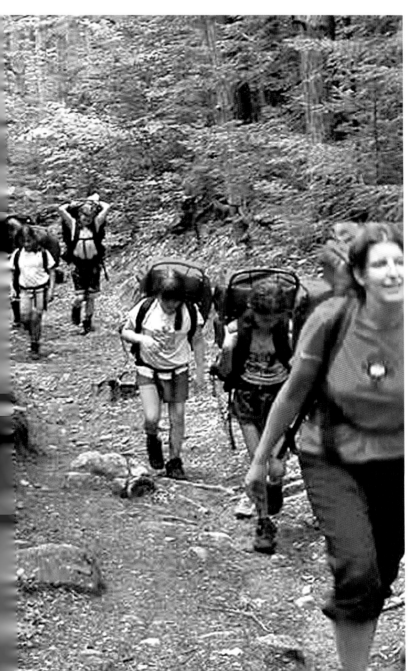

18

Summer Camps

Safe Haven or Unsupervised Disaster?

The fondest dream of the Nigerian family living in North Carolina was to give their children the American dream. So, the family saved its money to send off their nine-year-old son, Charles to a church-run summer camp in North Georgia.

The Abayas believed he would be safe and supervised, particularly after speaking with camp officials. One of the drawing cards for this summer camp was its lake and number of water-related activities like row boating and swimming. The family made it clear that their son did not know how to swim but was looking forward to learning. They made this statement both in person as well as on all of their application forms.

When the Abayas drove their son to the camp and said goodbye to him, they did not realize that they would be bringing him home in a casket.

Camp-safety experts are adamant that camps must administer a skills test to all children before permitting them to participate in any water activities. Unfortunately, this camp did not have a rigid skills test protocol. They didn't even have a lifeguard on duty while children played near the beach and lake area.

After unpacking their bags that first day, the campers were given free time to let them settle in. Many children, including Charles, went down to the lake. Urged on by older boys Charles walked slowly into the waters not wanting to appear that he was afraid. He decided to splash in the shallows, believing he would stay safe. One of the camp counselors saw the boy and assume he knew how to swim. Unfortunately, the lake's bottom had a massive drop-off near the shoreline. Charles fell into the open area of the lake and drowned.

LEGAL ACTION and OUTCOME

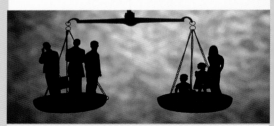

My firm was successful in compensating the family and bringing about change to this and other summer camps. The evidence reveals that while there were checklists and training protocols in place the staff was unaware until after the death. The safety experts we retained were all critical of the lack of supervision of the children and the failure to do pre-testing of all children before any activities were commenced. They all wonder why more deaths and serious injuries had not occurred. Our evidence also revealed several similar incidents that were never reported to the parents. This Georgia camp now has a rigid training program for its staff and warning signs posted at the lake. Additionally, they have instituted a buddy system of pairing skilled children swimmers with those with little or no skills.

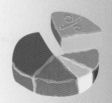

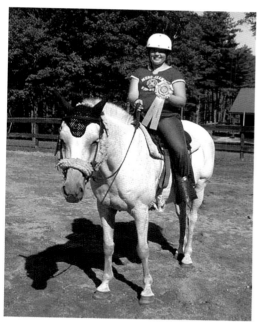

⇨ There are approximately 12,000 camps in the U.S. Of these, some 7,000 are resident camps and 5,000 are day camps.

⇨ Approximately 8,000 camps are operated by nonprofit entities like youth agencies and churches. The other 4,000 are privately owned by independent, for-profit operators.

⇨ Only about 25 percent of all U.S. camps are accredited by the American Camping Association (ACA).

⇨ Each year, more than 10 million campers, and nearly all of them children, attend camp.

⇨ The number of day camps in the U.S. has risen by nearly 90 percent in the last 20 years.

⇨ There are no federal injury and death reporting requirements for camps, so no one knows exactly how many campers die or are injured each year. But thousands of campers are injured- many seriously- and a few die each year. For example, there were eight deaths reported to the ACA in 2003. Statistics from the approximately 75 percent of camps that are not accredited by ACA are not available.

Source: American Camping Association.

Laws and Regulations

In 2001, U.S. Rep. Christopher Shays introduced legislation that would require recreational camps to report information concerning deaths and certain injuries and illnesses to the Secretary of Health and Human Services (HHS). The legislation would also require HHS to collect the information in a central data system and to establish a President's Council on Recreational Camps.

This legislation has been languishing in committee since late 2001.

And this is just a proposed law to report injuries and deaths. It will do nothing to prevent injuries and deaths. Considering the large number of camps and campers involved, we would like to see legislation that goes beyond a reporting requirement to the heart of the matter, which should be to prevent injuries and deaths in the first place.

Another federal law was proposed in 2001 that would have a stronger impact on campers' safety. Introduced by U.S. Rep. Robert E. Andrews, this law would require camps to conduct criminal background checks of all employees. And, citing the case of a camper who drowned while a lifeguard was on duty supervising 70 children, the law would mandate a minimum camper-to-lifeguard ratio. No action has been taken on this bill.

A University of Michigan study published in 2003 examined the current state of summer camp safety and health requirements in Michigan, one of the nation's more proactive states in camp safety. State laws require annual licensing, a dedicated camp health officer and first aid training for many camp staff.

Even so, the researcher found that, out of 129 Michigan camps, half had a health officer with paramedic training or less, and half had registered nurses on staff. Two-thirds of camps surveyed reported that ambulances responding to an emergency would go to a small or rural hospital, and more than a third said it would take an ambulance 10 or more minutes to get to their camp.

And bear in mind that this is one of the better states.

Use the following checklist to remove the hazards of **SUMMER CAMP**:

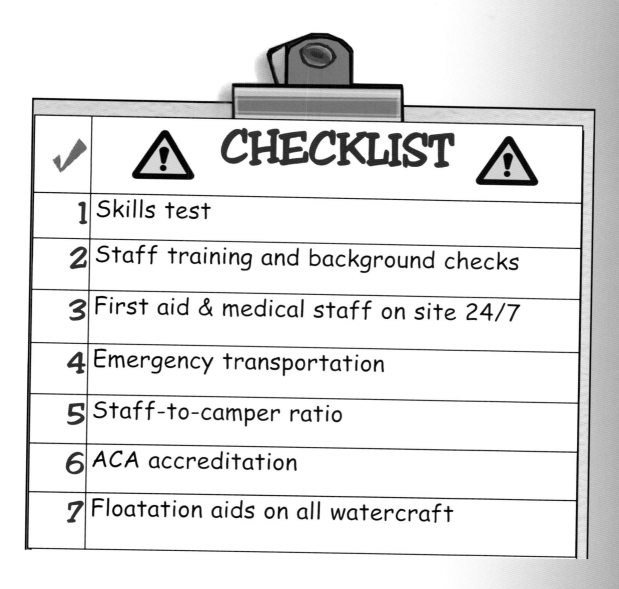

CHECKLIST

✔		
1	Skills test
2	Staff training and background checks
3	First aid & medical staff on site 24/7
4	Emergency transportation
5	Staff-to-camper ratio
6	ACA accreditation
7	Floatation aids on all watercraft

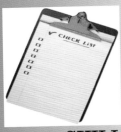

1. SKILLS TEST
A skills test is needed for swimming, diving, water sports, boating, rock climbing, repelling, horseback riding–any activity where skill is required. Even with skills testing, there should be a "buddy" system for swimming.

2. STAFF TRAINING AND BACKGROUND CHECKS
Check who provides training, how comprehensive it is and if there is adequate supervision of counselors. The American Camping Association (ACA) requires staff screening which may include criminal background checks where permitted by law. Ask about the screening process.

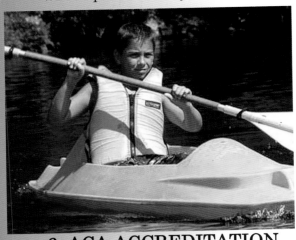

3. FIRST AID & MEDICAL STAFF ON SITE 24/7

4. EMERGENCY TRANSPORTATION
This should be available at all times.

5. STAFF-TO-CAMPER RATIO
Ratios differ for different age groups. Use common sense-one lifeguard for 70 swimmers is not reasonable by any measure.

6. ACA ACCREDITATION
Parents can expect a higher standard of safety from accredited camps. But even with ACA-member camps, a thorough investigation of any camp is advised.

7. FLOATATION AIDS ON ALL WATERCRAFT
As seen in the above photograph, floatation aids are needed on all watercraft, and if the watercraft has a stated occupancy, there should be a like number of floatation aids available on the craft.

19
Jet Skis

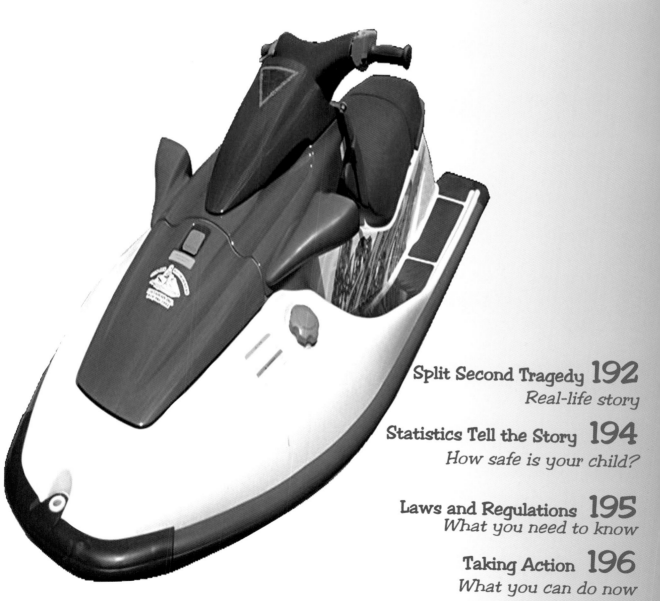

Split Second Tragedy

*C*andace and Richard followed the ambulance to the local trauma center, not knowing if their 11-year-old daughter, Alisa, would live or die. What was supposed to be a fun weekend outing on the lake turned -in a split second- to tragedy.

The family had taken the hour drive to the lake with one of Candace's co-workers, Josie, and her 14-year-old son, Brett. Brett's Jet Ski®- also known as a Personal Watercraft, or PWC- was in tow behind the SUV. Brett received the PWC for his 14th birthday and had taken it on the lake several times before. The group planned to locate a picnic area and enjoy a day on the lake, taking turns on the PWC.

After setting up in the picnic area, the group put the PWC in the water. All were aware of the basic rules: wear a life preserver, do not speed, and always observe the right-of-way. Never having ridden a PWC before, Candace and Richard were very cautious themselves, and especially protective of Alisa. The two watched intently as Brett maneuvered the PWC on his own before they became comfortable letting Alisa ride along with the teen. Although Alisa desperately wanted to drive, both parents emphatically said no.

The PWC made several passes, with Alisa smiling and waving to her parents. Candace and Richard began to feel more comfortable. They had seen television commercials, and even a movie or two, showing kids having fun on PWCs. With life preservers and a good driver, what was the harm? Richard started cooking the hot dogs for the picnic, while Candace kept a lookout. About half an hour later, Richard heard a blood-curdling scream as Candace called out Alisa's name.

Alisa had fallen off the back of the PWC as Brett hit a strong wave created by a speeding powerboat. The thrust was so powerful that as Alisa hit the water, immediate internal damage was caused, leaving Alisa lifeless. She was quickly swept up, revived and taken to the trauma center, where the family learned that her spleen was ruptured and her rectum severely torn.

After many days in the ICU and almost a month in the hospital, Alisa returned home to begin her rehabilitation. Three years later, she still walked with a noticeable disability. Because of the fragility of her internal organs, she was prohibited from participating in any sports play or strenuous activity. Her long-term prognosis is still questionable.

My law firm was hired to find the reason why this tragedy occurred. We quickly discovered that the PWC manufacturer - although aware of the high number of injuries resulting from passengers being thrown from the rear of the vehicle- failed to place warning labels on the PWC. In addition, they failed to take advantage of several low-cost design changes that could prevent, or at least minimize, these types of injuries.

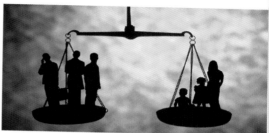

LEGAL ACTION
and
OUTCOME

During our investigation, we learned that the manufacturer failed to make the necessary changes because of financial considerations. After several years of litigation, the case was settled. Today, the manufacturer of these PWCs does place clear warnings on the vehicle itself, as well as on all of the literature. They still fail, however, to make the necessary design modifications to avoid these tragedies.

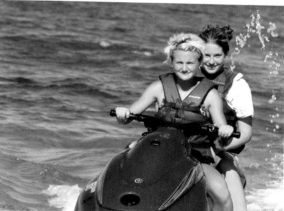

Of particular note is the litigation tactic of the manufacturer in alleging that they were virtually immune from fault because the law of admiralty applied to this case. Admiralty law is very restrictive, similar to workers compensation law. A defendant is responsible for only a small portion of the damages. Unfortunately, many courts around the country had granted PWC manufacturers such "admiralty" immunity, but in 1996, the U.S. Supreme Court (in the case of Yamaha Motor Corporation, U.S.A vs. Calhoun), decided that PWC manufacturers should not be able to hide behind admiralty law. Rather, they would be subject to the same law as anyone in the United States whose negligence causes harm.

Statistics Tell the Story

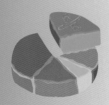

⇨ PWCs are the only recreational boats for which the leading cause of death is blunt trauma rather than drowning. (*American Academy of Pediatrics, February 2000.*)

⇨ PWC injuries to children are far more severe than those to adults, particularly the severity of head injuries, chest trauma, and spinal paralysis. (*Small Watercraft Injuries in Children, February 2000, the University of Florida Pediatric Surgery Department.*)

⇨ In 2002, 189 children under the age of 14 were injured in PWC accidents. This accounted for 14 percent of all PWC injuries. (*U.S. Coast Guard.*)

⇨ In 2003, 200 youth under the age of 14 were injured in PWC accidents, which accounted for 16 percent of the total injuries. (*U.S. Coast Guard.*)

⇨ In 2002, eight children died in PWC accidents. These children comprised 11 percent of all PWC fatalities. (*U.S. Coast Guard.*)

⇨ In 2003, 10 children died in PWC accidents, which accounted for 17 percent of all PWC fatalities. (*U.S. Coast Guard.*)

Shamefully, there are presently no national standards for the age of a PWC driver, the maximum speed limit, or any other actions relating to the safe driving of a PWC. No driver's test or show of competency is required from a PWC driver, despite the fact that the vehicles can achieve speeds of over 65 miles per hour. PWCs are marketed as thrill vehicles, with weaving between boats and buoys, spinning donuts, jumps and radical changes in course considered common practice.

Some states do require mandatory boater education. Although children do not have the reasoning skills to understand boating safety concepts, there are no age restrictions.

The Watercraft Industry (WI) has taken the responsible position that no child under 16 should operate a PWC. The American Academy of Pediatrics (AAP) also issued a policy statement advocating that no one under the age of 16 should operate a PWC (*Pediatrics*. February 2000. 195(2): 452-453.)

Likewise, the Coalition of Parents and Families for Personal Watercraft Safety advocate no children drivers (www.pwcwatch.org). Started by family members of children who died in PWC accidents, this highly respected group should be congratulated for their vigilance in this industry and their push for reforms. Particular credit should be given to Nita Boles of Plano, Texas, who lost her 16-year-old daughter in a PWC accident. According to Ms. Boles, "what I blame is ignorance. Clearly adults are not aware how serious and how frequent these accidents are."

Lack of experience is another important issue that has not been addressed. According to the Florida Department of Environmental Protection, a 1996 survey confirmed that one out of every three boating accidents involve PWCs. (This mirrors the national statistic.) Of these, 45 involve operators with fewer than 20 hours of experience driving a PWC. An additional 25 percent claimed 20 to 100 hours of operation.

Taking Action

The following is a helpful checklist to remove the hazards of **JET SKI** injuries and deaths:

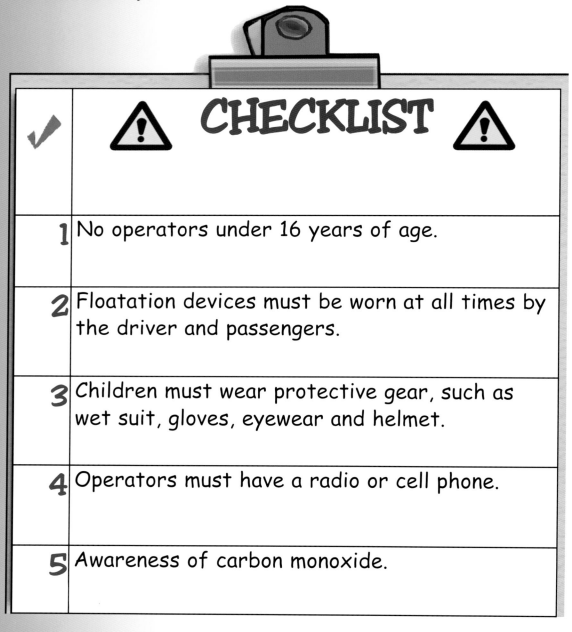

⚠ CHECKLIST ⚠

1. No operators under 16 years of age.

2. Floatation devices must be worn at all times by the driver and passengers.

3. Children must wear protective gear, such as wet suit, gloves, eyewear and helmet.

4. Operators must have a radio or cell phone.

5. Awareness of carbon monoxide.

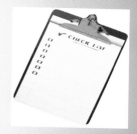

1. NO OPERATORS UNDER 16 YEARS OF AGE.

Although children under age 16 (and some reportedly as young as age six) currently operate PWCs across the country, the 16-year-old cut off is reasonable; this is the usual age allowed for driving a car.

2. FLOATATION DEVICES MUST BE WORN AT ALL TIMES BY THE DRIVER AND PASSENGERS.

The devices must be U.S. Coast Guard approved and age appropriate.

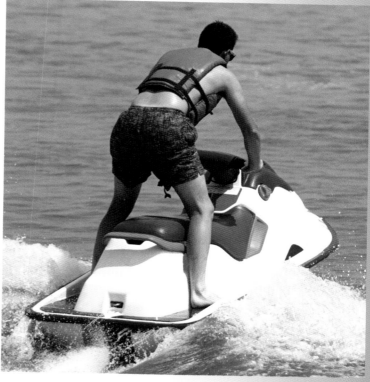

3. CHILDREN MUST WEAR PROTECTIVE GEAR, SUCH AS WET SUIT, GLOVES, EYEWEAR AND HELMETS.

The AAP has yet to take a position regarding which helmets are appropriate and promises to issue a position paper after careful study. Helmets not only protect against the full force of impact, but also prevent hair from being caught in the blades of motors in the event that a child is thrown overboard. Wet suits and gloves will help protect against cold, and eyewear will protect against obscured vision when water is sprayed in the face.

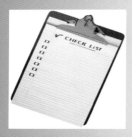

4. OPERATORS MUST HAVE A RADIO OR CELL PHONE.

Note that many cell phones do not operate on remote lakes.

5. AWARENESS OF CARBON MONOXIDE.

As discussed in detail in the houseboat chapter (following), water vehicles can have carbon monoxide traps. PWCs are no exception. These "dead zones" under some models pose a serious danger to unaware operators and passengers.

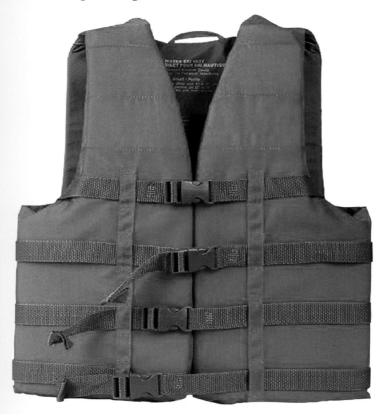

20

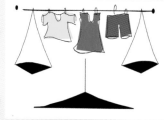

Houseboats

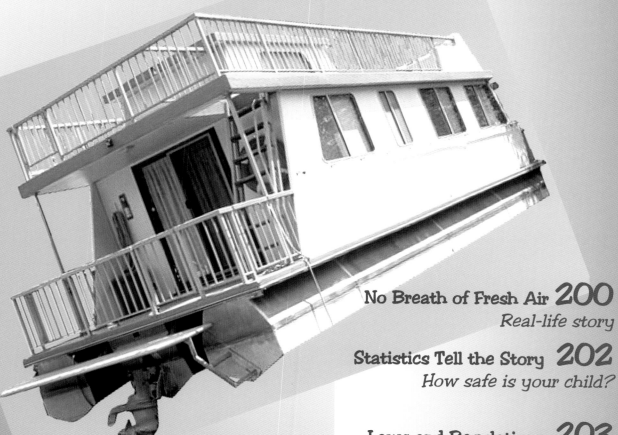

No Breath of Fresh Air

Michelle's parents found what seemed to be the formula for family fun: a hot summer weekend and a rented houseboat on a big lake. About an hour north of their major metropolitan area, the man-made lake offered all types of boat rentals, from paddleboats to speedboats to houseboats. They chose the houseboat- not too fast, no apparent safety hazards, perfect for a relaxed, safe time together.

The parents, Kimberly and Joe, were instructed in the basic operation of the boat at the rental company dock. They learned how to turn around, back and dock the houseboat for the night. They were also instructed in the operation of the stove, shower and the gasoline-powered generator that powered everything inside the boat, including the TV and the microwave.

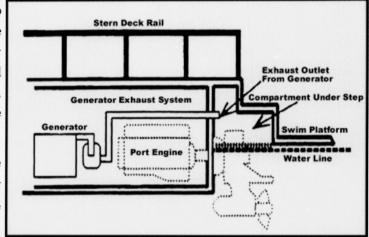

Cruising around the lake, the family spent a wonderful Friday night before finding a safe place to dock. On Saturday morning, they cruised the lake some more, and Joe found a safe, open area of water in which Michelle could swim. Joe parked the boat where his daughter could dive off the rear swim platform. He turned off the boat's engine, to be safe. Joe and Michelle went inside the boat to enjoy the Saturday football game in the comfort of the air-conditioned room. They didn't realize that although Joe had turned off the boat's motor, the generator that continued to run was a danger to their daughter. After about an hour, Joe decided to check on Michelle. To his shock, he found her floating face down in the water adjacent to the swimming platform. Joe dove in and retrieved Michelle's body. He administered CPR and rushed to the dock to meet the ambulance, which arrived within minutes.

It did not take long before the emergency room doctor informed Kimberly and Joe that their daughter had suffered extreme carbon monoxide poisoning.

For months following the incident, Kimberly and Joe worried that Michelle might have suffered some permanent damage, as her grades began to fall and her behavior became more aggressive. Concerned, they hired our law firm to investigate. We soon discovered that carbon monoxide poisoning was not rare with houseboats, particularly around the swimming platforms.

For years, we discovered, houseboat manufacturers routed the generator exhaust to the area adjacent to the swim platform. (In boating terms, this is venting through the transom into the stern cavity. See diagram, page 200). As a result, the carbon monoxide travels from this stern cavity under the boat, directly beneath the swim platform. Within seconds, life-threatening concentrations of carbon monoxide occur. Swimmers nearby the swim platform, or even persons sitting on the platform itself, can quickly be overcome. In past years, many people- including children sitting on the platform- died from carbon monoxide poisoning in this manner.

Fortunately, Michelle's parents' quick actions saved her life. The boat manufacturer and the rental company were fully aware of the danger. They were at fault in not correcting the problem and in not alerting the parents to the danger. Kimberly and Jo should have been told to turn off the gasoline-powered generator, particularly when the boat engine was off and the boat was not underway.

Doctors performed MRIs, PET scans, and neuro-psychological testing on Michelle as lawyers worked up the damage portion of the case. Happily, Michelle had not suffered any irreversible damage.

LEGAL ACTION and OUTCOME

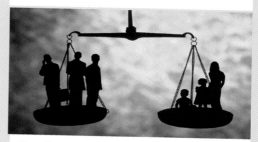

On behalf of the parents, we notified the manufacturer and rental company that if they would agree to two conditions we would not bring a lawsuit. The first condition was that all medical bills to date, including all of the medical evaluations, be paid in full and that a sum be set aside for future medical care, if needed. The second and most important condition was that the houseboat manufacturer and rental company agree to either discontinue use of that particular houseboat model, or take immediate steps to change and retrofit so that the houseboat would be safe. The manufacturer and rental company ultimately agreed to these terms and the case was settled out of court.

Statistics Tell the Story

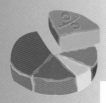

Unfortunately, there is no national database for carbon monoxide deaths on houseboats. There have been studies and individual cases, however, some of which we document here:

⇨ Between 1990 and 2000, in the Lake Powell area alone (in the southwestern United States), there were nine deaths and 102 serious illnesses requiring emergency room care caused by carbon monoxide on houseboats. *

⇨   In August 2000, fifteen people were hospitalized in Lake Cumberland, Kentucky, for being overcome by carbon monoxide poisoning on two rented houseboats. *

⇨   In June 2000, four people died from exposure to fumes from a houseboat in Missouri. *

*2002 National Park Service Study, in consultation with the National Institute for Occupational Safety and Health and the Morbidity and Mortality Weekly Report, December 15, 2000.

Keep in mind that exposure to engine fumes from any boat is potentially harmful. Note that other boats (like water skiing boats, for example) also present carbon monoxide poisoning danger; young people have suffered carbon monoxide poisoning while holding on to the backs of boats, or congregating near the area where fumes are being exhausted. One particular practice, called "teak surfing," or "drag surfing," involves holding onto the swim platform or transom of the motor boat, then letting go once the boat is up to speed. This is a very dangerous practice; the potential for carbon monoxide poisoning is very high, as is the potential for serious injury.

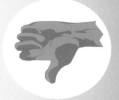

In 2004, the Centers for Disease Control (CDC) issued the following alert:

You probably know carbon monoxide poisoning is a danger when gasoline powered engines are run in enclosed spaces. What many people don t know is that severe carbon monoxide can also occur outdoors and most particularly with houseboats.

Gasoline-powered engines and generators on houseboats can produce deadly carbon monoxide, a colorless, odorless gas that can poison or kill. Carbon monoxide tends to build up above the water near the platforms in boats. **The amount of carbon monoxide that can build up in the air space beneath the stern deck on houseboats can be deadly within seconds to minutes. It can also reach life-threatening concentrations on or near the swim deck.**

Unfortunately, there are no national laws pertaining to houseboat design or mandatory carbon monoxide alarms inside houseboats, which could alert boaters in the event of dangerous carbon monoxide release.

In the year 2000, the United States Coast Guard issued a letter to the entire houseboat industry, advising of the danger of the design defect. Only six manufacturers agreed to recall all the boats with the defect. *(United States Coast Guard (USCG) Release December 21, 2000.)*

Because of the lack of overall industry responsibility, the Coast Guard issued a mandatory recall in 2001 of all houseboats which were built and equipped with swim platforms and electrical generator exhaust systems vented into the stern cavity. *(United States Coast Guard Release (USCG) February 28, 2001.)*

The Coast Guard noted, "We have made the manufacturers aware of the problem and that venting generator exhaust through the vessel side is an approved solution. We expect them to correct the problem quickly."

Critics believe that the carbon monoxide danger in houseboats still exists. The industry has not solved the problem on its new boat models. Nor has the industry effectively recalled all of the houseboats with the dangerous design. This is complicated by the fact that often houseboats are sold used, and manufacturers are unable to track down the new owners. The situation is further complicated by the fact that there have been a number of houseboat manufacturers who have gone out of business, and yet their products still float on many lakes and water bodies in the United States today.

Taking Action

Use the following checklist to insure safety on your **HOUSEBOAT** outing:

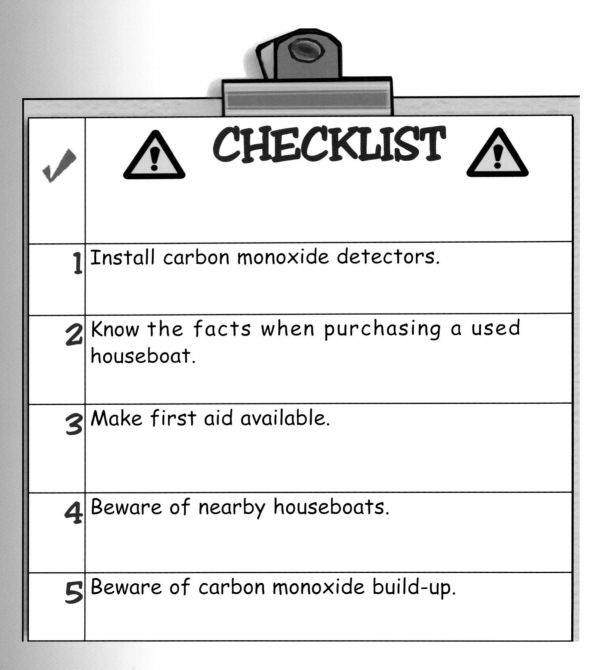

⚠ CHECKLIST ⚠

✔		
1	Install carbon monoxide detectors.	
2	Know the facts when purchasing a used houseboat.	
3	Make first aid available.	
4	Beware of nearby houseboats.	
5	Beware of carbon monoxide build-up.	

1. INSTALL CARBON MONOXIDE DETECTORS.

Because of the potential for carbon monoxide release inside the living space, carbon monoxide detectors are mandatory. It's important to note, however, that carbon monoxide detectors inside the houseboat will have no effect on the danger of poisoning in the swim platform area.

2. KNOW THE FACTS WHEN PURCHASING A USED HOUSEBOAT.

Know for certain whether the houseboat you are considering purchasing was manufactured with the dangerous venting design. Also make sure that all valves and other boat parts are completely checked and deemed safe from unintended carbon monoxide emissions.

3. MAKE FIRST AID AVAILABLE.

A radio or mobile phone must be available for immediate dispatch of emergency aid. A basic first aid kit must also be available at all times. In the event of a carbon monoxide accident, remember that establishing an airway and moving the person to fresh air quickly are crucial. Call for professional assistance immediately.

4. BEWARE OF NEARBY HOUSEBOATS.

According to a 2004 CDC proclamation:
Exhaust from another vessel that docked, beached or anchored beside your boat can send carbon monoxide into the cabin and cockpit of your boat. Your boat should always be at least 20 feet from the nearest boat that is running a generator or engine.

5. BEWARE OF CARBON MONOXIDE BUILDUP.

According to the CDC, traveling at slow speeds or idling in the water can cause carbon monoxide to build up in the cabin, cockpit and aft area, even in an open space. Wind entering from the aft section of the boat can also increase a buildup of carbon monoxide.

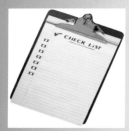

The "station wagon effect," or back drafting, can also cause carbon monoxide to build up inside the cabin, cockpit and bridge. This happens when operating the boat at a high-bow angle (with improper or heavy loading, for example), or if there is an opening that draws in exhaust.

IMPORTANT: IF THE ELECTRICAL GENERATOR VENTS THROUGH THE TRANSOM INTO THE STERN CAVITY, NEVER RUN THE GENERATOR IF SOMEONE IS SWIMMING IN THE REAR AREA OR SITTING ON THE STERN DECK.

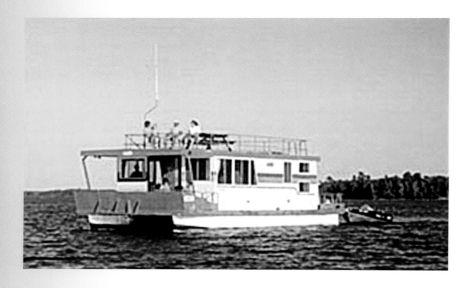

For a thorough review of all data on carbon monoxide houseboat dangers, go to
http://safetynet.smis.doi.gov/COhouseboats.htm

21
Snowmobiles, Skateboards & Go-Carts

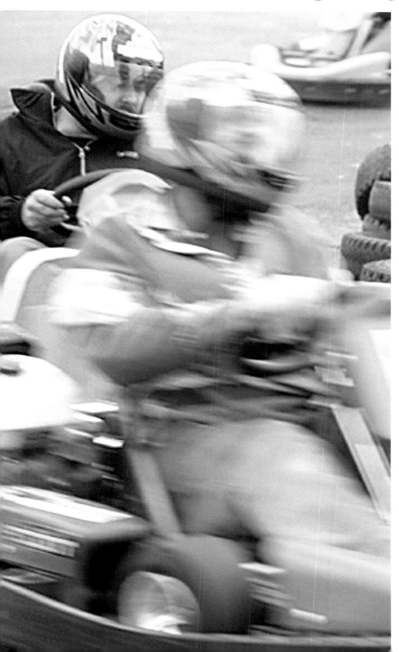

More Dangerous Than You'd Think

Gerald had been driving motorized go-carts since the age of five, so at 14 he was considered an experienced rider. While there were many riding areas in his rural community, the best was The Gravel Pit, a ten-acre, barren, bulldozed plot of farmland with many dunes, small hills and trails.

To the untrained eye, go-cart riding would appear extremely dangerous, because often the go-cart will flip onto the top of its metal cage and then return to a four-wheel ground position to resume its ride. Central to the safety of such activity is the four-point safety harness or belt, which keeps riders in place.

Unlike motorcycle scooters, the vast majority of go-carts are handmade. The Internet is full of dealers of various go-cart parts, but most of the carts are designed and assembled by the go-cart owners themselves. This was true of Gerald's go-cart, which he named The Pulverizer. Gerald and his dad had worked on the go-cart over the winter months, and they assembled what they believed was a safe vehicle. They had purchased a new four-point harness for the passenger side, but for the driver side Gerald removed the safety harness from his old go-cart and placed it on his new Pulverizer.

The summer months found Gerald and his friends at The Gravel Pit, riding up and down hills and occasionally flipping their vehicles. One day, Gerald's girlfriend, Katherine, with her parent's permission, came out to The Pit to ride with him. Like Gerald, she had been riding go-carts since she was a young child. She even brought her own helmet and gloves. After Gerald and Katherine were secured in the go-cart, with both safety harnesses intact, they set off for an adventurous ride. Several hours of riding didn't slow their enthusiasm. Until, that is, one final stunt. Gerald and Katherine ventured up a small hill only to tip upside-down over the side, rolling twice. This wasn't a new move; both of them had done it before. After the go-cart came to a stop, Katherine, laughing and full of the thrill, popped her belt off and exited the go-cart without a scratch. She quickly discovered, though, that Gerald was lying lifeless in the go-cart, with his belt undone. Gerald was quickly rushed to the emergency room of the rural hospital and then life-flighted to the metro trauma canter 100 miles away. That evening his parents learned the tragic news- two bones in Gerald's neck had been severed and he would be paralyzed for the rest of his life.

LEGAL ACTION
and
OUTCOME

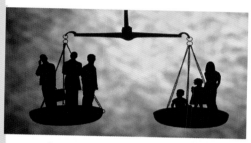

The family hired me to investigate the circumstances of this terrible accident. Clearly Gerald's harness had failed, but why? Had it been misuse on Gerald's part or a defect in the belt? We retained a noted seat belt expert, a former government official, who ran stress tests on the belt and discovered that it had a defect that caused it to unintentionally come open. It was Gerald's weight on the belt, particularly on the coupling, that caused it to pop at the point he was upside down. This sent Gerald's head directly to the ground, causing his broken neck. Examination of the other equipment showed no other defects. The helmet performed its job, and the go-cart itself was

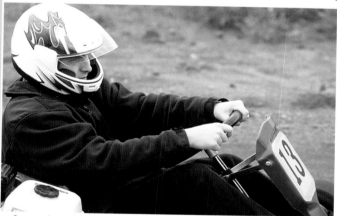

functionally safe. We undertook a lawsuit against the safety belt manufacturer, who immediately claimed that the removal of the belt from the first go-cart caused the creation of the defect.

Unfortunately for the company, we discovered a track record of failed safety belts that had nothing to do with multiple vehicle use. Further, our expert saw no post-production defects in the belt, but rather a defect at the point of initial manufacture. After many months of litigation, the case was ultimately concluded to the satisfaction of Gerald's parents.

Statistics Tell the Story

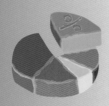

⇨ Traumatic brain injury (TBI) is the leading killer and disabler of children. Each year, 3,000 children are killed and approximately 29,000 are hospitalized due to traumatic brain injury, according to the National SAFE KIDS Campaign (www.safekids.org). The vast majority of these injuries occur on wheeled or moving vehicles; nearly 28,000,000 children between the ages of five and 14 ride bikes, scooters, skateboards and other wheeled sports vehicles.

⇨ According to the Consumer Products Safety Commission (CPSC), 30,000 emergency room injuries result from scooters (2002), with 40 percent involving children 15 years or younger.

⇨ The Toy Manufacturers of America lists the scooter as the top selling toy of 2003.

⇨ In March 2000, the *Journal of Pediatrics* reported the results of the Toledo, Ohio, Children's Hospital study, which found that nearly two-thirds of children's deaths from snowmobiling are due to head and neck trauma. Non-fatal injuries most often occur when the child is thrown off the snowmobile. The article reports that towing someone on an inner tube behind the snowmobile is also a source of injury.

GO-CARTS:

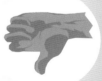

There are no federal or state laws regarding go-carts.

SNOWMOBILES:

There are a number of snow states-like Michigan, Vermont, Wisconsin, Minnesota and South Dakota- that have very detailed laws on snowmobile use and safety. These state laws vary from very strict to almost non-existent.

SCOOTERS:

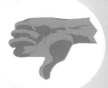

No federal or state law exists regarding scooters.

Taking Action

Because each of these vehicles is different in the injuries they produce as well as the hazards evident, please note different checklists.

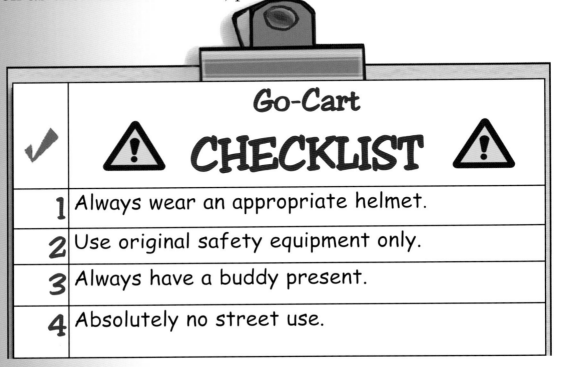

Go-Cart
✔ ⚠ CHECKLIST ⚠

1	Always wear an appropriate helmet.
2	Use original safety equipment only.
3	Always have a buddy present.
4	Absolutely no street use.

1. ALWAYS WEAR AN APPROPRIATE HELMET.
For specific helmet requirements and needs, see Chapter 24 of this book.

2. USE ORIGINAL SAFETY EQUIPMENT ONLY.
Although in the case we prosecuted, Gerald was successful in safely transferring h
seat belt from one go-cart to another, we learned the valuable lesson that safety equipmer
should not be used on more than one vehicle. While Gerald's seat belt did not alter
become defective when he transferred it to his new go-cart, there have been a numb
of reported cases where, in fact, the reuse of seat belts caused a defect that later led
a serious injury.

3. ALWAYS HAVE A BUDDY PRESENT.
Go-carting often occurs in remote places. In the event of an accident, there needs to
be an individual present who can coordinate medical treatment.

4. ABSOLUTELY NO STREET USE.

Ultimately all children have a natural inclination and desire to ride their go-carts on the street. This is absolutely prohibited.

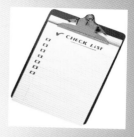

Snowmobiling
CHECKLIST

✔		
1	Always use an appropriate helmet.
2	Always have a buddy present.
3	Drive only on established trails.
4	Don't hurdle snow banks.
5	Avoid unknown waterways.
6	Always take a safety course.
7	Use a Global Positioning System(GPS).

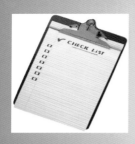

1. ALWAYS USE AN APPROPRIATE HELMET.

Please see Chapter 24 for the specifics on helmet safety and use.

2. ALWAYS HAVE A BUDDY PRESENT.

Snowmobiling often occurs in remote places. In the event of an accident, there needs to be an individual present who can coordinate medical treatment.

3. DRIVE ONLY ON ESTABLISHED TRAILS.

While the snow is a wonderful sight and provides a lot of fun, it also covers up defects and hazards in the land, such as barbed wire fences, pipes and other hazards that can instantly kill. Therefore, driving only on established trails should be the norm.

4. DON'T HURDLE SNOW BANKS.

Hurdling snow banks may be a fun activity, but it's a dangerous one. There are a number of serious injuries that have occurred from hurdling snow banks.

5. AVOID UNKNOWN WATERWAYS.

No one can be sure how thick the ice is or what hidden dangers it holds. Therefore, avoid unknown waterways.

6. ALWAYS TAKE A SAFETY COURSE.

In virtually every state, there are safety courses for driving snowmobiles. These are often available through snowmobile dealers and are as necessary as driver education is to the driving of an automobile by anyone, particularly a teenager.

7. USE A GLOBAL POSITIONING SYSTEM (GPS).

Snowmobilers are often out in freezing or near freezing weather, when the potential for hypothermia needs to be considered. A GPS unit can make it possible to find an injured or distressed rider.

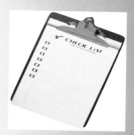

Scooters
CHECKLIST

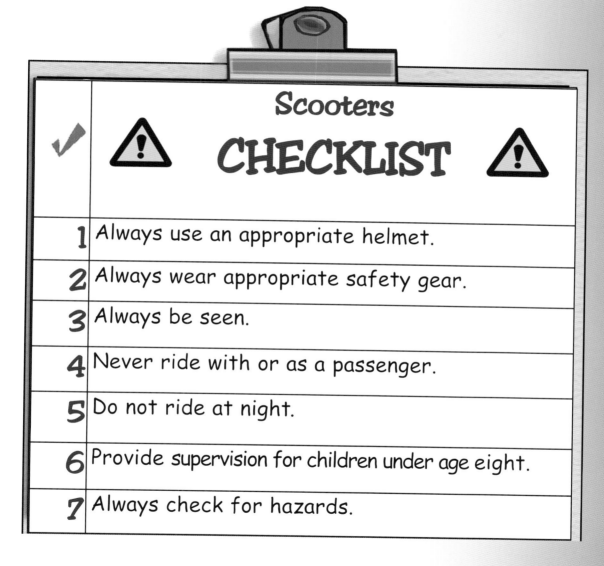

✔	
1	Always use an appropriate helmet.
2	Always wear appropriate safety gear.
3	Always be seen.
4	Never ride with or as a passenger.
5	Do not ride at night.
6	Provide supervision for children under age eight.
7	Always check for hazards.

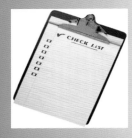

1. ALWAYS USE AN APPROPRIATE HELMET.
Please see Chapter 24 for the specifics on helmet safety and use.

2. ALWAYS WEAR APPROPRIATE SAFETY GEAR.
At minimum, this would include elbow pads, kneepads, wrist guards and gloves. Replace overly used, worn guards and pads.

3. ALWAYS BE SEEN.
One of the inherent dangers when riding a scooter is that you will not be seen by traffic. Always wear very bright colors, to be certain drivers will see you.

4. NEVER RIDE WITH OR AS A PASSENGER.
Virtually every association that has examined scooter safety has mandated a no-passenger rule. Unlike a go-cart or snowmobile, the passenger renders a scooter dynamically unstable, which can lead to a loss of control.

5. DO NOT RIDE AT NIGHT.
Hazards can be nearly impossible to detect at night, even with head lamps. It is best to ride only in daylight.

6. PROVIDE SUPERVISION FOR CHILDREN UNDER AGE EIGHT.
Various consumer groups have designated the age of eight as the cutoff for supervision. Children younger than eight simply do not realize the inherent dangers and can become so consumed in the use of the scooter that they will too easily place themselves in harm's way.

7. ALWAYS CHECK FOR HAZARDS.
Before using the scooter, the rider or parent should check the vehicle thoroughly for hazards such as loose, broken or cracked parts, sharp edges on the metal boards, slippery top surfaces and wheels with nicks and cracks. Scooters should be ridden only on smooth, paved surfaces that are free from traffic, sand, gravel and dirt.

22

Cheerleading

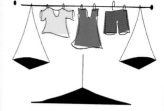

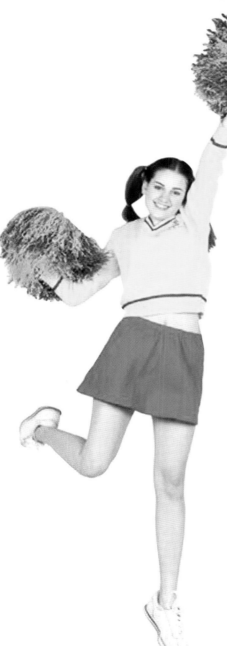

As Sport Develops, Injuries Increase

Gina's grandmother and mother had both been high school cheerleaders when the primary function of a cheerleader was leading the sideline cheers of the crowd with pompoms and limited dance routines. But cheerleading changed dramatically in the 1980s.

By the time the 15-year-old Gina became a cheerleader, the emphasis was on stunts and tricks, including basket throws, pyramids and, yes, gymnastics. No longer relegated to the sidelines, cheerleaders had now become a star attraction at games and participants in their own competitions. Today, the leading champi-onships are broadcast nationally and draw millions of viewers.

Unfortunately, the issue of safety has not kept pace with the transition of cheerleading to the status of a full-fledged sport.

Gina was delighted to have made the cut for the cheerleading squad. Her squad had two-hour after-school sessions to learn their new routines. Despite her own inexperience, Gina was paired with an equally inexperienced male partner.

Because of overcrowding at the school, the squad was required to practice in the school's hall-way directly adjacent to the cafeteria. Even worse, the coach spent about half of each prac-tice at the far end of the school in her office performing admin-istrative duties while the cheerleaders practiced unsupervised.

Near the end of a practice session, Gina and her partner were doing a liberty, which is a stunt in which the base partner extends his arms vertically and holds his partner overhead while she poses on one foot on the extended hand. Gina's partner slipped, causing them both to lose their balance. Gina fell approximately eight feet to the ground and broke her left ankle so severely that bone protruded from her skin.

Even after treatment, Gina will always walk with a noticeable limp. Approximately every 10 years she will require surgery to replace the metal plates in her foot and ankle.

LEGAL ACTION and OUTCOME

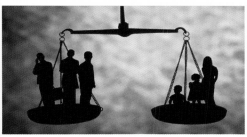

Her stunned family wanted my law firm to investigate whether this disabling injury could have been prevented. Her parents were surprised to learn that the school and coach had committed numerous safety lapses.

First, there were no mats in place to cushion Gina's fall. Second, the coach failed to train and insist on a mandatory spotter for a trick such as a liberty. Finally, the coach had never undergone any form of certification. The fact that the coach took more than 20 minutes to locate a first aid kit to help control Gina's bleeding shows how unprepared the school really was.

Because of the severity of Gina's injuries, a claim was made and the case was ultimately settled. However, this young girl has a lifetime of pain ahead of her. She will be reminded of her loss every time she takes a step.

Statistics Tell the Story

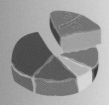

⇨ In 2001, there were 25,000 cheerleader injuries requiring emergency room care, according to the U.S. Consumer Products Safety Commission (CPSC).

⇨ Cheerleading injuries doubled between 1999 and 2001, according to the CPSC.

⇨ Between 1995 and 2000, eight high school cheerleaders suffered catastrophic injuries. This compares with seven catastrophic injuries for all of high school basketball, even though the number of basketball players is estimated to be eight times greater than cheerleaders.
(*Source: National Center for Catastrophic Sports Injury Research, 18th annual report.*)

⇨ In 2003, the *American Journal of Sports Medicine* studied cheerleading injuries and documented a rate of 1.95 direct catastrophic injuries per year. That translates to 0.6 injuries per 100,000 participants.

Note: The *American Cheerleader* Magazine (www.americancheerleader.com) and various cheerleading associations vigorously contend that compared to football and other contact sports, cheerleading is a low-injury sport. They also site that with increased safety, the injury rate will decrease.

Unfortunately, the law has not kept pace with the development of cheerleading. Only 12 states even recognize cheerleading as a sport. Safety laws and regulations vary greatly from state to state and even from school to school.

Often a law is passed immediately as a knee-jerk response to tragedy. A pyramid stunt that caused a cheerleader's death prompted both Minnesota and North Dakota to ban pyramids even at the college level. And Illinois banned basket tosses after a catastrophic injury occurred in that state. We prefer a legislative approach that focuses on prevention.

Be aware that there are groups with conflicting philosophies regarding safety. The most responsible group on safety has been the American Association of Cheerleading Coaches and Advisors (www.aacca.org). In 2003-2004, the AACCA issued a 6-page set of safety guidelines that cover all maneuvers and procedures in exhaustive detail.

These guidelines-based on extensive study of cheerleading injury patterns-are so thorough and well-documented that they should be adopted in all states. The thumbs-down symbol is not for the ACCA but rather for the state legislatures and schools that have failed to incorporate the AACCA's cutting-edge advancements in safety.

Taking Action

As the intensity of cheerleading increases and coaches and athletes place greater emphasis on gymnastics skills, we recommend that you grade your child's cheerleading squad on the following safety requirements. For any areas that receive a failing grade, petition the squad or school to enact changes as recommended below.

✔	⚠ CHECKLIST ⚠
1	Has your squad adopted the AACCAA safety guidelines?
2	Is your coach AACCA certified?
3	Does your coach have and refer to the sport's rule book?
4	Are all team members required to test their skills regularly?
5	Are mats in place at each practice?
6	Are trained spotters used?
7	Are there rules for appropriate footwear?
8	Are there medical screening requirements?
9	Is there an emergency plan?
10	Are safety standards mandatory at practices?

1. HAS YOUR SQUAD ADOPTED THE AACCAA SAFETY GUIDELINES?

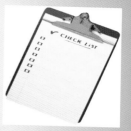

All squads should adopt the AACCA guidelines immediately. (See www.aacca.org for full details). The rest of this report card focuses on the AACCA's key recommendations.

2. IS YOUR COACH AACCA CERTIFIED?

All coaches should be certified. Once again, the American Association of Cheerleading Coaches and Advisors is leading the field with a certification process that is both thorough and complete.

3. DOES YOUR COACH HAVE AND REFER TO THE SPORT'S RULE BOOK?

All coaches should have a copy of the Spirit Case & Rule Book published by the National Federation of State High School Associations (www.nfhs.org). This resource contains detailed technical and safety information about all accepted stunts and tricks in the sport. Not only is it a must-read for coaches, the Rule Book should be present at all practices for easy reference by athletes and coaches alike.

4. ARE ALL TEAM MEMBERS REQUIRED TO TEST THEIR SKILLS REGULARLY?

Each team member should be required to demonstrate his or her skill level periodically in order to remain on the squad. One common mistake squads make is not requiring skill testing before allowing a new cheerleader to join the squad. This skill testing must be repeated periodically to ensure that no squad member is being allowed to perform beyond his or her level of accomplishment.

5. ARE MATS IN PLACE AT EACH PRACTICE?

Adequate mats must be used at each practice. Because of the sport's current nature, some falls and tumbles are inevitable. These falls must occur where the landing surface is adequately cushioned in order to prohibit severe injuries.

6   ARE TRAINED SPOTTERS USED?

Appropriately trained spotters are a must. Once again, because of the likelihood of falls, a spotter must be used each and every time a fall is possible. The squad should spell out a protocol that indicates when and how spotting should be done for each move.

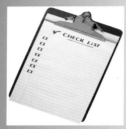

7. ARE THERE RULES FOR APPROPRIATE FOOTWEAR?

All cheerleaders should wear only appropriate athletic shoes for all practices and performances. Improper footwear is often a primary cause of falls and trips. "Gym slippers" should be prohibited and all athletes should be required to wear properly sized and fitted footwear.

8. ARE THERE MEDICAL SCREENING REQUIREMENTS?

Schools should insist on a proper medical screening of all cheerleaders. Physicians should look for any pre-existing injuries or conditioning deficiencies, a leading cause of over-use injuries. In addition, studies have shown that women involved in the so-called aesthetic sports of cheerleading, ice skating, dance and gymnastics are at increased risk of eating disorders. The physician should take a complete medical history that includes a discussion of eating habits. Parents and coaches should observe students' eating habits as appropriate.

9. IS THERE AN EMERGENCY PLAN?

Squads must plan for emergencies. Because cheerleading is a sport, the same emergency protocol should be followed as with other sports (see Chapter 16 Report Card). The emergency protocol should include:

- Immediate access to a telephone and first aid kit
- Instructions for how to summon ambulance service or other emergency assistance and
- Instructions for how to reach local hospitals.

10. ARE SAFETY STANDARDS MANDATORY AT PRACTICES?

The same non-negotiable safety standards must be upheld for all performances and practices. Based on anecdotal reports, we know that a higher number of injuries occur during practices than an actual game or performance. This is often due to a lack of supervision by the coach, inattention by the participants or such intense preparation that physical exhaustion leads to weakness and impaired judgment.

BOTTOM LINE: As cheerleading transitions into a separate sport and the maneuvers become more intense and complicated, safety practices must keep pace to avoid unnecessary injuries and even death.

Many thanks to the advocacy of former cheerleader Amy Davis of Utah. Amy suffered a serious, preventable injury and has taken that tragedy into a platform advocating needed safety changes. (www.livingthemoment.com)

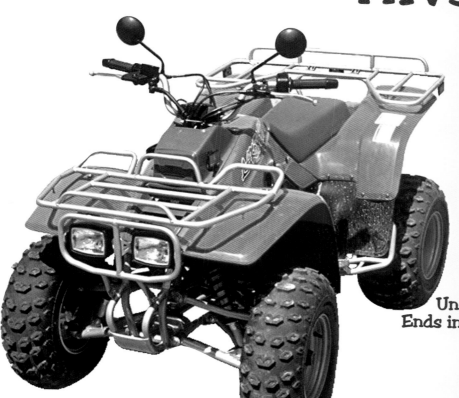

23
ATVs

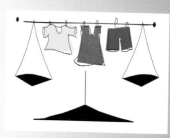

225

Unsupervised Off-Roading Ends In A Lifetime Of Paralysis

Despite their popularity, the three-wheel all-terrain vehicles (ATVs) once sold in the United States were banned in 1988 by the U.S. Consumer Products Safety Commission (CPSC) for safety reasons. The ATV industry then replaced the dangerous three-wheel ATVs with the four-wheel variety. There are now over eight million such vehicles in the US.

Unfortunately, the addition of that fourth wheel gave many Americans, including the Statler family, the erroneous belief that the four-wheel ATVs are safe. The Statlers, however, did refuse to buy one for their 15-year-old son Randy. Randy's parents did not base their rejection on any safety concerns, though. They told their son that their property was not big enough for an ATV and that the noise would bother the neighbors.

One of Randy's friends had a friend whose father had a weekend farm, complete with woods and a fishing pond. The friend's father also owned an ATV to use primarily as a farm machine to move around the property and to occasionally haul wood and sod.

Randy was invited by his friend's father to have a weekend on the farm with the assurance that he and six other boys would be supervised by the adult at all times.

On that weekend, the ATV predictably became the center of attention. The friend's father, who was the supervising adult, allowed each boy to take turns on the ATV on Friday night. Darkness cut their adventures short, but the boys could hardly fall asleep thinking about the next day and riding the ATV all day.

Early on Saturday morning, the boys became impatient with taking turns. Their "solution" was to ride double even though the ATV clearly displayed warning labels that only single riders would be safe and that in all instances helmets must be worn. The supervising adult felt that since the boys were small, would only be riding off-road and promised to ride slowly that it would be okay for them to ride double. Since it was a hot summer day, he also gave them permission to ride without helmets.

The boys took turns riding from the farmhouse down to the pasture, then looping around through the nearby woods where a winding path was evident in the worn ground. The trees and the winding path were simply irresistible to the adventurous boys.

All day Saturday the cycle was the same. Each rider started at the farmhouse, drove down to the pasture, twisted and turned his way through the woods, then headed back to the farmhouse for a change of riders.

In mid-afternoon, the supervising adult announced, "Boys, only 45 more minutes of riding." Although disappointed, the boys decided they could cram even more fun into their remaining time by riding faster.

With only 10 minutes left, Randy was riding on the back with his friend Jonathan driving. Jonathan raced through the pasture and into the woods, but then something unexpected happened. As the teen was making the last turn, he realized he was going too fast and slammed on his brakes.

The design experts call it "plowing." As the driver brakes too hard, pressure forces the ATV's rear wheels to slide in the opposite direction. Jonathan was able to cling to the handle bars, but the force flung Randy off the ATV headfirst into a tree trunk. The impact snapped his neck, causing instant and total paralysis.

LEGAL ACTION and OUTCOME

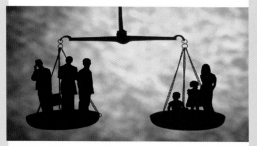

On Randy's behalf we filed a lawsuit against the homeowner's insurance policy of the supervising adult. We contended that he had failed to safely supervise the boys.

The case was eventually settled. Like many catastrophically injured children, Randy will almost certainly outlive his parents, perhaps by decades. The settlement has funded a life-care plan to take care of all Randy's future medical treatment and institutional needs, even after his parents are gone.

Statistics Tell the Story

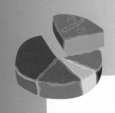

The following statistics outline the many tragedies that have been caused by four-wheeled ATVs.

⇨ From 1997 to 2001, injury rates increased 23 percent for children ages six to 12 and 233 percent for children younger than six years old.

⇨ In 2002, nearly 30,000 children 14 and under were treated in emergency rooms for ATV-related injuries. These injuries often include broken bones and head and facial injuries.

⇨ At least 44 children 14 and under died of ATV-related injuries in 2002. Children ages 10 to 14 accounted for more than 75 percent of these deaths. Most fatalities are due to head and neck injuries.

⇨ In 2001, 87 percent of the injuries to children under 16 occurred while they were riding on adult-size ATVs. The most common causes of injury are rollovers, falls from the vehicle and crashes with stationary objects.

⇨ Wearing a helmet while riding an ATV reduces the risk of fatal head injury by 42 percent and the risk of nonfatal head injury by 64 percent. But helmets can't protect against other common causes of ATV-related injury like spinal cord, chest and abdominal damage.

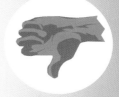

ATV manufacturers are self-regulated. The only federal requirements by the CPSC are warning labels on ATVs and engine size regulations for use by children under 16.

- Currently, 27 states have minimum age requirements for operation of an ATV.

- Three states require ATV operators to be 16 or older.

Taking Action

The following checklist is helpful in assuring safety of the child while using an **ATV**:

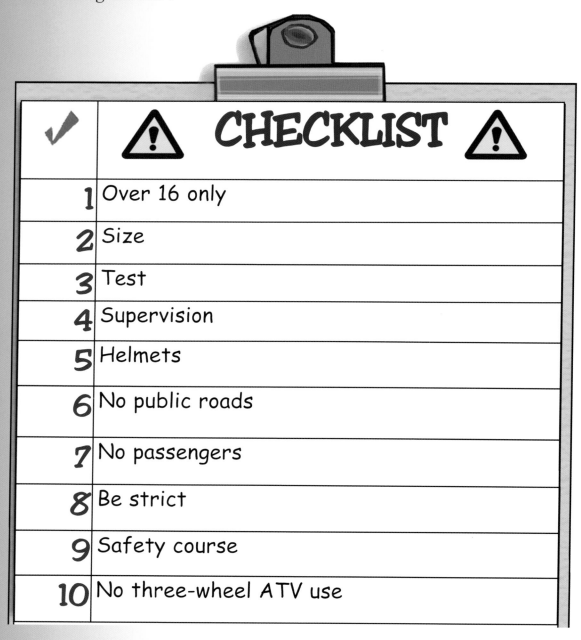

CHECKLIST

1. Over 16 only
2. Size
3. Test
4. Supervision
5. Helmets
6. No public roads
7. No passengers
8. Be strict
9. Safety course
10. No three-wheel ATV use

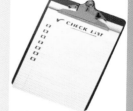

1. OVER 16 ONLY

Given the relatively high likelihood of catastrophic injury, we encourage you to prohibit all children under 16 years from riding an ATV.

2. SIZE

If you choose to let your child ride, limit all rides to youth-sized ATVs. Manufacturers' guidelines state that children under 16 should operate ATVs with engines smaller than 90 cc. Children ages six to twelve should operate ATVs with engines between 70 to 90 cc. Under no circumstances should a child less than age six ever ride an ATV.

3. TEST

Read and discuss the ATV's warning labels, instruction manual and training video with your child on multiple occasions. Quiz him or her periodically. If he answers any questions incorrectly, do not let him ride.

4. SUPERVISION

Always supervise all children operating ATVs. Over time, a handful of juries have found four-wheeled ATV manufacturers responsible for riders' catastrophic injuries and deaths. But in the vast majority of cases tried in front of juries, they have found that the child was not satisfactorily supervised and the injury was due to a clear misuse of the ATV.

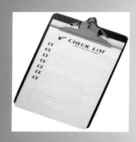

5. HELMETS

Insist on the proper protective equipment for every ride, no exceptions:

- U.S. Department of Transportation-approved helmet with face protection
- Goggles (if the helmet lacks face protection)
- Long-sleeved shirt and pants
- Boots with non-slip treads
- Gloves

6. NO PUBLIC ROADS

ATVs should only be used on designated trails, never on public roadways or paved surfaces.

7. NO PASSENGERS

Never permit your child to be or carry a passenger on an ATV.

8. BE STRICT

Issue strict punishments for any misuse of the ATV- three strikes, and it's sold.

9. SAFETY COURSE

Children and ALL adults who supervise ATV use should enroll in and successfully complete an approved ATV course.

10. NO THREE-WHEEL ATV USE

Although three-wheelers have been banned for several years as dangerous, there are still many three-wheelers in use, and therefore subject to be sold as used or given as gifts. Because of the severe injury and death track record of three-wheel ATVs, there should be no use of them.

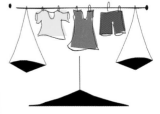

24

Helmets and Restraint Devices

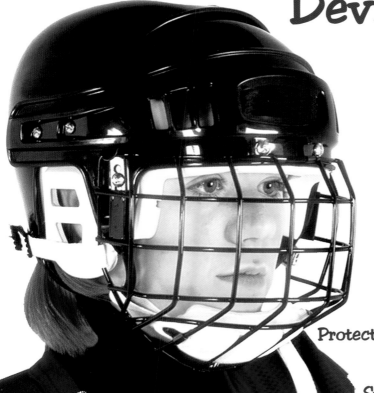

Protection That Did Not Exist

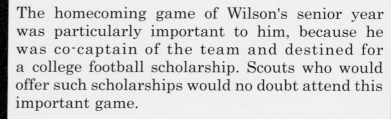

From early childhood, Wilson dreamt of being a football star. Every backyard scrimmage, annual football summer camp, and pee-wee league prepared the boy to fulfill his dream.

Stocky and low to the ground, Wilson was the perfect build for the defensive nose-man position. Stationed at mid-field, a mere two to three yards off the ball, Wilson formed the "brick wall" of the defense, the protection against the break-away offensive fullback run. Quick and aggressive, Wilson excelled in this position, single-handedly tackling many a pumped-up fullback destined for a touchdown.

The homecoming game of Wilson's senior year was particularly important to him, because he was co-captain of the team and destined for a college football scholarship. Scouts who would offer such scholarships would no doubt attend this important game.

Before each game, the team's equipment manager checked and spit-shined the five-year-old helmets, fitting each with a new strap and a foam insert.

In the third quarter of this important game, Wilson saw it coming. An unfortunate opening in the defensive line had the fullback steaming right in Wilson's direction. Just feet from the fullback, head down, Wilson charged and put his helmet right in his opponent's jersey numbers, dropping him on the spot. Tragically, Wilson dropped, too. His helmet had cracked almost down the middle, providing no protection from the severe impact. Unconscious, Wilson was taken to the hospital.

Initial CT scans revealed internal bleeding in the brain, and while the doctors tried as best they could to relieve the advancing pressure, it was this pressure that caused Wilson's permanent disability. Even after extensive rehabilitation, Wilson's IQ dropped approximately 20 percent, and his motor control ability was greatly diminished. Because of the severity and longevity of the injuries, The Keenan Law Firm was retained.

LEGAL ACTION and OUTCOME

After the lawsuit was filed and sworn testimony taken, it became clear that the type of paint used by the school on the helmets greatly affected the surface, making the helmets more susceptible to internal cracks. Unfortunately, the helmet manufacturer did not advise against the use of this type of substance, although clearly they knew from their own research that such use could cause cracks in their helmets. During the litigation, the helmet manufacturer contended that the type of crack evident in Wilson's helmet would clearly have been visible prior to the game. The

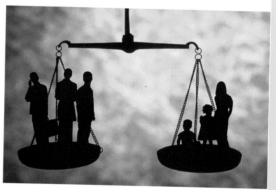

equipment manager and coach both denied any visual cracks; however, our expert agreed that given the severity of the separation, some cracks would have been evident on even a cursory examination of the helmet.

With the high school pointing the finger at the helmet manufacturer and the helmet manufacturer pointing the finger back at the school, I was content to let the jury decide who was ultimately at fault and to what degree. Because of the uncertainty of the outcome and the severity of injuries, both the helmet manufacturer and the school requested mediation. After several lengthy proceedings, the case was ultimately settled for sums ensuring the quality of Wilson's life and medical care for the rest of his life.

Statistics Tell the Story

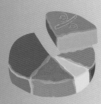

All safety experts agree: Helmets should be used in all contact sports and any activity where potential head injury can occur (except playground play, which will be discussed later).

⇨ Twenty-seven million children ages five to 14 ride bicycles (*Press Release*, May 2004, <u>www.safekids.org</u>)

⇨ Bicycles are associated with more childhood injuries than any other consumer products except the automobile. Nearly half (47 percent) of the children hospitalized for bike-related injuries suffer from traumatic brain injury, with head injuries accounting for up to 80 percent of all bike-related fatalities. (*National SAFE KIDS Campaign*)

⇨ According to the Bicycle Helmet Safety Institute (<u>www.bhsi.org</u>), bicycle helmets reduce the risk of serious injury to the brain by 85 percent.

⇨ More than 70,000 people need hospital emergency room treatment each year for injuries related to skateboarding, according to the Consumer Products Safety Commission.

⇨ Eighty-two thousand people suffer brain injuries each year while playing sports such as football and baseball, according to the Brain Injury Association of Alexandria, Virginia.

⇨ In 2002, about 23,000 skiers and snowboarders suffered head injury, according to the Consumer Products Safety Commission. *(reported by* <u>www.consumerreports.org</u>*)*

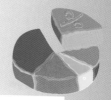

⇨ According to the Children's Safety Network, horse-related injuries sent 34,636 children to emergency rooms. More than 17 percent of these injuries were head injuries. (**www.childrenssafetynetwork.org** and National Electronic Injury Surveillance System (NEISS), 1992.)

*Important: Non-compliance a big factor.

⇨ In May of 2004, the National SAFE KIDS Campaign found, shockingly, that fewer than 41 percent of kids ages five to 14 wear helmets while participating in wheeled activities, and more than a third (35 percent) of the children who use helmets wear them improperly.

* Also important to note:

⇨ According to the National SAFE KIDS Campaign, helmet use is lowest (33 percent) in the areas where most bicycle accidents occur - residential streets.

⇨ In states with mandatory helmet laws, more child bikers wear helmets (45 percent) than in states without helmet laws (39 percent).

⇨ Girls (45 percent) are more likely than boys (33 percent) to wear helmets.

Laws and Regulations

Beginning in February 1999, all bike helmets manufactured or imported for sale in the United States must meet new federal safety standards set by the Consumer Products Safety Commission (CPSC). All helmets meeting this new standard will carry a label stating they meet CPSC safety standards.

Helmets used for all other activities must also be certified. Note, however, that a helmet is certified only for a specified use. Not all activities are the same, and so not all activities require the same helmet specifications.

According to the Snell standards (www.smf.org/stds), helmet standards and certifications are mandated according to the intended use. While one may think that activities such as bicycling and skateboarding are very similar, in fact the injury patterns from such activities vary greatly. For example, studies have shown that in injuries sustained by cyclists, most frequently the impact occurs from the front third of the helmet, down near the lower edge. The rider involved often cannot use his outstretched hands and arms to protect his head and face, because his hands are needed to maneuver the bike.

Skateboarders, on the other hand, have less active control of the skateboard than bicyclists do of their bikes. Unlike bicyclists, skateboarders and those who rollerblade and roller-skate are more likely to fall backwards, impacting the back of the head. In addition, the skateboarder or roller-skater has far more freedom with his arms and hands to naturally react and cushion impacts from the front. Therefore, while the main area of protection in a bike helmet needs to be in the front, in a skateboarder's helmet it needs to be in the rear.

The following seven points are recommended to remove the hazards from dangerous helmets or improper use of **HELMETS**:

CHECKLIST

✔		
	1	Make sure the helmet carries a certification sticker or label.
	2	Review the consumer report Web site before buying to discover safety malfunctions.
	3	If a child severely knocks his or her head once with the helmet, throw it away.
	4	Never use a damaged helmet.
	5	Only use manufacturer-approved paints, oils or other substances on a helmet.
	6	Follow the manufacturer instructions regarding the proper use of the helmet.
	7	No child under the age of one should ride in a vehicle requiring a helmet.

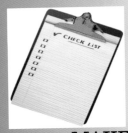

1. MAKE SURE THE HELMET CARRIES A CERTIFICATION STICKER OR LABEL.

Make sure that the helmet carries at least one of the following certifications: Consumer Products Safety Commission (**www.cpsc.gov**), Snell, ASTM or ANSI. Many helmets are made outside the United States and are brought into this country via eBay or other backdoor methods, so you cannot assume that all helmets meet current certifications.

2. REVIEW THE CONSUMER REPORT WEB SITE BEFORE BUYING TO DISCOVER SAFETY MALFUNCTIONS.

Surprisingly, even helmets that carry a certification (**www.consumer reports.com**) prove to be unsafe. For example, in July 2004, Consumer Reports tested a number of bike helmets- all of which met federal safety standards for impact and buckle-and-strap system strength. Yet, when tested, the buckles broke in multiple samples. With one toddler helmet, four of 12 samples failed; with one other helmet, three of 12 samples failed; with another, two of 12 failed. Specifically, the buckles used by the Nexus Company and the Ergo-Look by the National Motoricity Company failed.

Bike helmets are not the only helmets that met federal certification standards and failed testing; ski helmets likewise failed on inspection. In December of 2003, Consumer Reports found that the helmets of Boeri Axis Rage did pass the impact federal standards and ASTM standards. However, the shells of seven of the 10 high-gloss Axis Rage helmets tested by Consumer Reports shattered when they were dropped from about six feet directly on an anvil surface. Therefore, Consumer Reports rated the Boeri Axis Rage helmet not acceptable.

Further, there were two helmets that failed the chinstrap retention test. The plastic rings on two helmet snaps broke on inspection. Those helmets were the W helmets, including W ski helmets with slider airflow vents, and the Boeri Axis Rage helmets.

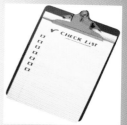

3. IF A CHILD SEVERELY KNOCKS HIS OR HER HEAD ONCE WITH THE HELMET, THROW AWAY THE HELMET.

In fact, when notified of a severe head impact without injury, many manufacturers will replace the helmet for free. It is good public relations for them, and they realize that the integrity of the helmet has been compromised by the impact. Replacement avoids future liability for the helmet manufacture.

4. NEVER USE A DAMAGED HELMET.

Always check for cracks, splinters or unreasonably weak portions of a helmet. When in doubt, throw it out.

5. ONLY USE MANUFACTURER-APPROVED PAINTS, OILS OR OTHER SUBSTANCES ON A HELMET.

According to the National Operating Committee on Standards for Athletic Equipment Recertification Program (www.nocsae.org), one of the most important areas of concern is the use of manufacturer-approved external finishes. Their guidelines indicate as follows: "Only paints, waxes, decals and cleaning agents approved by the manufacturer are to be used on any helmet. It is possible to get severe and delayed reaction by using unauthorized materials, which could permanently damage the helmet's shell and affect its safety performance."

6. FOLLOW THE MANUFACTURER INSTRUCTIONS REGARDING THE PROPER USE OF THE HELMET.

Against the backdrop of many bicycle injuries, the National SAFE KIDS Campaign, together with Bell Sports, instituted a national campaign to teach children the "eyes, ears and mouth" checklist to ensure proper helmet fit. The following is cited directly from the National SAFE KIDS Campaign (www.safekids.org):

EYES: The rim of the helmet should be one to two fingers' width above the eyebrows.

EARS: The straps should form a "V" just beneath the earlobe.

MOUTH: The buckles should be flush against the child's skin under the chin. When the rider opens his or her mouth, he or she should feel the strap snug on the chin and the helmet hugging the head.

According to Dr. Shannon Scott-Vernaglia of Massachusetts General Hospital for Children, the "**MVP**" process should be used:

"**M**" means **MOVE** it down over the forehead. The helmet should be sitting straight and on top of the head. It should not be pushed back at all. It is not a cap; it is a helmet.

"**V**" is the way the straps should fit over the ears. Center the straps so the buckles fall down right below the ears.

"**P**" is for **PULL** the chinstraps snug so the helmet will not slide off.

7. NO CHILD UNDER THE AGE OF ONE SHOULD RIDE IN A VEHICLE REQUIRING A HELMET.

According to the Bicycle Helmet Safety Institute (**www.bhsi.org**), a child of any age needs protection while riding, but a toddler's neck may not support the weight of the helmet. For this and other reasons, nobody in the injury prevention community recommends riding with a child under the age of one. If in doubt, take the child and helmet to a pediatrician for advice.

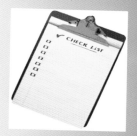

SPECIAL CONSIDERATIONS

FOOTBALL HELMETS

In May of 2002, the Bicycle Helmet Safety Institute issued a release announcing a "revolutionary" new football helmet. Manufactured by Riddell (www.riddell.com), the helmet is far thicker than any helmet now being sold and has a design that is intended to shift the force within the helmet. No tests are available.

HORSEBACK RIDING

The horse-riding community has been at the forefront of equestrian helmet use by children. A wonderful Web site, produced by the Children's Safety Network, issues safety concerns and even specifies the approved helmets on the market (http://www.marshfieldclinic.org/nfmc/pages/default.aspx?page=nccrahs_resources_facts_sheet_4). CSN Rural Injury Prevention Resource Center prepared the excellent resource publication, "A Guide to Promotion of Helmet Use For Riding Clubs and Communities."

IMPORTANT: Playgrounds and helmets do not mix.

The Consumer Products Safety Commission is on record as warning against children wearing bike helmets when playing, especially on playground equipment. The CPSC has reports of two strangulation deaths of children whose bike helmets became stuck in the openings of playground equipment. Further, the Troxel Company, a major U.S. bicycle helmet manufacturer, reported in 1997 that one of their helmets snagged on a swing and nearly caused the choking of the child who was wearing it. Since that time, Troxel has placed warnings on their helmets specifying that they should not be used in playgrounds. In Norway and Sweden, there were six documented cases between 1984 and 1992 of playground injuries that were caused by helmet use, according to the Bicycle Helmet Safety Institute warning.

Part Four

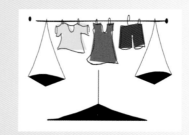

Schools/Daycare

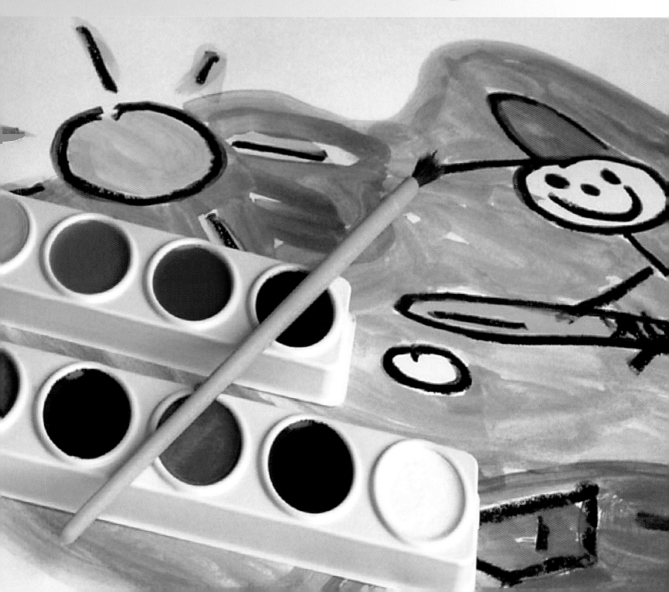

25

School Safety

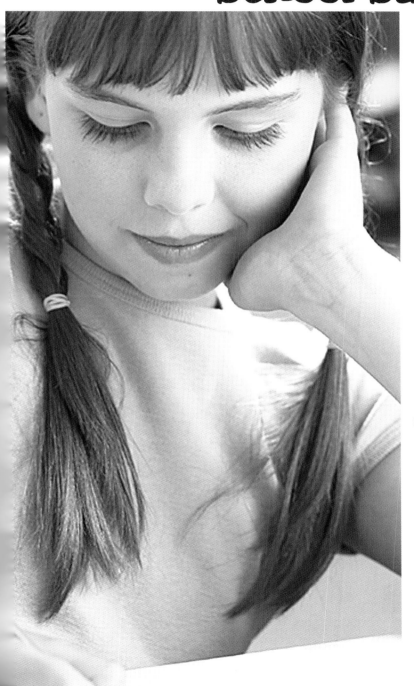

Your Child's School: No Place for Violence

Anne and Steve Porter were living the American dream with good jobs and a comfortable home in an upper-middle-class suburban neighborhood. They chose it so that their 10-year-old gifted daughter, Melanie, would be able to attend a public school district consistently ranked as one of the best in the state.

As the family ate breakfast together one February morning, they did not know that in a matter of hours their lives would change forever and that their "perfect" daughter would struggle with irreversible brain damage each day thereafter.

The family also did not know that a year before, almost to the day, a mentally deranged intruder had entered the front door of their daughter's elementary school and roamed the halls freely until confronted by a teacher. The stranger proclaimed to the teacher that he was there to "hurt a little girl." Although he was asked to leave, he was not arrested.

Following this incident, the school administrator announced a sign-in system at the front door. Strangely, while the side doors were locked, the front door, the one the intruder had entered, was left unlocked.

Months passed uneventfully. But one day, the school employee who enforced the sign-in procedure was called away on other administrative duties. Since no one took that employee's place to supervise visitor sign-in, the school's front door was left unlocked and unattended.

Another mentally deranged man, unrelated to the first, entered the front door and moved freely down the hallway. He approached a group of fourth-grade girls at their lockers. Without warning, the intruder pulled a claw hammer from his coat pocket, swung it over his head and plunged it into the back of Melanie's skull.

When the paramedics arrived, they were aghast, realizing the best they could do would be to stabilize Melanie for air transport to the trauma center with the hammer still embedded in her head. The admission X-rays confirmed the grim news: The hammer had indeed clawed its way deep into Melanie's brain. The question the medical staff kept asking over and over: How did this little girl manage to survive at all?

The next day, the school system built a wall at the cost of $800 that would block any intruder from coming in the front door into the hallway. Instead, the wall diverted visitors directly into the principal's office, where no entrance to the hallway would be permitted unless the visitor was authorized by the staff.

While Melanie struggled for her life, district officials decided they would only make improvements to this one school. They left the other 60 schools in their district unchanged, ignoring the fact that intruders can target any school.

As a result of the attack, Melanie suffers permanent cognitive and emotional damage that affect her every day of her life. Because a lawsuit against the school is in progress, no further details are available about her prognosis and life care needs.

Statistics Tell the Story

It is an unfortunate fact of life that "stranger danger" in American schools has been on the rise for several years. Here is just a small sampling of cases:

In May 2001, Jason Pritchard used a fillet knife to attack four children in an Anchorage, Alaska school. He was charged with four counts of attempted first-degree murder. The same year in Felton, Pennsylvania, an intruder who lived 400 miles away in Tennessee used a machete to attack six school children.

The year of Melanie's attack also saw two intruder-violence cases in Colorado. In Greenwood Village, a 34-year-old intruder assaulted one middle school and one high school student. Later, in Westminster, a man with a gun entered a middle school and was intercepted before harming anyone.

And, in late 2004, metro Atlanta schools were stalked by Phillip Brooks, a man with a lengthy arrest record, who was wanted for identity theft. He gained entrance to seven DeKalb County elementary schools in seven weeks, each time identifying himself as a parent. He was caught stealing in at least one school; thankfully, nothing worse happened. Yet, in a county with a seven million dollar school security budget, one wonders how he was able to gain entrance to these schools and wander their corridors unchecked.

Consider these statistics:

1. In the 2001-2002 school year, 17 school-aged youth were victims of a school-associated violent death.

2. In 1999-2000, there were 32 school-associated violent deaths. Of these, 24 were homicides and eight were suicides.

3. From 1992-2000, 390 school-associated violent deaths occurred on campuses of U.S. elementary or secondary schools. Of these, 234 were homicides and 43 were suicides. Statistically, children are at least 70 times more likely to be murdered away from school than at school. However, we believe most schools' security systems are far too lax.

(Source: U.S. Department of Education, National Center for Education Statistics.)

Laws and Regulations

For the first time, the federal government has begun scrutinizing the number and severity of crimes in all public schools nationwide because of the *No Child Left Behind* Act. This law permits students to transfer out of their school if they have been the victim of a serious crime at school or if their school is found to be "persistently dangerous."

But the definition of "persistently dangerous" is slippery enough that, according to the Cleveland Plain Dealer, 46 states claim to have no persistently dangerous schools. The problem is that each state is allowed to craft its own definition of what a dangerous school is. Only 38 schools in the country were classified as persistently dangerous in 2004. And of those, 27 were to be found in Philadelphia, whose public schools enroll about 200,000 students.

In contrast, the Chicago public schools, with 438,000 students, had no persistently dangerous schools. This, despite the fact that the school system records showed 66 robberies, 26 guns found on school property and 36 teacher assaults in one school year.

It is fair to assume that both these districts, as well as countless others, have all too many unsafe schools. But at least Philadelphia is honest about its problem.

And *No Child Left Behind* has an even more basic weakness: Assume, for a minute, that a student is able to transfer from his or her "persistently dangerous" school to a safer one. That transfer does nothing to improve the safety of the dangerous school's other students. No child left behind, indeed.

So, we grant the federal government a "thumbs down" on the school safety issue, both for not requiring improvements at dangerous schools and for allowing individual states so much flexibility in crafting their own definitions of what a dangerous school is as to become meaningless.

We grant the state governments a "thumbs down" on safety for taking advantage of the federal loopholes to avoid the "persistently dangerous" label, thereby all but guaranteeing that large-scale improvements will not occur.

NOTE: Research shows that the three most common school accidents involve (a) playgrounds, (b) sports and (c) school buses. The following Report Card omits these top three potential hazards because they are covered in separate chapters: playgrounds in Chapter 14, sports in Chapter 16 and school buses in Chapter 30. Cheerleading is covered in Chapter 22.

REPORT CARD

	SUBJECT	GRADE
1	Fire detection system	
2	Specific fire drill plan in place	
3	Building access controlled	
4	Internal communications network	
5	Awareness that over crowding causes problems	
6	Adequate interior and exterior lighting	
7	Secure storage, mechanical and electrical areas	
8	Adequate exterior grounds maintenance	
9	Designated pick-up and drop-off areas	
10	Safety plan in place for all emergencies	

1. FIRE DETECTION SYSTEM

According the Centers for Disease Control, more than 6,000 structure fires occur in schools every year. Half of these occur in schools without any working smoke or fire alarms. Automatic sprinkler systems exist in only 23 percent of the schools where fires occur. At minimum, all schools should have smoke alarms. Sprinkler systems should also be mandatory.

2. SPECIFIC FIRE DRILL PLAN IN PLACE

Emergency/Fire drills must be conducted regularly. Besides the complete evacuation of all staff and students, fire safety includes proper fire extinguisher maintenance. All fire extinguishers must be inspected monthly and serviced annually, with the attached tags properly dated and initialed each time. Also:

⇨ All smoke/fire detectors must be in place and operational.
⇨ Adequate first aid supplies must be available in sufficient quantity, and their location must be known to all teachers, staff and administrators.

3. BUILDING ACCESS CONTROLLED

As described in the sample case, and other cases around the country, stranger danger is a ticking time bomb. Statistics are sketchy as schools do not report stranger danger intrusions on a regular basis. At minimum, the following must be in place:

a) All access doors must be closed to the outside during school hours. Persons inside can easily exit but no one from the outside can gain access. This can be accomplished by two alternative, CHEAP, one-time measures.

⇨ First, schools can install a buzz intercom system that goes directly into the principal's office. One's identity and lawful purpose are verified before the visitor is buzzed inside. The cost is about $300 to $500.
⇨ Second, most schools have the principal's office positioned right inside the school door, as in the case I handled. The school simply erected a wall that would divert a person who enters the school directly into the principal's office. As with the intercom system, one's identity and purpose is verified before the outsider is granted access to the school.

b) Badges and/or ID s for teachers, staff, visitors and students (as age appropriate). Drills must be performed to train teachers and staff to stop those without ID badges.

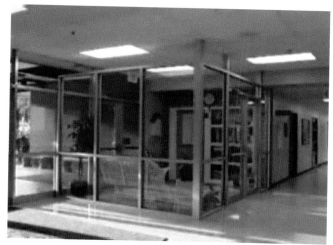

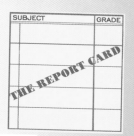
The photograph is from the case story at the beginning of this chapter. It shows the glass barrier erected which requires all those entering the front door to first go through the principal's office.

4. INTERNAL COMMUNICATIONS NETWORK

Staff members must be able to maintain contact between classrooms and office via in-house phones, intercoms, or two-way portable radios.

5. AWARENESS THAT OVERCROWDING CAUSES PROBLEMS

While statistics are sparse, the overcrowding of schools, particularly the use of trailers, appears to be central in districts where there is an increase in student-on-student violence and student-on-teacher violence. While trailers may be a necessary evil with rapid school growth, administrators must pay specific attention to the stress created. A school system that does not recognize the correlation is asking for trouble.

6. ADEQUATE INTERIOR AND EXTERIOR LIGHTING

In many of the premises security cases I have handled, including apartment abductions, ATM murders and hotel armed robberies, there is often inadequate lighting involved. Wrongdoers are naturally attracted to areas of low or inadequate lighting. The same is true of violence in schools, thus mandating that proper lighting is an important step to safety.

7. SECURE STORAGE, MECHANICAL AND ELECTRICAL AREAS

Ask if these areas kept locked. Also ask if shelves/shelving units are anchored firmly to the walls. Finally, ask if items are properly shelved (e.g. heavy items shelved on bottom, items not stacked on floor creating trip hazards).

8. ADEQUATE EXTERIOR GROUNDS MAINTENANCE

Is all foliage properly trimmed to eliminate hiding places for people who can not penetrate the school but will wait till the children are outside? Are poisonous/toxic plants removed? There have been several reported cases where younger children not possessing their full immune system have been overcome with toxic landscape chemicals.

9. DESIGNATED PICK-UP AND DROP OFF AREAS

Although simple to put in place, schools all too often modify the students' pick-up and drop-off areas. For safety's sake, parents and children need to develop a firm habit; thus, these areas should remain constant and not change unless absolutely necessary.

10. SAFETY PLAN IN PLACE FOR ALL EMERGENCIES

Support Services must be available: Counselors, school security officers, adequate number of staff trained in basic first aid are available.

Signage: All exits must be clearly marked, emergency evacuation maps must be posted in each room, and notices describing procedures to be followed in the event of emergency must be posted.

Drills: These must be in place for ALL emergencies and sign off sheets assuring that all personnel have been trained and refreshed.

MAJOR TRUTH: HOPE FOR THE BEST BUT PLAN FOR THE WORST.

Many thanks to school safety expert Edward Dragan for his advocacy in making schools safer for children.

26
Daycare Safety

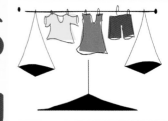

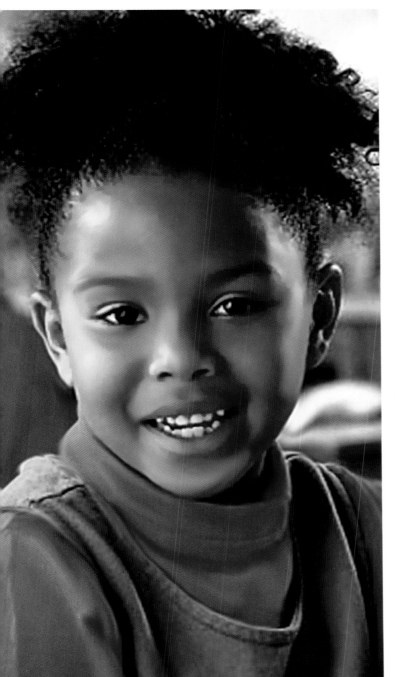

When Caregivers Fail

Part of a national chain, the daycare center appeared to be a friendly place. Panda bears, ducks and happy faces greeted one-and-a half-year-old Jason when his parents, Gary and Natalie, dropped him off on their way to work. They had no idea that this daycare choice would be fatal. Less than 500 days after his birth into their lives, Jason was taken from his family by a childcare worker's violent actions.

The assistant director of the center ultimately pled guilty to involuntary manslaughter in Jason's classic case of shaken baby syndrome. "The baby just would not stop crying, and I shook him to make him stop," she said. "I never thought that would kill the baby." Child abuse experts hear this statement all the time, and in cases all over the country. Yet the brutal force of the shaking can hemorrhage the baby's brain, causing swelling and brain pressure; this is what led to Jason's death.

LEGAL ACTION and OUTCOME

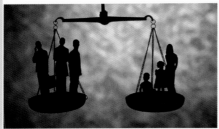

No parent should lose his or her child in the supposed safekeeping of a national daycare center. The center Jason was killed in provided no staff training on the life-threatening dangers of shaking a baby. Also, despite the huge sum of money spent by the company on advertising, they budgeted no money for employee background checks. Had they checked, the center would have discovered that the guilty employee had been fired from two other daycare centers.

As Gary and Natalie sought justice, they were met with a series of appalling incidents. The national corporation stated that they were not responsible for the center. The franchise said that the act of the employee was so outrageous that it was "beyond the scope of her employment." In other words, they were not responsible either. And the insurance company asserted that they were denying coverage, because the underlying act was criminal and therefore excluded by the coverage.

Shocked and dismayed, the family pressed their lawsuit. The insurance company lost the coverage issue; the judge ruled that the act was covered because the employee did not intend to kill. The franchise was held accountable because they didn't perform background checks. The chain was held responsible in the suit because it failed to provide the necessary training.

Statistics Tell the Story

In 1997, about 31,000 children four years-old and younger were treated in U.S. hospital emergency rooms for injuries at childcare/school settings.*

At least 56 children have died in childcare settings since 1990. Twenty-eight of these children died from suffocation related to soft bedding or nursery equipment. *

*According to the Consumer Products Safety Commission (CPSC). (www.cpsc.gov)

A study by the Consumer Products Safety Commission revealed that two-thirds of childcare settings exhibit at least one safety hazard. The targeted hazards included: cribs, soft bedding, playground surfacing, playground surfacing maintenance, child safety gates, window blind cords, drawstrings in children's clothing and recalled children's products.

⇨ Between 40 and 50 babies die each year in accidents involving cribs, yet eight percent of the facilities examined by the CPSC had cribs that didn't meet current safety standards.

⇨ As many as 900 babies die of Sudden Infant Death Syndrome (SIDS) each year, and soft bedding is one of the risk factors. Yet nineteen percent of the settings had cribs that contained soft bedding.

⇨ Over 100,000 children under the age of five went to emergency rooms with stair-related injuries in 1997. Thirteen percent of the childcare settings didn't use child safety gates where needed.

⇨ Every month, on average, one child dies by strangulation from a window covering cord. At least two children have died in childcare environments after standing in their cribs and becoming tangled in a window blind cord. The CPSC found that 26 percent of childcare settings had loops on the window-blind cords in which children could become entangled.

⇨ At least 22 children have died and 47 have been injured by drawstrings since 1985. Yet children wore clothing with drawstrings at the neck in thirty eight percent of childcare settings.

⇨ Since 1990, at least three children have died in childcare facilities in incidents involving portable cribs and playpens that have been recalled, yet five percent of child care settings still had products that had been recalled by CPSC.

Laws and Regulations

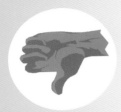

Almost 13 million children under school age attend childcare programs during some portion of the day in this country. Twenty-nine percent are in center-based care, and the remaining 71 percent of the programs are in non-center based facilities, including in-home childcare and care by a relative. There are no federal regulations for daycare facilities. Instead, daycare is regulated on a state-by-state basis. A review of state licensing requirements by the CPSC showed that most of the hazards they identified were not addressed in these requirements. For example, while cribs are covered by federal regulations, states don't always require daycare centers to use cribs that are up to these standards. And while all daycare centers use equipment like strollers, cribs and high chairs, many have no state requirements for dealing with recalled equipment.

Some state non-profit groups successfully conduct their own auditing of childcare facilities. A private group in Denver recently did just that, checking facilities statewide with over twelve million dollars in private funds. The group examined training standards, with an emphasis on advancing education.

Audits like these are important, but they will not replace the need for both federal and state governance. Parents need to know that if a childcare facility is open for business, it means that it is a safe place to bring their children. Obviously, this is not currently the case.

Taking Action

Parents and other concerned adults can use this report card to help determine the safety of a daycare facility.

PASS/FAIL
ALL OF THE FOLLOWING SHOULD BE AVAILABLE FOR YOUR REVIEW:

REPORT CARD

	SUBJECT	GRADE
1	Proof of licensing	
2	National accreditation	
3	No or low number of complaints	
4	Proof of insurance	
5	Toy safety and use procedure	
6	Pedophile surveillance procedures	
7	Emergency medical treatment procedure	
8	Documentation of health screens for all children in attendance	
9	Background and health checks of all employees	
10	An up-to-date training procedure for employees	

1. PROOF OF LICENSING

In many states, faith-based centers, such as churches, and health clubs, including national chains, are not subject to state licensure. Without this licensure, the facility is free to hire any personnel it desires, supervise children in any manner it sees fit and maintain whatever facility health conditions it chooses.

View your state's licensure requirements at **www.ncedl.org** (click "products," then go to "policy briefs-vol.2, no.1"). Remember that licensure only means that the facility meets minimum standards. You may disagree with the minimum standards. Check everything out for yourself. There are vast differences from state to state. The ratio of staff workers to children in Texas, for example, is one adult to twenty children while in New York it is one to eight.

2. NATIONAL ACCREDITATION

Because many states have no or very low standards for licensure, you must demand that there be accreditation by one or more national associations, such as the National Association for the Education of Young Children. These organizations set minimum standards regarding age, staff training and safety standards.

3. NO OR LOW NUMBER OF COMPLAINTS

Several states now provide public access to complaints filed against daycare facilities, either over the telephone or via the Internet. This trend mirrors the public access to nursing home complaints, which was mandated by federal law and has now become a major element in increasing the safety of the nursing home industry. Hopefully, this trend in daycare facility access information will likewise increase the safety of daycare facilities.

Also, check with the Better Business Bureau to see if any complaints have been filed with them regarding the facility. You can access this information via the Internet, or in writing.

A "low number of complaints" may simply mean that the filed complaints are not of a serious enough nature to discourage use of the facility. Each complaint must be judged independently. Of course, only one complaint that is major or life-threatening should be enough to discourage use.

Complaints that result in a civil lawsuit are of a serious nature. For a small fee, many databases (such as **www.knowx.com**) provide access to filed lawsuits. Information regarding the actual lawsuit itself and the ultimate outcome are often available on the Internet.

Your local court system may also be accessible directly via the Internet, as are most metropolitan court dockets. Begin by calling the court clerk in the county in which the facility is located. The clerk will either direct you to the Internet site, or, in many instances, he or she will retrieve the information for you. The clerk may also request a written letter.

4. PROOF OF INSURANCE

The maxim "hope for the best but plan for the worst" applies to many sections of this book, including daycare facilities. If tragedy strikes and your child is catastrophically injured, you must know that the facility has adequate insurance coverage to guarantee payment of full medical bills and treatment. You also want the facility to be able to provide a quality of life for your child and family. Currently, a minimum of one million dollars coverage per claim is considered adequate.

Review the insurance policy itself. Note the coverage period (start and ending dates). If you continue to use the facility beyond the "end date" of the policy you review, request to see a copy of the updated policy.

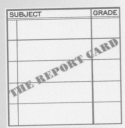

Simply having an insurance policy does not guarantee coverage, however. As noted in the sample case, there is often a denial of coverage. The insurance company states that the acts of the daycare facility are outside those covered by the insurance policy. This is not a hypothetical argument, but rather reality. A case in point is the 2003 opinion in South Carolina regarding Tender Loving Care Daycare Center. The center was sued when a baby in its care died from "shaken baby syndrome." The family contended that the facility was negligent in hiring and supervising the employee who was the perpetrator of the child's death. The South Carolina Appeals Court, however, ruled that "child abuse" is excluded from the insurance policy. In other words, the insurance company was let off the hook and the family received no justice.

5. TOY SAFETY AND USE PROCEDURE

At a minimum, the facility should follow all of the safety points contained in Part 3, Chapter 15 of this book regarding toys. Be aware, however, that many facilities do not follow these guidelines. Particularly negligent are centers that exclusively or substantially use donated toys; often, the center assumes that someone else did the safety checking.

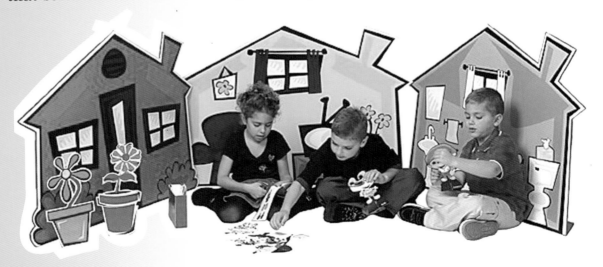

Many toys are rated for age appropriateness: see item six on the "Toy Safety Report Card." Centers often have one central toy depository, however, to which all children have free access. Instead, toys should be segregated according to age appropriateness, and children should not be able to choose toys beyond their skill or safety level.

Lack of sanitation, which can lead to the spread of dangerous organisms and even injury and death in children, is an important issue in daycare centers. Toy sharing, which often accounts for the spread of infection, is of special concern, so make sure that the facility has some procedure regarding the cleaning of toys. Specifically, the washing, bleaching and air-drying of toys should be done every two weeks, more frequently during periods of increased communicable diseases.

6. PEDOPHILE SURVEILLANCE PROCEDURES

Willie Sutton, the famous bank robber, was once asked why he robbed banks. He replied, "That's where the money is." There are a number of reported cases where convicted pedophiles have moved into apartments in direct proximity to daycare centers. That's because while many states prohibit registered sex offenders from living close to a school or even a church, there is no provision in most states concerning living next door to, or across the street from, a daycare facility.

Virtually all states now have a sex offender registry, which lists at least the home address (and often the work address) of the sex offender. If the registry is up-to-date, it is a simple matter to know whether a sex offender is living or working in your child's environment. Please note, however, that many of the government-maintained databases are hopelessly out of date. At minimum, the daycare facility and you, as a backup, should check the sex offender registry at least four times a year.

7. EMERGENCY MEDICAL TREATMENT PROCEDURE

The facility should have health insurance information for each child. This information should include the family's insurance company, policy number and contact phone numbers. The facility should also know where the nearest emergency room hospital is located and specifically whether that hospital accepts the child's insurance coverage. Many children have been catastrophically injured and died while an ambulance transported them from emergency room to emergency room in search of a hospital that would accept the child. This is in clear violation of federal law, but it happens all the time.

Additionally, the facility staff should know the children's hospital or children's trauma center located nearest the daycare facility. While normal emergency rooms may be sufficient for the average injury, a catastrophic injury dictates direct transport to a children's hospital or trauma center.

8. DOCUMENTATION OF HEALTH SCREENS FOR ALL CHILDREN IN ATTENDANCE

Vaccination records should be kept up-to-date for all children in attendance. In Philadelphia, 23 children got seriously ill with chickenpox in 2001 because one child had not been vaccinated. (This was not discovered until after the fact.) Children are very susceptible to the spread of disease in childcare facilities. Therefore, the facility should have clear health criteria requirements for all children who attend. And if a facility accepts children with mild illnesses, it should have a method of segregating these children from the healthy children.

9. BACKGROUND AND HEALTH CHECKS OF ALL EMPLOYEES

Unfortunately, low wages and high staff turnover exist in many facilities. High staff turnover clearly reflects negatively on the quality of a daycare program, according to the National Center for Development & Learning. In addition, without background checks, there is no guarantee that your child is not being taken care of by an ex-con just released from prison, by a nurse whose license has been revoked or suspended, or even by a sex offender. So the facility must have strict background checks on all employees, and it must conduct annual updates.

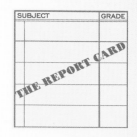

The workers must also possess a statement from a doctor stating that they are in good health and have no communicable diseases. This statement is a good safety net, because a doctor will not want to sign such a statement exposing him or her to liability unless the worker is truly healthy. This is not an insignificant requirement- there have been reports of employees with highly contagious diseases who work hands-on (in play activities and food preparation) with kids in daycare centers.

10. AN UP-TO-DATE TRAINING PROCEDURE FOR EMPLOYEES

A good daycare facility will have a detailed employee training manual and a "checklist" properly displayed in the facility. Take time to review the training manual and checklist; they assure that safety is the number-one priority of the center. Does it make sense to you? Do you agree with its contents? Do you feel comfortable with the environment that is defined and the methods that will be used with your child? Make sure there is not only an employee training procedure, but testing as well. Testing assures two important things: that employees actually read the manual and checklist, and that, more importantly, they understand them.

Keep in mind that staff training should be specific to each age grouping in the center. Guidelines should detail procedures for caring for infants, babies, toddlers, preschoolers, and grade-schoolers. In the guidelines for infants, for example, a litmus test for proper training and updating is whether the facility teaches the staff the correct positioning procedure. As noted in a 2000 study by the Children's National Medical Center in Washington, D.C., 25 percent of licensed childcare centers in the metro area were unaware of the American Academy of Pediatrics' ten-year-old recommendation that infants be placed in a non-prone position while sleeping in order to reduce the risk of sudden infant death syndrome (SIDS). The study indicated that 28 percent of all centers still position infants in the prone position; shocking, against the statistic that at least 20 percent of reported cases of sudden infant death syndrome (SIDS) occur in daycare centers.

NOTE: The author was interviewed extensively on this subject in the May 2003 issue of *Smart Money*, pages 69-71.

Part Five

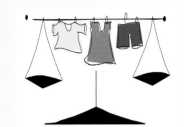

Transportation

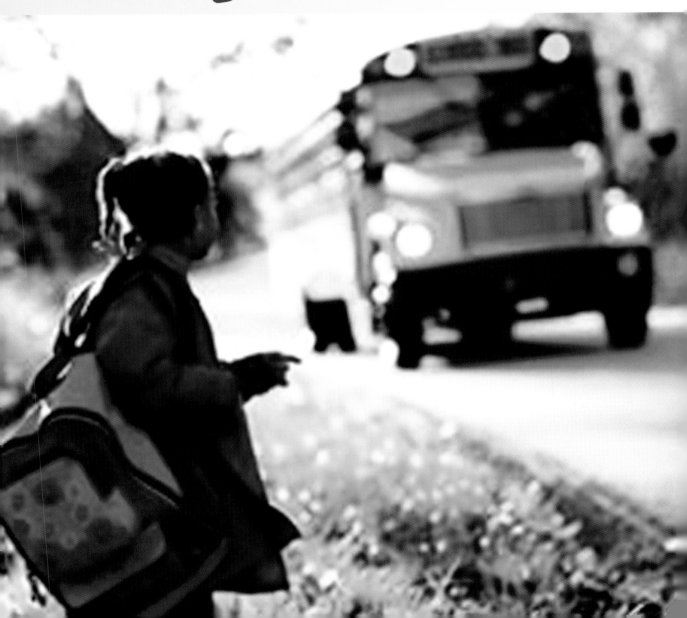

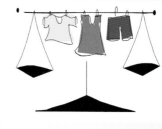

27

Auto Design

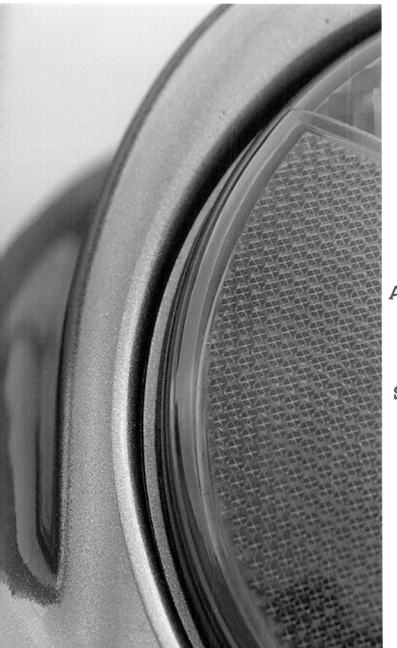

A Safety Device Proves Deadly

Jessie, age 16, was working part-time for her father's office supply company in order to make some extra money. Her father had purchased a new car, but she was required to furnish the gasoline and insurance. After completing her work after school, her dad told her to go on home and that he would follow in a few minutes.

What happened next was a parent's worse nightmare. Jessie's dad, Ralph, made the 11 mile journey home to discover that Jessie was not there and had not called as she always does advising of any side trips. He became concerned and went back down the nearly straight rural road in search of his daughter. This time he discovered some metal debris on the side of the road and pulled over to investigate. What he found was unimaginable; his daughter's new car, with less than 5,000 miles on it, was in a dozen pieces. Her body was literally strewn in all directions. After calling the police and the emergency technicians, her father also discovered another vehicle that contained two obviously dead occupants and one clinging to life.

The survivor told police at the hospital that he was in the back seat of the other vehicle and saw Jessie's vehicle approaching in the opposite direction. For no reason Jessie's vehicle, which had been traveling a safe speed according to the witness, crossed the center line and hit the witness's vehicle head on, killing the other two occupants and nearly killing him.

Jessie's dad pondered what could possibly have caused his little girl to cross the center line and cause such a tragedy?

The only clue was several months earlier, when Ralph had received a form letter from the auto manufacturer advising that there was an electrical hazard inside the steering wheel harness that needed to be fixed. Jessie's dad promptly took the vehicle to the dealership and assumed that everything was fixed. Somehow Jessie's father believed this letter had something to do with his daughter's death.

LEGAL ACTION
and
OUTCOME

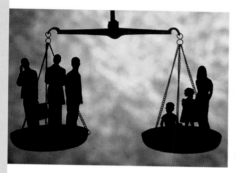

Armed only with the manufacturer form letter, the parents hired my law firm to undertake an investigation and to obtain the answers. After taking possession of Jessie's vehicle, we delivered it to a forensic team of engineers to recreate the accident and examine every aspect of the vehicle. According to the black box analysis, the driver airbag had deployed before Jessie hit the brakes. The black box, of course, includes coded information, which tells a great deal about the functioning of the vehicle at any time. The engineers then examined the contents of the steering harness and discovered that the wiring into the steering wheel, which went to the volume controls of the radio (radio volume could be turned up or down through a button on the steering wheel) was without protective covering immediately adjacent to where the airbag was housed. Through scientific formulas, the engineers were able to prove that the vibration in the steering harness, particularly from the radio controls and the lack of guarding, had caused the premature release of the airbag. Jessie must have been adjusting the volume on the radio and triggered the release of the airbag, which caused her to lose control of the steering wheel, only able to hit the brakes. Because of the premature release of the airbag and her loss of control, she unintentionally crossed the center line of the highway at 45 miles per hour, striking the other vehicle, killing herself and the two occupants in the vehicle.

After filing the lawsuit and engaging in subpoenaing of documents, we discovered that Jessie's father had been right all along. There had been a premature release of the airbag which prompted the manufacturer to recall all of the vehicles and have the local dealerships make necessary corrections. Unfortunately, Jessie's local dealership did not follow the manufacturer retrofit instructions, and thus her vehicle continued to be a ticking time bomb ready to explode.

After months of litigation and the sworn testimony of many technical personnel at the manufacturer's headquarters and the testimony of our experts, the case was ultimately concluded favorably for the family. Sadly, the airbag that was intended to protect Jessie's life caused her death.

Statistics Tell the Story

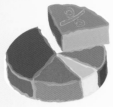

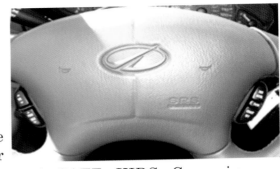

Motor vehicle crashes are the leading cause of unintentional deaths of children under the age of 14, according to the National SAFE KIDS Campaign. (www.safekids.org)

➪ In 2003, 1,639 children died in vehicle crashes, according to the Insurance Institute for Highway Safety. (www.iihs.org)

➪ In 2002, a quarter million children under the age of 14 were injured as occupants in motor vehicle-related crashes, according to the National SAFE KIDS Campaign.

➪ According to the National SAFE KIDS Campaign, 25 percent of all children involved in motor vehicle-related crashes were later diagnosed with post-traumatic stress disorder, double the percentage of adults.

➪ As of January 2004, 141 children have been killed by passenger airbags, according to the Nationa SAFE KIDS Campaign.

➪ Although rollover crashes constitute only three percent of motor vehicle crashes, these crashes represent one-third of all deaths, over 10,000 deaths annually, according to Public Citizen. (www.citizen.org)

➪ Fourteen of 16 small cars were rated poor in a test that simulates a crash with an SUV at a side impact angle. None of the 16 were rated "good," according to a March 2005 report by the Insurance Institute for Highway Safety. (www.iihs.org)

➪ 100 children are killed, and 2,500 are injured a year by unintentional vehicle backing maneuvers, according to www.cdc.gov and www.kidsandcars.org

RULE: The bigger the vehicle, the bigger the blind spot.

Laws and Regulations

While there are volumes of Federal laws and regulations addressing the safety requirements of vehicle manufacturers, the case of Claire Duncan, a 26-year-old woman, illustrates how the auto industry side steps the intent of regulations.

The auto industry and the government have known for years that deaths and serious injuries can be prevented by strengthening the structures surrounding the roof compartment. In the early 1970's, the American car manufacturers made a concerted effort to minimize the standards proposed for roof strength. Standard 216 was ultimately adopted, requiring that the strength-to-weight ratio be a minimum of 1.5, a very low and dangerous condition.

Initially, all manufacturers strived to have the ratio much higher, thereby making the vehicles much safer. Unfortunately for Claire Duncan, she was driving a 2000 Ford Explorer that suddenly rolled over while she was traveling on Interstate 95, in Virginia. She had attempted to pass another vehicle and suddenly lost control of the Explorer; it rolled over five times, fracturing her skull and ultimately killing her.

Ironically, in 1995, the strength-to-weight ratio in the Ford Explorer was 1.72, a ration sufficient enough to have saved her life. Instead, in 1999, Ford decided to downgrade the strength to only a fraction above the minimum, 1.56. During the Jacksonville, Florida civil jury trial against Ford Motor Company, it was revealed through Ford's company documents that Ford engineers had on multiple occasions objected to the reduction of the roof strength ratio in 1999 and had strongly advocated that the 1995 ratio of 1.72 should even be increased to make the vehicles as safe as possible.

Because of Ford's deliberate indifference to the safety of its consumers, the jury delivered a large verdict.

Also, on this topic, a report issued in March of 2005 indicated that the auto industry had been misleading the government concerning overwhelming data that supported a link between roof strength and injuries, according to the report of Martha Bidez, a professor of biomechanical engineering at the University of Alabama at Birmingham. Further, Public Citizen, a national group founded by Ralph Nader, issued a press release in March of 2005 documenting the particulars of the false and misleading information the industry supplied to the government (www.citizen.org).

As to backing deaths and injuries, there are no regulations regarding the blind spot.

Bottom line: Do not believe for a minute that the Federal government or the auto industry is looking out for your child's safety.

Taking Action

Because of the enormity of the subject matter of vehicle safety, we will depart from the normal one-checklist approach used throughout the book. Instead we will provide a general checklist followed by three specific checklists for airbags, roof strength and side impacts.

IN GENERAL:

Not all vehicles are created equal; some are much safer than others. To assist in finding the safest vehicle for your family please consider the following checklist:

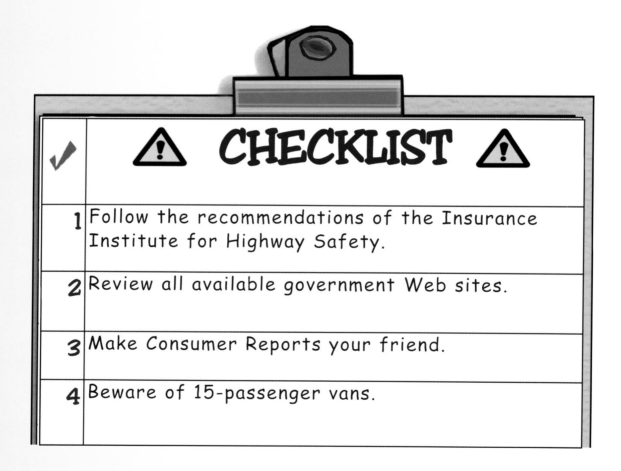

✔	⚠ CHECKLIST ⚠
1	Follow the recommendations of the Insurance Institute for Highway Safety.
2	Review all available government Web sites.
3	Make Consumer Reports your friend.
4	Beware of 15-passenger vans.

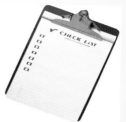

1. FOLLOW THE RECOMMENDATIONS OF THE INSURANCE INSTITUTE FOR HIGHWAY SAFETY.

The Insurance Institute for Highway Safety is a non-profit organization funded by the auto insurance industry, which has a vested interest in decreasing deaths and serious injury. The institute provides the most comprehensive vehicle ratings. Go to **www.iihs.org/ratings/default.aspx**. There are a number of categories such as 40 mile-per-hour frontal offset crash tests, side-impact crash tests and a number of other important features. Check out the database before you buy your next car.

2. REVIEW ALL AVAILABLE GOVERNMENT WEB SITES.

The National Highway Traffic Safety Administration (**www.nhtsa.dot.gov**) also has a complete database on vehicles concerning crash tests going back to 1991. Simply go to the home page and follow the prompts, or go directly to **www.nhtsa.dot.gov/cars/testing**.

3. MAKE CONSUMER REPORTS YOUR FRIEND.

Consumer Reports is a non-profit organization which does not accept any money from any company for whom they rate a product. They publish a monthly magazine and also have an extensive Web site (**www.consumerreports.org**) which requires a password to obtain key information...well worth the small yearly fee. The magazine and Web site contains valuable information on vehicles and ratings. IMPORTANT: the testing done by Consumer Reports far exceeds the safety tests conducted by the government.

4. BEWARE OF 15-PASSENGER VANS.

When 15-passenger vans are lightly loaded with little cargo and only a few passengers, the vehicle has the driving characteristics of a basic SUV. However, with increased passengers, the center of gravity moves higher and towards the rear, which increased the vehicle's propensity to over-steer and decreases its stability.

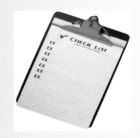

Therefore, the risk of rollover in a loaded 15-passenger van is greatly increased. The National Highway Traffic Safety Administration (**www.nhtsa.dot.gov**) has issued 15-passenger van warnings in 2001, 2002 and again in 2003 given the large number of rollover crashes involving religious groups and civic groups on trips:

According to the NHTSA warning, the following precautions need be observed:

⇨   Require ALL occupants to wear their seat belts or the appropriate child restraint. Nearly 80 percent of those who died nationwide in 15-passenger vans were not buckled up. Wearing seat belts dramatically increases the chances of survival during a rollover crash.

⇨   If possible, seat passengers and place any cargo forward of the rear axle. Also avoid placing any loads on the roof. By doing so, you will lower the vehicle's center of gravity and lower the chance of rollover.

⇨   If your organization owns a 15-passenger van, check the van's tires once a month for proper inflation and tread that is not warn down. Excessively worn or improperly inflated tires can lead to a loss of control situation and rollover.

⇨   Use caution on both interstates and rural roads to avoid running off the road. If your van's wheel should drift off the roadway, gradually slow down and steer onto the road when it is safe to do so. Most 15-passenger van rollovers occur at high speeds as a result of a sudden steering maneuver, such as an over-correction.

⇨   As a driver, ensure you are well rested and alert. Always maintain a safe speed for weather and road conditions. The agency recommends that only trained and experienced drivers should operate 15-passenger vans.

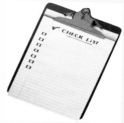

The following checklist should assist in the proper use of **AIRBAGS**:

⚠️ CHECKLIST ⚠️

✔	
1	Never place an infant in a rear-facing child seat in the front seat.
2	Children under the age of 12 should be properly restrained in the back seat.
3	To minimize injury risk, children should not lean or rest against chest only or chest/head combination side airbags.
4	In the event there are no available rear seats, follow acceptable procedures.
5	Turn off passenger front airbag.
6	Discover if your vehicle's side airbags were designed to minimize risk to children.

NOTE: This entire checklist was adapted from the National Highway Traffic Safety Administration.

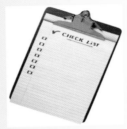

1. NEVER PLACE AN INFANT IN A REAR-FACING CHILD SEAT IN THE FRONT SEAT.

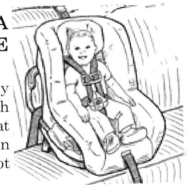

The hazards of placing the child in the front seat are tragically well-known, given the number of children deaths. Although there have been attempts at creating a weight adjusting front seat trigger for the airbag, an airbag that would know a child was in the front seat and thereby not deploy, that technology has not been fully developed.

2. CHILDREN UNDER THE AGE OF 12 SHOULD BE PROPERLY RESTRAINED IN THE BACKSEAT.

The age and size of the child will dictate what type of backseat restraint is proper, i.e., safety seat, booster seats, or the traditional seat belts. For greater explanation of the age and size dictates, go to www.nhtsa.dot.gov/people/injury/airbags/airbags03/page7.html. The Web site has phone numbers and email addresses for the procedure of how to add an on/off switch.

3. TO MINIMIZE INJURY RISK, CHILDREN SHOULD NOT LEAN OR REST AGAINST CHEST ONLY OR CHEST/HEAD COMBINATION SIDE AIRBAGS.

4. IN THE EVENT THERE ARE NO AVAILABLE REAR SEATS, FOLLOW ACCEPTABLE PROCEDURES.

5. TURN OFF PASSENGER FRONT AIRBAG.

6. DISCOVER IF YOUR VEHICLE'S SIDE AIRBAGS (SABS) WERE DESIGNED TO MINIMIZE RISK TO CHILDREN.

Unfortunately, the federal standards relating to safety design for children regarding SABs are entirely voluntary. Consequently, some manufacturers do design safely for children and others do not. NHTSA provides this information to consumers at www.safercar.gov. If your vehicle meets safety standards for children, it will have an "M" in the appropriate column. If your vehicle does not have an "M," you should check your owner's manual or contact the vehicle manufacturer to find out whether or not your car's SABs are safe for children.

The following checklist should assist in minimizing the danger of **ROLLOVERS**:

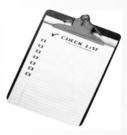

✔	⚠️ CHECKLIST ⚠️
1	Keep tires properly inflated.
2	Use proper loading allocations.
3	Run government databases for the rating of your vehicle.
4	If possible, purchase a vehicle with an electronic stabilizing control (ESC).

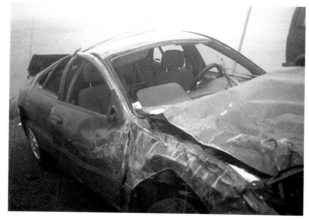

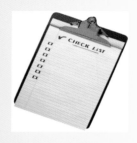

1. KEEP TIRES PROPERLY INFLATED.

Analysis of many rollover occurrences indicate that the vehicle was either not in good mechanical condition or, quite often, the tires were not properly inflated, thus causing a rollover at higher frequencies.

2. USE PROPER LOADING ALLOCATIONS.

Consult your manufacturer's handbook for proper loading. If you have added a roof rack, then consult the manufacturer's guide regarding proper positioning of cargo.

3. RUN GOVERNMENT DATABASES FOR THE RATING OF YOUR VEHICLE.

The roof crush vulnerability rating is well known to government and independent testing agencies. Therefore, please consult the three sources set forth in the "General" checklist.

4. IF POSSIBLE, PURCHASE A VEHICLE WITH AN ELECTRONIC STABILIZING CONTROL (ESC).

According to the American Automobile Association Foundation for Traffic Safety, (www.aaafoundation.org), the use of the electronic stabilizing control (ESC) can greatly reduce the occurrence of a rollover. Studies from the Insurance Institute for Highway Safety have found ESC to dramatically reduce the involvement of equipped vehicles in single-vehicle crashes involving injury or death. The ESC devise is designed to keep the vehicle "on track" thus preventing it from under-steering (i.e., the front tires lose traction and the vehicle turns less than you intend) or over-steering (i.e., the rear tires lose traction and the vehicle turns further than you intend).

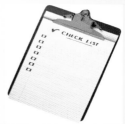

The following checklist can greatly reduce death and serious injuries with **SIDE-IMPACT COLLISIONS**:

⚠ CHECKLIST ⚠

✔	
1	If possible, purchase a vehicle with side head airbags.
2	If possible, purchase a larger vehicle.
3	Run a data search on your current vehicle.

1. IF POSSIBLE, PURCHASE A VEHICLE WITH SIDE HEAD AIRBAGS.

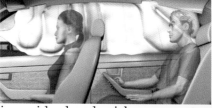

Many vehicles today are equipped with the side head airbags, which, according to statistics of the National Highway Traffic Safety Administration, greatly reduces the occurrence of serious injury and death. For further information regarding side head airbags, go to www.nhtsa.dot.gov/people/injury/airbags/airbags03page9.html.

2. IF POSSIBLE, PURCHASE A LARGER VEHICLE.

As noted in the "Statistics Tell the Story" section. when the Insurance Institute for Highway Safety ran side impact analysis, they found that 14 of 16 small cars were rated poor. (www.iihs.org)

3. RUN A DATA SEARCH ON YOUR CURRENT VEHICLE.

Both the NHTSA and the IIHS contain on their Web site detailed analysis of side impact safety on various vehicles.

A special thanks goes to the courageous leadership of Brian O'Neill of the Insurance Institute of America, Joan Claybrook and Ralph Nader of Public Citizen, the leadership of the American Automobile Association and the staff of Consumer Reports. Together, these groups provide valuable information necessary for consumers to understand the degree of safety, or lack thereof, for their children.

Buying a Car for a Teenager

The first three recommendations found in the "General" checklist on page 270 apply to buying a car for a teenager.

1. Follow the recommendations of the Insurance Institute for Highway Safety.
2. Review all available government Web sites.
3. Make Consumer Reports your friend.

Please read the narrative sections of these recommendations for further detail. Also, apply the fourth recommendation on the **ROLLOVER** checklist on page 275: *"If possible, purchase a vehicle with an Electronic Stabilizing Control,"* and read the narrative for explanation. Finally, use recommendation No. 1 on the **SIDE IMPACT COLLISION** checklist, page 277: *"If possible, purchase a vehicle with side air bags,"* and read the narrative instruction that follows.

In addition to the previously made recommendations, two specific recommendations apply to buying a car for a teenager:

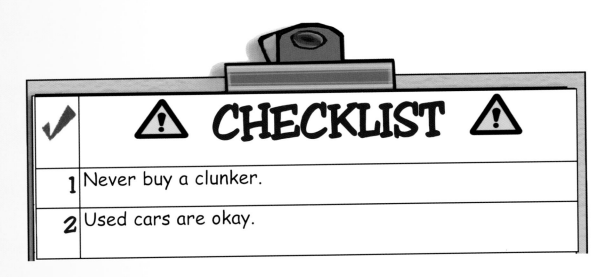

✔	⚠ CHECKLIST ⚠
1	Never buy a clunker.
2	Used cars are okay.

1. NEVER BUY A CLUNKER.

Cost is often an issue with buying a teenager a car, and there is an inclination to get a clunker. Clunkers are most often the worst safety vehicles on the highway. They do not have any of the modern safety technology and are prone to break down on the highway. Your child's life is too important to entrust it in an unsafe clunker. Better to save up for a good car than to purchase an unsafe one.

2. USED CARS ARE OKAY.

Often, parents believe that only a new car is a safe car. However, this is not always true. Even the highly safety-conscious Consumer Reports (www.consumersreports.org) recommends buying a used car for a number of reasons: Late model vehicles are often better values and just as safe as or safer than many new vehicles. Obviously, used vehicles have a lower purchase price and often lower insurance rates. Also with the cost savings, you can obtain a safer car if you shop carefully..

Consumer Reports has two valuable used vehicle lists: "Reliable" and "Used cars to avoid." As noted previously in this text, to obtain specific vehicle recommendations, you must be a Consumer Reports subscriber. (Currently the price is $26 a year, or you can subscribe to the monthly online service of $4.95 per month, which can be cancelled at any time.)

Both the "Reliable" and the "Used cars to avoid" lists have price categories beginning below $4,000 and increasing in $2,000 increments (i.e., $4,000 to $6,000; $6,000 to $8,000; $8,000 to $10,000). Each of these categories has between four to 15 specific models listed under each. These lists can be a lifesaver. Use them.

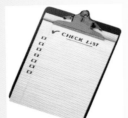

The following checklist should be used to prevent deaths and serious injuries from **BACKING MANEUVERS**:

✔	⚠ CHECKLIST ⚠
1	Visualize...walk around.
2	If possible, equip with rear camera.
3	Sensors have problems.

1. VISUALIZE...WALK AROUND.

Seventeen small children can be positioned behind an average minivan and be outside the view of the driver. The average vehicle has a 12-foot blind spot, an SUV or minivan 15-feet and a pick-up truck 30-feet, according to **www.comsumerreports.org**. With a shorter driver, the blind zone increases to 17 feet with an average vehicle, 24 feet with a SUV or minivan and 51 feet with a pick-up track. **THERE IS NO SUBSTITUTE FOR WALKING AROUND AND SEEING FOR YOURSELF**.

2. IF POSSIBLE EQUIP WITH REAR CAMERA.

Currently, eight vehicles have the camera as standard equipment, and 17 vehicles offer it as optional equipment.

3. SENSORS HAVE PROBLEMS.

Once believed to be the answer to the backing death and injury epidemic, the Web site **www.consumerreports.org** documented that after extensive testing, the sensors sounded too late for action and often failed to detect small objects such as a child on a tricycle.

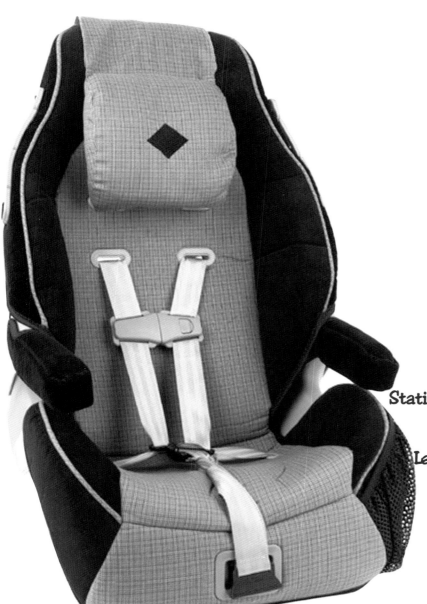

28

Car Safety Seats

281

Safety Seat Kills Child

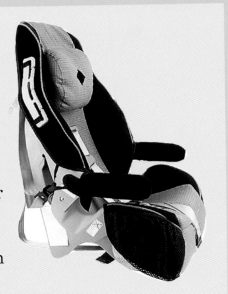

Delilah, age two and a half, had outgrown her rear-facing child car seat. So her parents, Paul and Sandra, went to the local department store to buy another car seat. There were prominent displays in the aisle next to the children's car seats, placed there by one of the nation's largest manufacturers of children car seats, proclaiming the safety of its new shield booster seat. The seat had a plastic shield around the torso portion of the front-facing car seat.

Paul and Sandra did not know at the time they purchased this new car seat that, since 1987, 40 children have died or were seriously injured by the same or similar shield booster seat manufactured by this company. Nor did they know that, in 1983, Canada had completely outlawed the shield booster configuration as being unsafe for children. And they had no way of knowing that Australia had always prohibited the sale of these types of seats.

They left the store believing that they had a safe product that would protect their child. It was only two months later that they realized the car seat's danger, when they were involved in a serious car collision caused by the other driver, so severe that it broke both of Paul's legs and sadly killed young Delilah.

The parents could not understand why a device that was intended to protect their child had, in fact, killed her.

Unfortunately, the reckless history of this manufacturer's conduct was well-known to my law firm when the parents called for help. I informed them at our first conference that we had handled several of these cases and could not understand why the federal government had not stopped the manufacture of this dangerous product. Although virtually every country has banned the shield booster seat and every reputable child safety group in the United

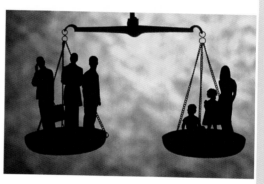

LEGAL ACTION and OUTCOME

States blasted the unsafe design of this car seat, it was not until 2003 that the U.S. government banned the design. Thus, there was a mountain of evidence supporting the fault of this major company. Sadly, the company was well familiar with the litigation we were about to file and invited a pre-lawsuit mediation. We had already hired a biomechanical engineer to analyze the force of the trauma to the child as well as a noted car/child safety designer. Both experts attended the two day mediation. The case was concluded to the satisfaction of the parents.

Statistics Tell the Story

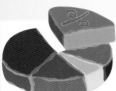

⇨ Since the campaign to remove all children from the front seat began in 1996, at least 200 child lives have been saved EACH year. (*Journal of Safety Research, August 2005*)

⇨ Motor vehicle crashes are the leading cause of death for children ages two to 14, according to the National Highway Traffic Safety Administration Fatality Review Fact Sheet, 2002. (www.nhtsa.dot.gov)

⇨ Nearly half the 774 children ages four to seven who died in car crashes from 1999 to 2003 were not restrained, according to the National Highway Traffic Safety Administration.

⇨ Children passenger restraints save lives. Child safety seats reduce risk of death by 71 percent for infants (less than one year-old) and by 54 percent for toddlers (one to four years old) in passenger cars, according to NHTSA.

⇨ More than 81 percent of child restraints are used incorrectly, including 88 percent of forward-facing toddler seats, 86 percent of rear-facing infant seats, and 85 percent of safety belts, as determined by Child Passenger Seat Inspection Stations across the country, according to a study done by the National SAFE KIDS Campaign. (National SAFE KIDS Campaign. February 2002. *Child Passengers at Risk in America: A National Study of Restraint Use.*)

⇨ A third of children (33 percent) ages 14 and under ride in the wrong restraint-type for their age and size, according to the the National SAFE KIDS Campaign survey.

SPECIFIC BOOSTER SEAT STATISTICS

⇨ Children ages four to seven who use booster seats are 59 percent less likely to be injured in a crash than children who were restrained only by safety belt, according to the *Journal of American Medical Association* (*JAMA Study of June 2003, "Belt Positioning Booster Seats and Reduction in Risk of Injury Among Children in Car Crashes"*).

⇨ A recent study also found that only a few children who should be riding in booster seats are doing so, according to the study conducted by the National Highway Traffic Safety Administration (NHTSA). Nearly 21 percent of children ages four to eight are "at least on occasion," riding in a booster seat while traveling in passenger vehicles. Another 19 percent of children in this age range were restrained "at least on occasion" in a front-facing child safety seat.

⇨ According to the Children's Hospital of Philadelphia (CHOPS), booster seats reduce the risk of serious crash injuries to children ages four to eight by about 60%. The hospital, along with State Farm Insurance, has long advocated the mandatory use of booster seats.

Laws and Regulations

In 49 states, including the District of Columbia, there are mandatory seat belt laws. New Hampshire is the only state that does not have such legislation. Sadly, in 31 states, the law only applies to occupants of the front seat. The following 18 states do require back seat occupants to wear seat belts as well: Alaska, California, Delaware, District of Columbia, Idaho, Kentucky, Maine, Massachusetts, Montana, Nevada, New Mexico, New York, Oregon, Rhode Island, Utah, Vermont, Washington and Wyoming.

Every state, including the District of Columbia, has some form of child restraint laws; however, the age and type of restraint mandated varies greatly from state to state. Child restraint laws are standard for all children covered except in Colorado, Nebraska and Pennsylvania. In Colorado, the law is secondary only for children ages four and five years who must be kept in booster seats. Nebraska's law is secondary only for those children who may be in safety belts and standard for those who must be in a child restraint device. In Pennsylvania, the law is secondary only for children ages four to seven who must be kept in booster seats.

The responsibility to abide by these laws also differs from state to state. In most states, the law applies to any driver of a vehicle wherein a child is an occupant. However, there are five states where the law only applies to parents or guardians, children of residence or children in vehicles registered in those states: Alabama, Illinois, Indiana, Iowa and Louisiana.

BOOSTER SEATS LAWS:

In April of 2005, New York became the 27th state, including the District of Columbia, to require booster seats for children four to six. Seven states and the District have laws that require booster seats until kids turn eight; Tennessee and Wyoming require them until age nine. Several other states also have height or weight requirements that could force slightly built, older children to continue using booster seats.

Further, in 2005, tougher standards for booster seats went into effect. At the same time, lap and shoulder belts are required for the center rear seats of new vehicles so that booster seats can be properly and more easily secured. The new laws are named for Anton Skeen, and referred to as "Anton's Law." He was a four-and-a-half-year-old who died in Washington State due to a faulty restraint system. Courageously, his parents, Autumn and Tom, fought for tougher standards for booster seats.

Taking Action

As with the previous chapter on auto design, because of the enormity of the subject matter, we will employ a number of general checklists:

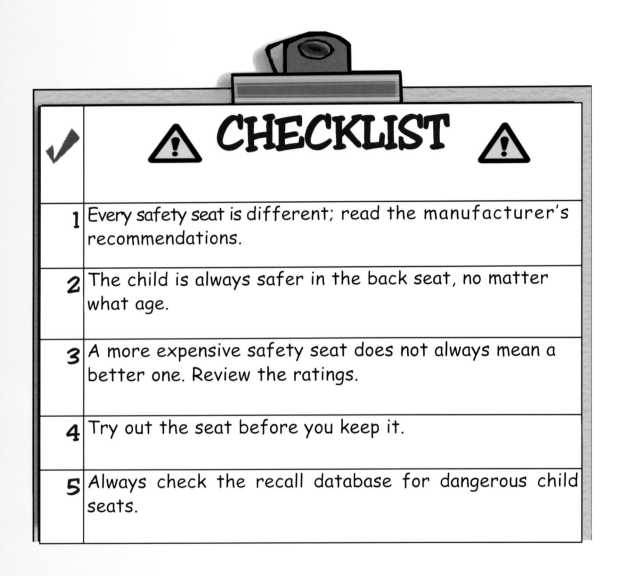

⚠ CHECKLIST ⚠

1	Every safety seat is different; read the manufacturer's recommendations.
2	The child is always safer in the back seat, no matter what age.
3	A more expensive safety seat does not always mean a better one. Review the ratings.
4	Try out the seat before you keep it.
5	Always check the recall database for dangerous child seats.

1. EVERY SAFETY SEAT IS DIFFERENT; READ THE MANUFACTURER'S RECOMMENDATIONS.

Be aware that outside box instructions may differ from those inside the box. Read the fine print, it's important.

2. THE CHILD IS ALWAYS SAFER IN THE BACK SEAT, NO MATTER WHAT AGE.

According to Consumer Reports (CR), when possible, position the car seat in the center of the back seat, the safest place in a vehicle, even if that means attaching the car seat with the car safety belt and not the LATCH system.

3. A MORE EXPENSIVE SAFETY SEAT DOES NOT ALWAYS MEAN A BETTER ONE. REVIEW THE RATINGS.

The Consumer Reports organization (**www.consumerreports.org**) conducts the most rigorous safety testing of any organization including the Federal Government; therefore, always get their rating of the seat before purchase. As for price, in May of 2005, CR found that the best convertible seat was $70, and the number two recommended seat was $200; clearly price doesn't always assure a safer seat.

Further, the CR testing in 2005 found serious problems with many very popular car seats. All seats come with a maximum weight-bearing limit. But when CR crash-tested rear-facing car seats at manufacturers' claimed weight limits, several had significant problems.

The attachment broke on the **Combi Avatar convertible seat**, sending it flying off the test rig, at a crash speed lower than that which the government requires car seats to withstand. Thus, CR rated the Combi Avatar as "Not Acceptable" and urged the manufacturer to fix the problem.

The **Evenflo PortAbout 5** infant seat flew off its base at a crash speed just above the federal standard, a margin of safety that is too small, in the judgment of CR. Thus, they rated it poor for crash protection. These are only several examples of the detailed work provided by CR.

4. TRY OUT THE SEAT BEFORE YOU KEEP IT.

The choice of a car safety seat is too important. Try it out: Practice installing the seat. If anything doesn't work or is difficult to work...return the seat and get a better seat.

5. ALWAYS CHECK THE RECALL DATABASE FOR DANGEROUS CHILD SEATS

As we have noted many times in this text, just because a product has been recalled does not mean that it is off the shelves in some retail store, on eBay or given to you as a gift by an unsuspecting friend or relative. Of all the recalled products, child safety seats are some of the most frequent recalls. ALWAYS, ALWAYS check the NHTSA Web site (**www-odi.nhtsa.dot.gov/cars/problems/recalls/childseat.cfm**) for recalls. The recall database goes back to 1990 and also contains information concerning ongoing investigations. Also, to subscribers of Consumer Reports, there is also a database of recalled children car seats (**www.consumerreports.org/cro/consumer-protection/recalls/car-seats.htm**).

Let us now turn our attention to the Checklists for the six types of children's car seats. The following checklists were derived from the NHTSA, (www.nhtsa.dot.gov/CPS/safetycheck/typeseats/index.htm):

REAR FACING SEATS (use with children up to one year old and who weigh less than 20 lbs)

Use the following checklist for safe use:

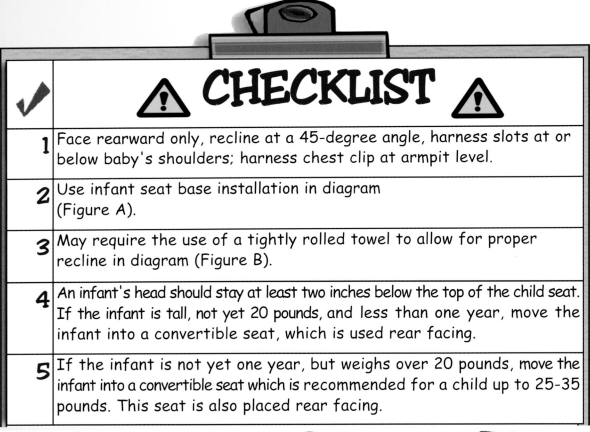

✔ ⚠ CHECKLIST ⚠

1	Face rearward only, recline at a 45-degree angle, harness slots at or below baby's shoulders; harness chest clip at armpit level.
2	Use infant seat base installation in diagram (Figure A).
3	May require the use of a tightly rolled towel to allow for proper recline in diagram (Figure B).
4	An infant's head should stay at least two inches below the top of the child seat. If the infant is tall, not yet 20 pounds, and less than one year, move the infant into a convertible seat, which is used rear facing.
5	If the infant is not yet one year, but weighs over 20 pounds, move the infant into a convertible seat which is recommended for a child up to 25-35 pounds. This seat is also placed rear facing.

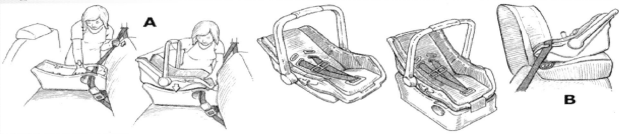

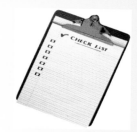

CONVERTIBLE SEATS: Rear Facing

(Birth to 40 lbs)
Use the following checklist for safe use:

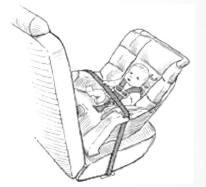

⚠️ CHECKLIST ⚠️

✓	
1	All are recommended for use by infants less than one year and up to about 20 pounds.
2	Some are recommended for use by infants less than one year who are heavier than 20 pounds (30-35 pounds).
3	Harness straps should be at or below infant's shoulders when used rear facing.
4	Harness chest clip should be at infant's armpit level.

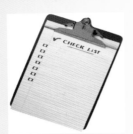

CONVERTIBLE SEATS: Facing Forward

Use the following checklist for safe use:

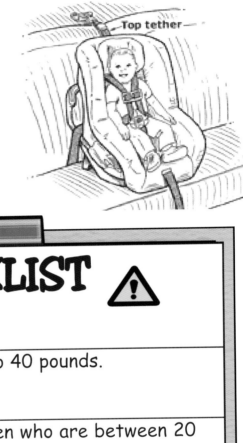

Top tether

✓ ⚠ CHECKLIST ⚠

✓	
1	All are rated for children up to 40 pounds.
2	Used forward facing by children who are between 20 and 40 pounds, and over one year.
3	Harness straps should be at or above child's shoulders. Use top harness slots of safety seat.

FORWARD FACING SEATS (Children 20 to 40 lbs...some up to 60)

Use the following checklist for safe use:

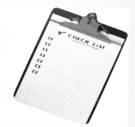

⚠️ CHECKLIST ⚠️

✔		
1	Harness straps should be at or above child's shoulders.	
2	Harness chest clip should be at armpit level.	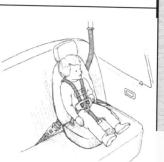

Additional Information:

The Lower Anchors and Tethers for Children (LATCH) System is designed to make installation of child safety seats easier by requiring child safety seats to be installed without using the

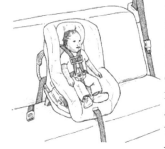

vehicle's seat belt system. As of September of 1999, all new forward facing child safety seats (not including booster seats) have to meet stricter head protection requirements, which call for a top tether strap. This adjustable strap is attached to the back of a child safety seat. It has a hook for securing the seat to a tether anchor found either on the rear shelf area of the vehicle or, in the case of mini-vans and station wagons, on the rear floor or the on the back of the rear seat of the vehicle. As of September of 2000, all new cars, minivans, and light trucks have this tether anchor.

As of September 1, 2002, two rear seating positions of all cars, minivans and light trucks come equipped with lower child safety seat anchorage points, located between a vehicle's seat cushion and seat back. Also, all child safety seats now have two attachments which will connect to the vehicle's lower anchorage attachment points. Together, the lower anchors and upper tethers make up the LATCH system.

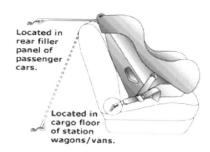

Located in rear filler panel of passenger cars.

Located in cargo floor of station wagons/vans.

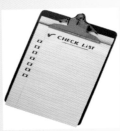

High-Back Booster with 5-Point Harness:

Forward Facing (20 to 40 lbs)

Use the following checklist for safe use:

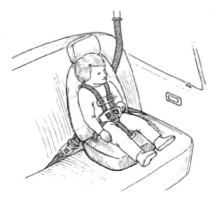

✔	⚠ CHECKLIST ⚠
1	Harness straps should be at or above child's shoulders.
2	Harness chest clip should be at child's armpit level.
3	Remove harness when child reaches 40 pounds and use the vehicle's adult lap and shoulder belt across child (belt-positioning booster).

All diagrams courtesy of the U.S. Department of Transportation National Highway Traffic Safety Administration

Belt Positioning Booster Seats:

FORWARD FACING ONLY

A belt-positioning booster seat should be used until the child can sit with his/her back against the vehicle seat with knees bent over the seat cushion edge, and feet on the floor, approximately four feet nine inches.

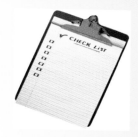

Use the following checklist for safe use:

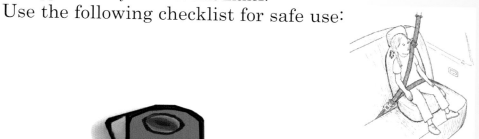

✔	⚠ CHECKLIST ⚠
1	All children who have outgrown child safety seats should be properly restrained in booster seats until they are at least eight years old, unless they are over four feet nine inches tall.
2	Can only be used with the adult lap and shoulder belt. **Never with a lap belt only.**
3	Provides the child a higher sitting height, which allows the adult lap and shoulder belt to fit properly.
4	The shoulder belt should cross the chest, resting snugly on the shoulder, and the lap belt should rest low across the upper thighs, never up high across the stomach.
5	Styles include high-back, no back, and base only. A high-back booster provides head support not provided by vehicle seats with low backs or no head restraints.
6	A belt-positioning booster seat should be used until the child can sit with his/her back against the vehicle seat back cushion with knees bent over the seat cushion edge, and feet on the floor, approximately four feet nine inches tall.
7	The mid-point of the back of the child's head (ear level) should not be above the vehicle seat back cushion or the back of the high back booster.

FREQUENTLY ASKED QUESTIONS

Q *Can I use a car safety seat after it was involved in a crash?*

A If the crash was moderate or severe, the seat needs to be replaced. If the crash was minor, it does not necessarily need to be replaced; however, if any of the following occurred, the crash was not minor:

    (a)   The air bags went off.

    (b)   The car could not be driven away from the crash.

    (c)   The vehicle door closest to the car safety seat was damaged.

Q *What about using a used car safety seat?*

A First, make sure the car safety seat was not recalled. Call the Auto Safety Hotline, (888) 327- 4236, or go to the www.nhtsa.dot.gov Web site, which has a complete list of recalls. Even if it is not a recalled safety seat, do not use if it has any cracks or breaks on the frame or seat, does not come with instructions, has any missing parts, or simply looks too old.

Q *What if my child has special healthcare needs?*

A Many states have special programs for special needs children. That information can be obtained by calling the Automotive Safety Program at (317) 274- 2977, by visiting their Web site at www.preventinjury.org, or by calling Easter Seals at (800) 221-6827.

Q *What if my baby weighs more than 20 pounds but is not one year of age yet?*

A Many babies reach 20 pounds well before their first birthday. However, just because your baby weighs more than 20 pounds does not make the child ready to ride face forward. Use a convertible seat that can be used rear-facing for children greater than 20 pounds.

Q *What if my baby is premature?*

A Use a car safety seat without a shield harness. Shields are often too high and too far from the body to fit correctly. A smaller child could hit a shield in a crash.

The above answers came from the American Academy of Pediatrics' Web site at www.aap.org/family/carseatguide.htm.

SPECIAL THANKS:

The Consumer Reports organization should be highly congratulated for their vigorous testing and call for tougher standards (www.consumerreports.org). Further, Public Citizen (www.citizen.org), the group founded by Ralph Nader and operated by former National Highway Traffic Safety Administration chairwoman, Joan Claybrook, should likewise be commended for their vigorous push for safer regulations. Additionally, the CP Safety organization, a non-profit organization dedicated to safely transporting children, should also be congratulated for their efforts.(www.cpsafety.com) Finally special thanks to Joe Burton, M.D, former medical examiner for DeKalb County, Georgia who has conducted pioneering research in the understanding of how injuries and deaths from defective car seats can be prevented.

Power Windows

29

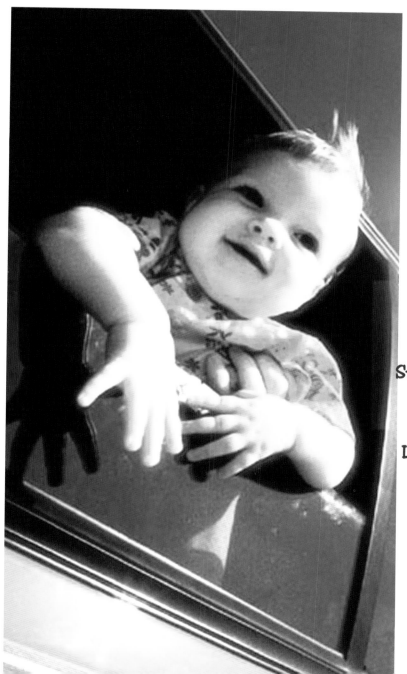

Unthinkable Tragedy

Phil jumped into his late-model automobile to pick up his son, Alan, from football practice at the high school. Holly, his three-year-old daughter, begged to come along. She loved her daddy and also had a very special relationship with her older brother. Holly loved to see Alan all dressed up in his football uniform.

The evening air was a little chilly when they arrived at the practice field, so Phil told Holly to stay in the vehicle, where she'd be warmer. As practice ended, Alan headed off the field to the locker room for a shower, waving to his baby sister on the way. Phil walked 10 yards from his vehicle to chat with the coach. To keep Holly from getting cold, he left the car on, but placed it in the parking position with the parking brake on.

Phil finished his five-minute conversation with the coach and returned to the car. Shockingly, he saw Holly's head lodged outside the window, with the window in the up position, trapping her neck. He ran as fast as he could to his daughter and lowered the window. Holly was lifeless. The EMTs arrived in an instant. At the hospital, the emergency room doctors did all they could, but Holly was gone.

LEGAL ACTION and OUTCOME

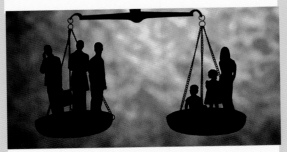

I was hired by Holly's family to determine if this terrible tragedy had been preventable. First we hired a human-factors expert, who reenacted Holly's death. The expert told us that Holly had lowered the window when she saw her brother; Alan had told him that he remembered Holly's bulky winter jacket and hood as she waved at him through the window. The expert believed that Holly was bringing herself back in the car when her foot activated the power-window switch, accidentally sending it up and then pinning her neck, causing her strangulation. Most power-window motors produce 50 to 80 pounds of force, although only eight to 10 pounds of force are needed to lift the window. The testing of Phil's vehicle indicated it had used 65 pounds.

The second expert we hired was a safety design engineer, who told us that Holly's death at the hands of a power window was not the first such death. Virtually all U. S. auto manufacturers use a rocker or toggle switch for their power windows. The opposite is true for foreign manufacturers, who do not use the rocker or toggle switch, but rather a push up/push down switch. The expert told us that the American method makes it far easier for a child to unintentionally or intentionally activate the switch. Additionally, the expert later testified that even if the manufacturer wanted to use the toggle switch, it could be made safe by installing an auto-reverse device along with it. This device could have prevented Holly's death, because the window would have stopped when it came in contact with her neck.

For several years, the auto manufacturer vigorously defended the claim we filed. The company argued primarily that it was doing exactly what all of the other American manufacturers were doing. As parents, how often have we heard our child proclaim, "All the other kids do it, why can't I ?" For the same reason the child's excuse fails, so should the outrageous excuse of the American auto industry.

After several failed mediations, the case was eventually settled. The company knew that the evidence regarding the safer practice used by the European auto manufacturers would be admissible before the jury. They also knew that the jury would learn how they had chosen not to use a different switch, despite company knowledge of deaths due to toggle switches like the one they had chosen.

Although the case was concluded satisfactorily for Holly's family, there has been little change in the U.S. auto industry on the issue of dangerous power windows.

Statistics Tell the Story

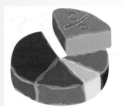

According to Kids and Cars executive director Janette Fennell, there have been 43 child deaths due to entrapments and strangulations from automobile power windows (www.kidsandcars.org). In June 2004, the group released details of the following occurrences:

On June 6, 2004, a Dallas woman stopped her 2001 Ford pickup and was talking to her husband through the driver's side window, according to press reports. Without the woman's knowledge, her three-year-old daughter had leaned out of the passenger's side window, and her knee or foot hit the rocker switch, causing the window to close on her neck. The mother noticed after a few moments, but the girl died from strangulation.

On June 3, 2004, in Walworth County, Wisconsin, a mother left her four-year-old son in her 1991 Lincoln Continental while she ran into the house of a friend. According to county police spokesman Captain Scott McCory, the boy leaned on the power switch and got his neck caught in the power window. He was dead when his mother returned to the car.

Another Wisconsin case occurred in April 2004 in Dane County. A mother left four children, ages two to six, in a 1996 Mercury Sable while she applied for a job at a golf resort. According to Captain Tanya Molony, the car was off, but the key was in the accessory position so the radio could play. The two-year-old child worked the window controls and caused the six-year-old to get his neck caught in a rear window. The children eventually lowered the window, but when the mother returned to the car, in less than 15 minutes, the boy was not breathing. He was later pronounced dead.

Ford spokeswoman Kristen Kinley says the company intends to replace all switches with the lift-up type, but that the change will take time. The company is also considering putting bounce-back windows on more models. But ultimately, Kinley says, "there's only so much automakers can do to prevent these tragedies. At some point, the parents have a responsibility to make sure children are supervised."

But even if parents are present, they cannot always prevent such accidents from happening.

In June 2003, Becky Hergatt pulled into her driveway in Mansfield, Ohio and rolled up the windows on her 1992 Buick because rain seemed imminent. She and her teenage daughter got out of the front seat and walked toward the house. Becky's daughter looked back at the car and screamed. Her five-year-old brother, Mac, was 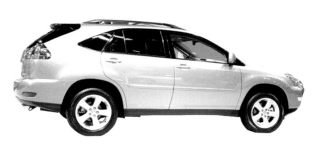 hanging from the car's rear window, his neck caught between the glass and the doorframe. "He was blue and limp," Hergatt said. Her daughter lowered the window and Becky, a registered nurse, performed mouth-to-mouth resuscitation. In three breaths, the boy was revived.

In 1968, Ralph Nader urged the National Highway Safety Board to issue public advisory warnings on the dangers posed to children by electric power windows in automobiles. Unfortunately, Nader's request was rejected.

Much credit and praise should be given to Janette Fennell and her group, www.kidsandcars.org, for their outstanding advocacy on this important issue.

Laws and Regulations

Once again, the government's response has been "too little, too late." In September of 2004, the Administrator of the U.S. Department of Transportation's National Highway Traffic Safety Administration (NHTSA) announced a regulatory upgrade to enhance the safety of power window switches and, according to the agency, prevent child deaths and injuries caused by the inadvertent closing of car windows. Unfortunately, the new regulation does not go far enough.

To understand why, one must understand the ways a child can get injured or die as the result of a power window. The dangerous activation of the power window switch happens in three distinct ways: 1. When a child leans on or bumps against a rocker or toggle switch; 2. When a child plays with a power switch, pushing or pulling up on the switch; or 3. When adults unintentionally close a power window on a child. The new NHTSA upgrade minimally addresses only the first situation, in which the switch is accidentally activated. It will not prevent all accidental or unintentional power window closings that cause serious injuries or deaths. In fact, only power window auto-reverse systems can put an end to these tragic deaths and injuries.

Sadly, NHTSA's rule does not require automatic reverse technology for all new passenger vehicles. Automatic reverse technology stops a power window from closing when a child is in harm's way. This requirement should be standard, just like the federal government's mandated safety requirement on all garage doors that close automatically-they must reverse to prevent deaths and injuries.

IMPORTANT:

Power window auto-reverse technology is included as standard equipment on 80% of European and many Japanese vehicles.

Unfortunately, this is a hazard where the only thing that can be provided is information, so please consider the following checklist:

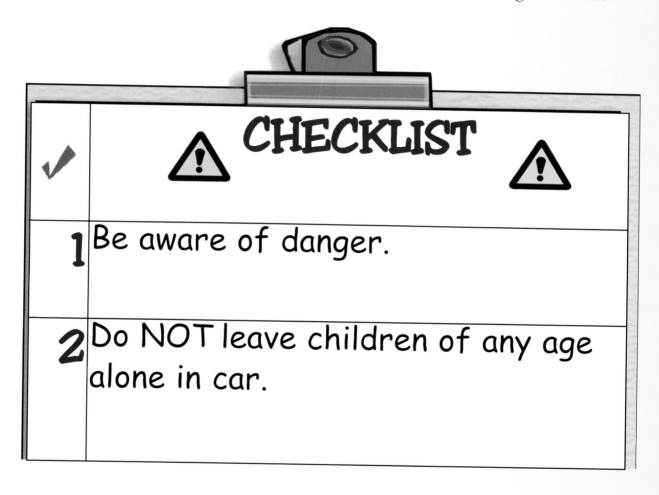

CHECKLIST

✔	
1	Be aware of danger.
2	Do NOT leave children of any age alone in car.

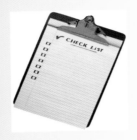

1. BE AWARE OF DANGER.

We obviously cannot advocate not buying American automobiles. But as we have pointed out, your chances of buying a foreign car with a power window safety feature are far greater than those of buying an American-made automobile with safe power windows. The only way to be sure is to ask before purchasing, regardless of where the car was made. And check out for yourself how the power windows work in the vehicle you are considering.

If you do not believe the danger, simply take a foam pillow and put it at the top of the power window encasing, and watch the window pierce the pillow. Then repeat the procedure with a small board and see for yourself how much power there is in the window.

2. DO NOT LEAVE CHILDREN OF ANY AGE ALONE IN A CAR.

There are many reports of children who are 15, 16 and 17 years old dying the same way that Holly did, so it is not accurate to say that the danger pertains only to small children.

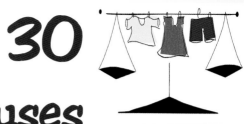

30

School Buses

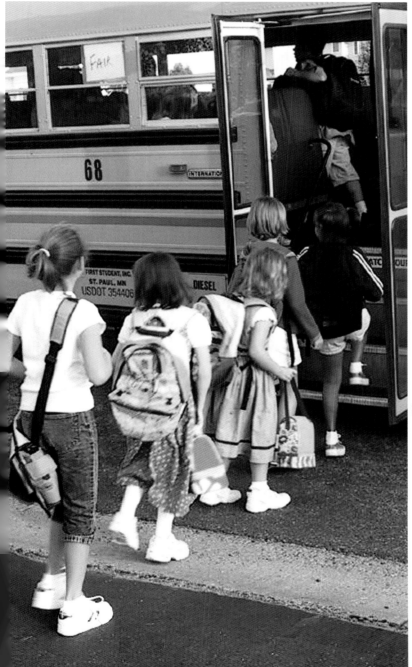

Incompetent Driver Transports Children

Jonas and Carolyn received the call from the emergency room saying that their oldest girl, Caroline, was involved in a tragic accident. The parents sped to the hospital, where they were informed that the school bus Caroline had been riding left the road and crashed into a tree. All the test results were not yet back, but it was already clear that Caroline had suffered head trauma and severe internal injuries.

For two weeks, Caroline labored in and out of consciousness in the hospital's intensive care unit. Her spleen was removed and emergency surgery was performed on her stomach because of a rupture. She also sustained a broken arm and a broken foot.

Two years later, the child still felt the effects of the injury. While she is fortunate not to have sustained permanent brain damage, Caroline will have disfigurement and a permanent loss of range of motion in her arm and leg for life.

Slowly but surely, the facts of the accident emerged. The bus driver recounted a phantom vehicle traveling head-on at the bus. She swerved to miss the vehicle and lost control of the bus, careening off the road and striking the tree broadside, she said.

None of the children, nor either of the two eyewitnesses, saw the phantom car. Both witnesses, one who was traveling toward the bus, the other who was traveling behind it, stopped when they saw the school bus leave the road. Thanks to their quick action and heroic efforts, children's lives were saved.

LEGAL ACTION
and
OUTCOME

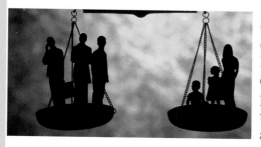

Because of the suspicious nature of the accident, I was asked by the family to file a lawsuit to obtain the truth under oath. We soon discovered that while the driver had a clean driving record at the time of her hiring five years before, no checks were done after her hiring. If checks had been performed, they would have revealed two reckless driving charges and one damage to personal property charge when the bus driver, using her personal car, left the roadway and hit two mailboxes and a gate.

We also discovered that the bus driver had been undergoing psychiatric counseling for depression and was on mega-dosages of anti-depressant medications. None of these facts were known to the school district. Although a random urine test procedure was in place, this driver had never been tested during her five-year employment.

Suspicions were also raised about the bus. In researching five prior bus accidents, we learned that all of the injured children had struck a metal reinforcement that was located on the backs of all the seats. This reinforcement was, in fact, precisely what Caroline's head and arm hit on impact. Because the bus company knew of the problem and did nothing to correct it, they were included in the lawsuit.

Ultimately, the case was concluded satisfactorily for the family. The school board vowed to conduct annual checks of the driving records of their drivers and to enforce their drug policy. In addition, all new models of the bus have been changed to eliminate the point-of-impact problem.

Statistics Tell the Story

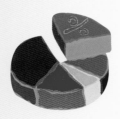

According to the latest statistics by the National Highway Traffic Safety Administration (NHTSA) (www.nhtsa.dot.gov), since 1993, 191 school-aged pedestrian children have died in school transportation-related crashes. Nearly two-thirds (65 percent) were killed by school buses, four percent by vehicles functioning as school buses and 31 percent by other vehicles. More than one-half (51 percent) of all school-age pedestrians killed in school transportation-related crashes are between ages five and seven.

An average of 22 school-age children die in school transportation-related traffic crashes each year: six are occupants of school transportation vehicles and 16 are pedestrians.

In 2005, the nation learned of the death of Lilibeth Gomez and Harrison Orosco, third-graders in Arlington, Virginia. The new school bus they were riding was broadsided by another vehicle, causing their deaths. The bus had no seat belts. Experts believe both deaths would have been prevented if seat belts were installed.

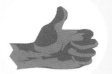

General

Statistically, school buses are the safest form of transportation, according to The National Coalition for School Bus Safety (www.ncsbs.org).

Modern school buses, including those manufactured after April 1, 1977, are equipped with more safety equipment than any other vehicle on the road, according to the School Bus Information Council (www.schoolbusinfo.org). In addition to safety features, the size of the school bus alone gives it an important advantage in all but the most catastrophic circumstances.

There are two sets of regulations issued under different Acts of Congress that relate to the safety of school buses. The first of these is the Motor Vehicle Safety Standards, issued by the National Highway Traffic Safety Administration under Public Act 1966. The NHTSA also administers recommended guidelines for the use of state highway safety funds, referred to as Section 402 funds, mandating certain safety criteria for state and county operated school buses.

Seat Belts

The effectiveness of safety belts on school buses has been an issue of much research and discussion since the mid 1980s. While volumes have been written on the subject, the bottom line is that the National Highway Traffic Safety Administration has not required the use of safety belts. While many reasons have been given, safety groups remain outraged. The government has been defensive about its position, and has launched several public relations campaigns to explain their views. Consumer groups contend that children are being sent a mixed message: "Wear seat belts in cars, but you don't need seat belts on school buses." Consumer groups fear a "carry over" effect that will cause children to not wear seat belts in cars. The NHTSA has even challenged the "carry over" arguments in DOT Report 806 965. Consumer groups have common sense on their side: if only one child's life is saved by seat belts on buses, then seat belts should be required.

Doctor Alan Ross of The National Coalition for School Bus Safety, (www.ncsbs.org), is the most vigorous advocate for seat belts on all school buses. He has challenged the testing done by the NTSB as seriously flawed. His advocacy at the grass roots level has caused over 300 communities over the last year to add seats belts to their school buses. Many thanks go to Alan and the NCSBS.

Interestingly, safety belts are required for pre-school age children. Contrary to their decision about safety belts not being required for school-age children, the government has mandated that safety belts are mandatory for pre-school age children. See the report and standards issued February of 1999 by NHTSA at www.nhtsa.dot.gov/people/injury/enforce/protectingchildren/protecting%20children.pdf.

Van use requires seat belts. Because vans (under 10,000 pounds gross weight) are much smaller than school buses, the government requires belting in these vehicles.

Charter Buses

Charter buses are different. Many children are transported on charter buses, to away football games and school outings, for example. From time to time, charter companies are also used to fill in for the traditional school bus system. These companies are regulated by a different agency, the Federal Motor Carrier Safety Administration (FMCSA)(www.fmcsa.dot.gov). According to a *Fox News* report on WAGA in October of 2004, a recent study found that only 47 percent of charter bus companies had a satisfactory rating. More alarming, only two percent of the 600,000 charter companies actually undergo safety inspections. The Atlanta news station reported that one local charter company had not been inspected in eight years. After a serious accident, it was revealed that the driver did not have a license to drive a school bus, although the company was accepting school charter assignments. School officials, who received their information from the news reporter, were shocked.

The following checklist should be employed to supervise the safe transportation of children:

⚠️ CHECKLIST ⚠️

✔	
1	Get to know the driver.
2	Know the specific driver-screening and audit system.
3	Know the specific drop off neighborhoods on the route and key people in the neighborhoods.
4	Make sure all pre-school children have seat belts.
5	Make sure all vans have seat belts.
6	Urge your school to modernize buses.
7	Check out the safety of any charter bus services used.

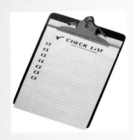

1. GET TO KNOW THE DRIVER.

The gut feeling you have about a driver is quite important. Is he or she reliable? Do you notice any abnormal behavior? What type of conduct and behavior does your child report? All of these are important in assessing the fitness of the driver. After all, the driver has your child's life in his or her hands during critical times, and the slightest inference of irregularity should require further investigation.

2. KNOW THE SPECIFIC DRIVER-SCREENING AND AUDIT SYSTEM.

As we see from this chapter's case tragedy, it is important that a driver's record be checked periodically. Although the driver's record in our sample case was checked upon hiring, no subsequent checks were performed. Such a check would have revealed that the driver clearly was unfit to be driving a school bus.

3. KNOW THE SPECIFIC DROP OFF NEIGHBORHOODS ON THE ROUTE AND KEY PEOPLE IN THE NEIGHBORHOODS.

A number of reported cases indicate great danger of children being dropped off at the wrong stop. This happens more often than we want to believe. Plan for that mistake and know the drop-off neighborhoods as well as the key people in them. Most importantly, instruct your child what to do if he is dropped off at the wrong point; tell him or her to go to the key home or to seek out an adult and ask the adult to phone you immediately.

4. MAKE SURE ALL PRE-SCHOOL CHILDREN HAVE SEAT BELTS.

Federal law requires seat belts for pre-schoolers, but that does not guarantee automatic compliance. Many school bus administrators either do not know about this law or have chosen, for any number of reasons, to disregard it.

5. MAKE SURE ALL VANS HAVE SEAT BELTS.

Because of the increased dependency on van transportation, particularly in fast-growing school districts, seat belt compliance must be stressed. School bus safety records depend in large part upon the large size of the vehicle. This is not the case with vans; seat belt use is mandatory in vans.

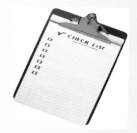

6. URGE YOUR SCHOOL TO MODERNIZE BUSES.

As with all areas of our life, technology brings safety advances. The following innovations in school bus design are worth noting:

a) Snub-Nose School Buses:

In the past, many children were hit by buses after exiting and walking around the front of them; the size of the engine hood kept the driver from seeing the children. New, snub-nose designs (see photo), however, keep children in full view of the bus driver after they exit the vehicle.

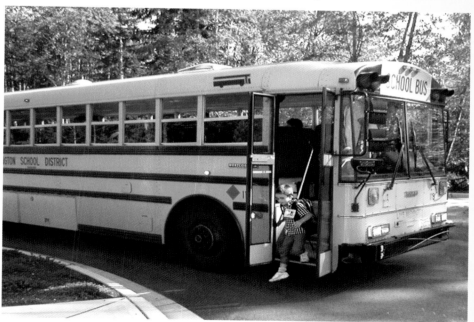

b) Gate Arm Extenders:

Modern buses have gate arms that are bigger and more visible and provide greater safety than the old arms.

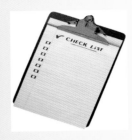

c) Video Cameras On Board:

Video cameras were initially installed primarily to record the conduct of children riding the bus as well as the bus driver. In the case of a school bully or bus driver acting inappropriately or unsafely, the video camera can act as an effective deterrent. It can also disclose after an event just how the circumstances developed. But the video camera has also come in quite handy in other, unintended ways. For example, I handled a case in which a child who was in his father's custody after a divorce disappeared after being dropped off at his bus stop. A study of the video showed a vehicle trailing the school bus and disappearing after the child exited the bus. When the father reviewed the tape, he quickly identified the vehicle as that of his ex-wife, who had a history of mental illness and was prohibited from visiting the child unsupervised. She had abducted the child and taken him to a local motel. An All Points Bulletin was put out for her vehicle, and the child was quickly and safely returned home to his father, while the mother was taken into custody.

d) Safety Belts:

While the Federal government does not mandate safety belts, we are convinced by the advocacy of Doctor Ross and his group. If seat belts save only one life, seats belts are worth the effort. Additionally we send a mixed message to children that they have to buckle up in every vehicle but a school bus. Let's not create confusion in the mind of an impressionable child.

7. CHECK OUT THE SAFETY OF ANY CHARTER BUS SERVICES USED.

As noted before, the Federal Motor Carriers Safety Administration (FMCSA) (www.fmcsa.dot.gov) regulates charter companies. Many school systems simply assume that the charter companies are safe and do no checking of their own. You must insist that someone check any charter bus services used and check them often.

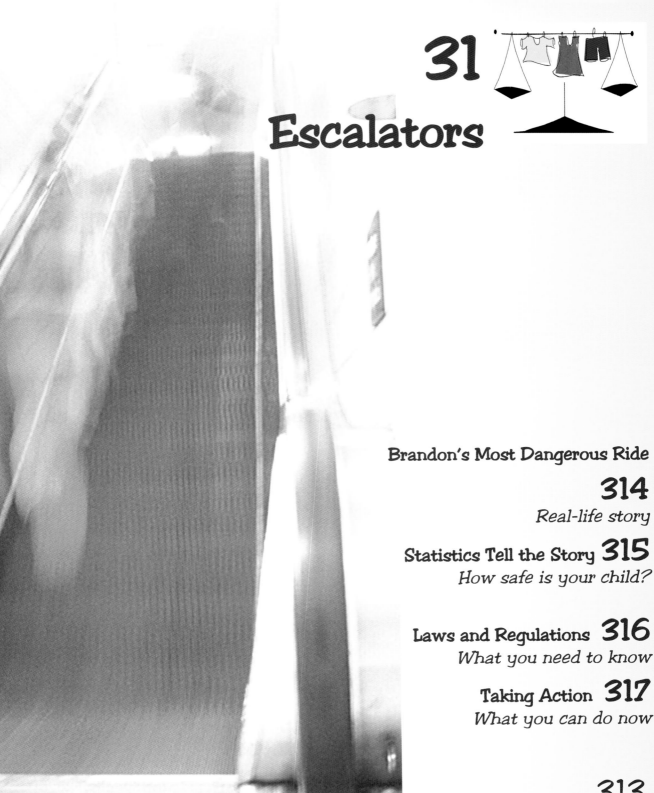

31

Escalators

Brandon's Most Dangerous Ride

Just back from a dream Disney World vacation, the Wallace family landed safely at the airport and proceeded up the nearly 80-step escalator to baggage claim. Eight-year-old Brandon excitedly ran several steps ahead of his parents and placed his knapsack on the stair ahead of him. As instructed, Brandon held tightly onto the moveable rail beside him. About to reach the top- half a dozen stairs from stepping off- Brandon let go of the railing to retrieve his knapsack. At that very instant, the escalator machinery buckled, jerking to a stop and then abruptly starting again. Brandon lost his balance and fell backwards on the escalator, the back of his head hit the jagged edge of the steps below him. Witnesses reported that Brandon instantly went lifeless.

The impact of Brandon's fall on the escalator caused a severe laceration and subdural hematoma- the medical term for the pressure that results from blood collecting in the space between the outer and middle layers of the brain. Surgeons worked in emergency mode to relieve the pressure in Brandon's head, but the impact had already caused irreversible brain damage.

LEGAL ACTION and OUTCOME

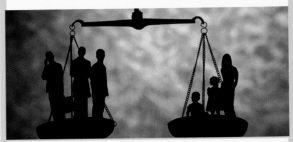

The Wallace family asked my law firm to investigate. We quickly discovered that two prior maintenance checks of the escalator had been missed. We also discovered that, despite receiving multiple complaints from airport passengers about the buckling of the escalator, no steps were taken to fix the problem. In an effort to help with Brandon's tremendous medical bills and lifetime of damages, our law firm filed a lawsuit on behalf of the child. During the proceedings, a nationally recognized escalator expert testified to the many maintenance failures; he also testified that the buckling that had caused Brandon's fall would never have occurred had proper maintenance been performed on the escalator.

Escalators are the proverbial two-edged swords for children. They often view an escalator as an amusement ride, a way to have fun. Kids don't recognize- in fact, many parents don't recognize- the dangers posed by escalators. But, as the Elevator and Escalator Safety Foundation points out, an escalator is a six-ton moving machine. Passengers like Brandon fall when the equipment malfunctions. Others get their fingers and toes entrapped in the steps or sucked into the gap between the sides of the steps and the sidewalls. Injuries range from pinched fingers and toes to abrasions, lacerations, fractures, permanent disability and death.

In 2003, 1,902 children under the age of 14 were injured by escalators, according to the U.S. Consumer Products Safety Commission (CPSC).

⇨There are over 6,000 escalator injuries treated in hospital emergency rooms each year in the U.S., including three deaths. (CPSC 2001.)

⇨ There is one hospitalization every year for every four escalators in service in the U.S. Eighty-five percent of these are preventable. (CPSC.)

⇨ Between 1992 and 2001, there were 20 deaths due to escalator accidents. (CPSC, National Injury Surveillance System and the Bureau of Labor Statistics.)

⇨The CPSC estimates that 75 percent of escalator injuries are due to falls, and 20 percent are due to entrapment. The remaining five percent are categorized "other."

⇨ One-half of all escalator entrapment injuries involve children under the age of five (CPSC: 2004 CDC Report, The Center to Protect Workers' Rights). Most are caused when footwear (including shoelaces) or fingers get caught at the top or bottom steps or sides of the escalator.

Laws and Regulations

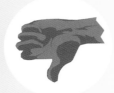

State and local governments usually require regular inspections of elevators and escalators, but enforcement of these requirements can be irregular. The American Society of Mechanical Engineers (ASME) and the American National Standards Institute (ANSI) Escalator Committee established voluntary guidelines for the safe construction, maintenance and operation of escalators; these guidelines have been promoted by the CPSC since 1990. Yet many of these recommendations have yet to be commonly accepted. For example, they require that escalator steps be painted with footprints or borders, to highlight them; that sidewalls be low-friction so that shoes can't get sucked into the gap between the step and the wall; that warning signs be posted at each escalator; and that skirt obstruction devices, which shut off the escalator if an object gets caught, be installed.

Many injuries on escalators occur as the result of maintenance failures and design flaws.

But even when the equipment is functioning safely and all maintenance checks have been met, catastrophic accidents can happen on escalators. In most cases, these injuries can be prevented with proper supervision of the child.

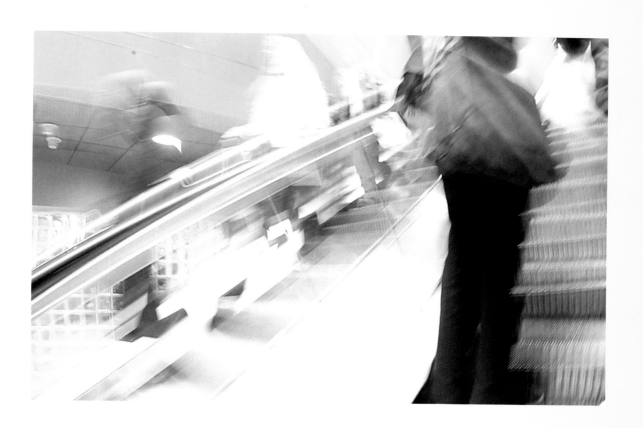

When you and your child take an **ESCALATOR**, use this checklist to make sure your child is safe.

CHECKLIST

✔	⚠ CHECKLIST ⚠
1	Adults: One hand on the handrails.
2	Taller Children: One hand on the handrails.
3	Smaller Children: Hold on to adult's leg or belt loop.
4	No loose objects on the child.
5	Do not carry any objects.
6	Children must stand still.
7	Adults need to be diligent.
8	No strollers.
9	Children must face forward.
10	Lift off small children from the last step.

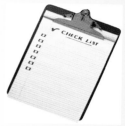

1. ADULTS: One hand on the handrails.

The adults must set the example for children and have one hand on the handrails at all times. The stability gained will allow the adult to quickly and safely react to any danger posed to the child.

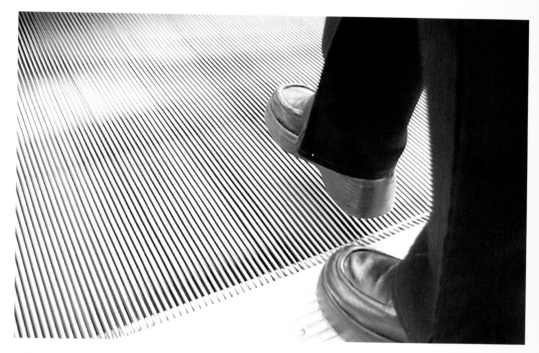

2. TALLER CHILDREN: One hand on the handrails.

The one hand placement is the best way to provide stability in case the child loses balance or the escalator suddenly jerks.

3. SMALLER CHILDREN: Hold on to adult's leg or belt loop.

Holding on to a fixed object provides maximum safety.

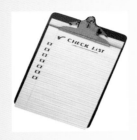

4. NO LOOSE OBJECTS ON THE CHILD.

Loose shoe laces or long pant legs can easily get caught in the moving parts of the escalator machinery.

5. DO NOT CARRY ANY OBJECTS.

The child should carry no suitcases or food and beverages. These objects will permit instability of the child.

6. CHILDREN MUST STAND STILL.

By instinct the child will want to run or move from stair to stair. Such movement will permit dangerous instability on the escalator.

7. ADULTS NEED TO BE DILIGENT.

In a split second, a tragedy can occur, and the adult must be ready to prevent instability and prevent the harm which can occur.

8. NO STROLLERS.

Virtually every escalator has a local or state law requiring that an elevator be in close proximity for the use of strollers and wheelchairs. **Be Safe: Use the elevator**.

9. CHILD MUST FACE FORWARD.

The natural instinct of the child is to face or look backwards, it's more fun. The child must be taught to always face forward.

10. LIFT OFF SMALL CHILDREN FROM THE LAST STEP.

Statistically many tragedies occur on the last step. Small children do not have the motor skills to get off the moving object; thus, simply lift the child off the last step and safely on the solid ground.

32

Shopping Carts

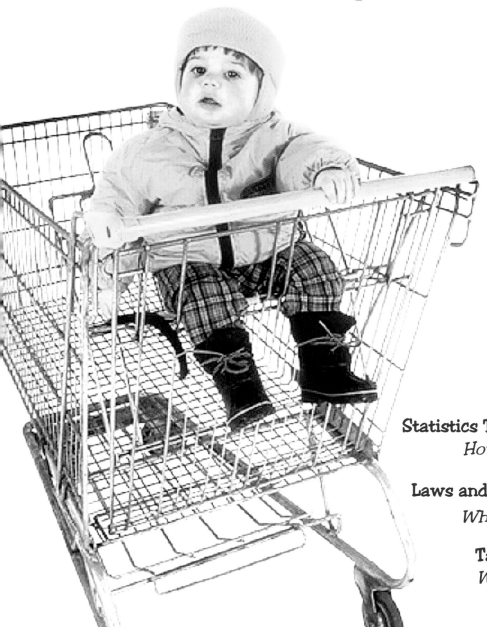

Advertised Hazard

Troy had alternate-weekend custody of his four-and-a-half-year-old son, Kendall, and he looked forward to their time together. At the start of one visit, Troy decided it would be fun to take Kendall to the grocery store to buy the food necessary for their weekend. Together, they had watched advertisements of a father and son racing through this popular grocery store- child riding below the cart, father pushing. In fact, once at the store, a life-size cardboard poster of the father, hands on the grocery cart, his young boy smiling from beneath, greeted Troy and his son. Kendall was excited to recreate the poster, so he climbed under a cart.

Half way through the shopping spree, Troy stopped the cart and walked 10 steps ahead to ask a sales clerk where to find an item on his list. At that moment, another shopper came by the pair's grocery cart and pushed it aside, not realizing that Kendall was below. At the moment of the push, Kendall had his small hand wrapped around the inside of the wheel. When the cart got pushed, his index finger was moved against the outer shield of the wheel; it was immediately severed. Kendall screamed, and his dad turned around to see blood covering the floor beneath the cart. The paramedics were quickly summoned; well trained, they picked up the amputated finger and took it to the hospital with the boy.

Surgeons worked tirelessly to reattach Kendall's finger, and the boy was discharged from the hospital several days later, in guarded condition. Although a second surgery was performed, Kendall regained only 20 percent of the movement in his dominant-hand index finger.

LEGAL ACTION
and
OUTCOME

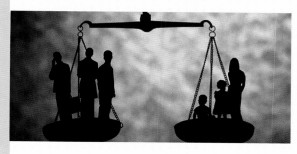

Troy thought about the television advertisements and cardboard cutout that prominently displayed a child under the grocery cart. Without this encouragement, his son would have been sitting in the upper portion of the cart, or walking beside him, not riding below. Troy retained me to bring suit in order to claim recovery of the medical expenses and the loss of movement in Kendall's hand. After subpoenaing documents and learning more about the history of the cart- including the fact that one prior claim resulted in a similar injury- we added the manufacturer of the cart to the suit. Kendall's injury, we learned, could have been prevented by the placement of a very low-cost safety guard on the inside of the wheel well.

Shockingly, the grocery store defended the case, stating that they never believed that anyone would put their child underneath the grocery cart. The advertisements, they argued, simply symbolized "the excitement one gets going grocery shopping." They believed it was unnecessary to warn patrons of the danger of the activity because "anyone would know not to put their child in that location." The cart manufacturer filed an action against the store, contending it was their conduct that caused the child's injury.

Ultimately, after many depositions were taken, the case was settled to the satisfaction of the family.

Statistics Tell the Story

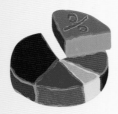

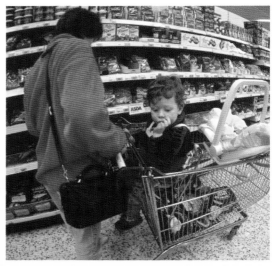

⇨Falls from shopping carts are among the leading causes of head injuries to young children. The U.S. Consumer Products Safety Commission (*CPSC*) estimated that in recent years, there were about 12,800 hospital emergency room-treated injuries annually to children five years and under associated with shopping carts. Of those, 5,700 were head injuries. About 25 percent were more serious head injuries such as concussions and fractures.

⇨Shopping cart accidents result in 650 hospital admissions per year. (*Pediatric Emergency Care* October 2004.)

⇨In 1999, nearly 23,600 children were treated in emergency rooms for shopping cart accidents. Most of them were under four years of age. Injuries include cuts, bruises, lacerations and concussions.

Many years ago, a number of children died from strangulation when their heads became entangled between the spokes of shopping carts. As a result, legislation was passed to reduce the space between the spokes of the wheels, virtually eliminating such strangulations.

There has been other legislation regarding shopping carts, as well. Some consumer groups have argued the following requirements for shopping carts must become law:

1. Lower the center of gravity or widen the wheel base of the shopping cart to prevent tipping.

2. Existing carts must have the equivalent of training wheels.

3. Children must be able to be strapped in when riding the carts.

None of these recommendations have been passed into law.

Taking Action

In order to protect your child from unfortunate, preventable **SHOPPING CART** injuries, please follow the checklist below:

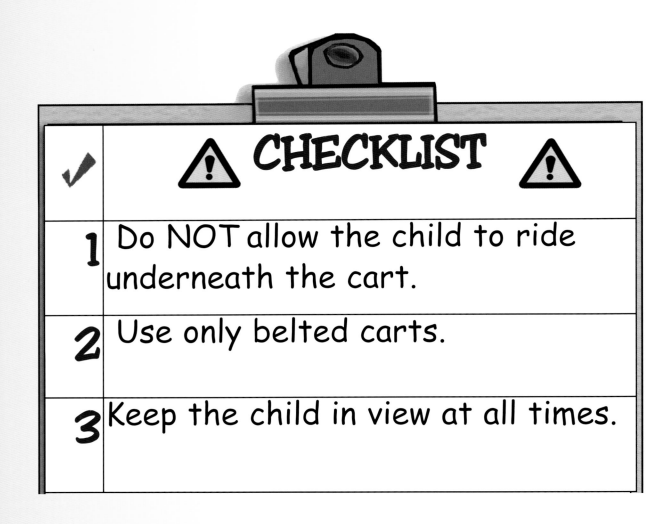

✔	⚠ CHECKLIST ⚠
1	Do NOT allow the child to ride underneath the cart.
2	Use only belted carts.
3	Keep the child in view at all times.

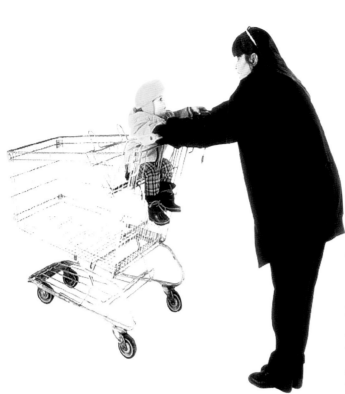

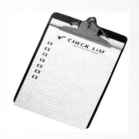

1. DO NOT ALLOW CHILD TO RIDE UNDERNEATH THE CART.

As we have seen in the tragedy recounted in this chapter, the space underneath a grocery cart is not designed for children. Although it may look like fun, under no circumstances should a child be permitted to ride in this location.

2. USE ONLY BELTED CARTS.

Virtually every major national retailer using shopping carts now has a belt in each cart so that all children can be safely secured. Several retailers, such as Kmart and Wal-Mart, have greeters at the front of the store, instructed to encourage customers to buckle up children in the carts.

As we see from the statistics above, the highest proportion of injuries occur when children fall out of the cart. Proper belting will help eliminate this potential life-threatening injury.

Fasteners can be fun to play with, so make sure that the child does not unsecure the safety belt. Also make sure than an older child does not disconnect the belt of a younger child.

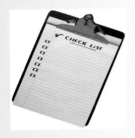

3. KEEP THE CHILD IN VIEW AT ALL TIMES.

As we will discuss in Chapter 34, there are many children abducted from retail establishments, particularly those where the surrounding circumstances cause the adult to be easily distracted and preoccupied. Therefore, if for no other reason than to prevent abduction, have the child in your view at all times.

Monitoring the child in the cart at all times can also help prevent accidents.

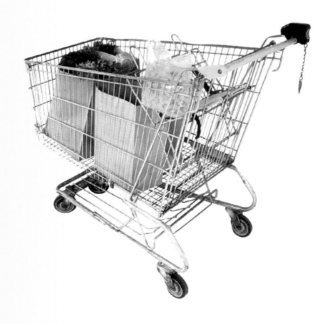

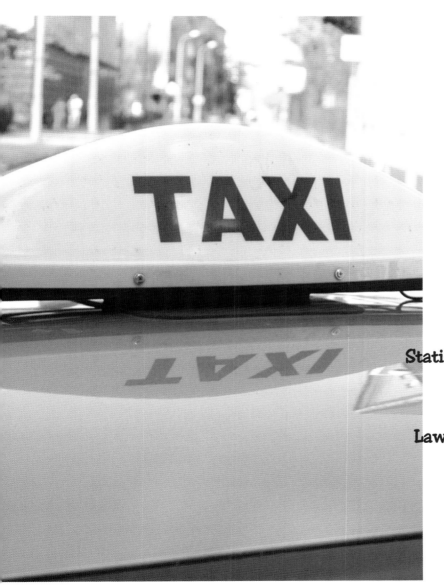

33
Taxis

Dangerous Ride

Betsy had an exciting year with the birth of her daughter, Angel. Around the time of Angel's first birthday, Betsy accepted an invitation to visit her sister at college. Betsy knew that taxicabs were common in the major metropolitan area where she'd be visiting, so she knew she'd have transportation when needed, starting with the trip from the airport to her sister's apartment complex.

The flight went well, and the baggage, including Angel's stroller, arrived on time. Bags in hand, Betsy pushed Angel to the taxi stand, where a shiny cab rolled up. In the usual hustle and bustle at airports, they were encouraged to move along quickly.

Betsy collapsed the stroller, and the taxi driver placed it and the bags in the trunk. Betsy jumped in the back seat of the cab with Angel. About 200 yards outside the airport pickup, Betsy realized that the seat belt connector had been pushed behind the seat, so she was unable to fasten it. That left both Angel and Betsy without restraining devices. Twice Betsy asked the driver, who was driving recklessly, to slow down.

Aggravated, the driver jammed on the brakes too close to the traffic ahead. Betsy and Angel crashed into the metal partition that divided the front and back of the taxi. Angel's head hit a small protruding drawer that is intended for passing money from passengers to the driver. (This drawer is used mostly at night, when a driver does not wish to roll down his window, but prefers to remain protected by the bulletproof glass that separates the front seat of the cab from the rear.)

Angel spent 10 days in the hospital and was released in guarded condition.

LEGAL ACTION
and
OUTCOME

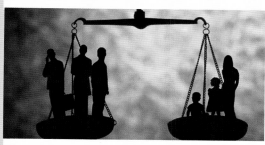

Because of the high cost of Angel's medical bills and the uncertainty of her future disability, I was asked to file suit against the taxicab company. The company claimed that the driver was an independent contractor, and they simply rented the car to him for 10-hour shifts. The driver said he was an employee of the taxi company and therefore did not have his own liability insurance. Ultimately, however, we obtained a document proving that the taxicab company was covered by insurance, regardless of whether the accident was caused by an employee or an independent contractor driving their vehicle.

We subpoenaed records of complaints regarding unavailable seat belts and were surprised to find that the city's taxi commissioner received over 30 complaints of back seats with no usable seat belts. The company maintained that the seat belts were provided, but passengers kept pushing them down behind the seat.

We also uncovered a memo from the company's vice president in charge of accident investigation, advising that the company should provide car seats for children. This advice had gone unheeded.

Because of the mounting information we obtained through the discovery period of the lawsuit, the case was settled to the satisfaction of Betsy.

Statistics Tell the Story

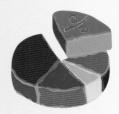

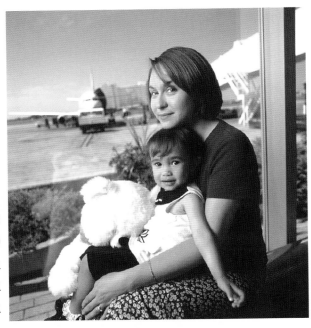

⇨ According to the 2000 census, there were 230,000 taxi and limousine drivers in the United States, an increase of 18 percent from 1990.

⇨ Taxi passengers are three times more likely to sustain relatively serious injuries than passengers in other vehicles. (Schaller, Bruce. February 28, 2001. *Taxi and Livery Crashes in New York City: 1990-1999.* Schaller Consulting.)

⇨ In New York City alone there were over 2,600 children injured in the 17,000 taxi-related accidents, according to a 2000 report. (*USA Today* April 2005.)

Sadly, virtually every jurisdiction exempts taxis from the requirement of having restraint devices and car seats for children. In contrast, in places like Prince Edward Island, British Columbia, car seats and seat belts are mandatory in all taxicabs.

In our sample case, Betsy only encountered the problem of not being able to secure her child in the taxi while visiting her sister. But many parents live in cities where a taxi ride is a daily occurrence. What is a parent to do to insure his or her child's safety when car seats are not provided? It would be quite a burden to carry a car seat on every outing with a child.

This conflict is seen in an interesting message board exchange on the Berkeley Parents Network (http://parents.berkeley.edu/recommend/where2buy/carseats/taxi.html). The message board has approximately 20 posts from mothers answering the question, "What will I do with my child in a taxi?" One woman advises to use a "travel vest." Another woman says only use a "mini car seat." Several advise not taking a taxi at all, but instead using only mass transit. The message board clearly documents the dilemma parents have when taxis do not provide for the safety of children.

Taking Action

The following checklist should be employed to supervise the safe transportation of children:

CHECKLIST

✔	
1	Always use a car seat. For specific car seat and booster seat safety recomendations see Chapter 28.
2	Use a multi-purpose seat.
3	Pay for wait time to prevent hurrying.
4	Practice, practice, practice.
5	Do not get in a taxi without seat belts.
6	Take mass transit if you can.
7	Be aware of protruding and sharp edges in the taxicab.
8	Complain of driver's speed or reckless driving.

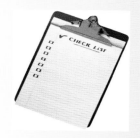

1. ALWAYS USE A CAR SEAT.

As we saw in the tragic retold in this chapter, holding your child in your arms in the back seat of a taxi is extremely dangerous. A car seat should always be used for a child traveling in a taxi.

2. USE A MULTI-PURPOSE SEAT.

Triple Play Products, a major manufacturer, makes a three-way safety seat. It functions as a baby stroller and then collapses to become a car seat. It also carries FAA certification so that it can be used safely on commercial air travel. There are other manufacturers of similar products. Look for these at http://brands.babycatalog.com.

3. PAY FOR WAIT TIME TO PREVENT HURRYING.

It takes time to properly install a car seat and safely secure a child in it. Some taxi drivers become aggravated by this "downtime," for which they are not paid. In fact, some drivers will not pick up passengers with car seats because of the lost time. For the driver who does stop, it would be helpful to tell him or her immediately that you are willing to pay for the wait time, in order to properly secure your child's car seat.

4. PRACTICE, PRACTICE, PRACTICE.

While you may be experienced at using the car seat in your automobile, using it in another vehicle may present a bit of a challenge at first. Practice installing the car seat in a family member's car or a neighbor's car, so that you will be aware of the problems you may experience in a taxi.

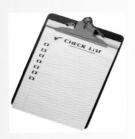

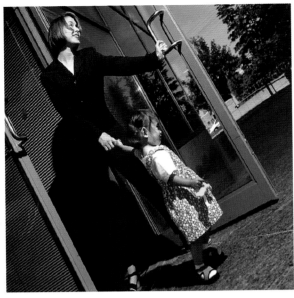

5. DO NOT GET IN A TAXI WITHOUT SEAT BELTS.

Many taxicabs don't have seat belts available. In fact, one driver explained that because passengers complained of the protruding ends of the seat belts, the drivers-"as a favor"-turn them around and push them back into the seats so that passengers could ride more comfortably.

Unfortunately, taxi drivers are correct when they point out that most people do not wear seat belts, even when provided. In 2001, the City of New York commissioned a study of taxis and taxi accidents in New York between 1990 and 1999. The study, conducted by Schaller Consulting, found that less than 17 percent of riders used available seat belts.

Do not get into a vehicle unless you can see both ends of the seat belts, and always fasten yours and your child's before the taxi moves.

6. TAKE MASS TRANSIT IF YOU CAN.

After going through the multiple posts on the Berkeley Parent Network, sometimes it is a lot easier to take mass transit than a taxicab.

Hauling a car seat around when you're not in the taxi can be a major inconvenience. Instead, consider taking mass transit.With mass transit, you can actually use a stroller that can then be used on the street. Thus, mass transit may be the answer.

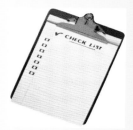

7. BE AWARE OF PROTRUDING AND SHARP EDGES IN THE TAXICAB.

It never occurred to Betsy that the pass-through drawer would be a hazard to her child. But hazards such as these do exist and are worth noting. Place yourself and your child in a position so that, in a forward-motion accident, neither of you will strike these protrusions.

Note: Because of the increasing awareness of the dangers to children in taxis, the Morgan Stanley Children's Hospital of New York is spearheading a drive to mandate booster seats in all taxis. Several car seat companies have donated a number of free booster seats. (*USA Today* April 2005)

8. COMPLAIN OF DRIVER'S SPEED OR RECKLESS DRIVING.

While it may seem simple to complain of the driver's speed or recklessness, the occupant of a taxicab has clear leverage to motivate the driver. Simply say, "I'm not going to give you a tip if you don't slow down." These simple but powerful words can correct dangerous driving.

Part Six
Hidden Predators

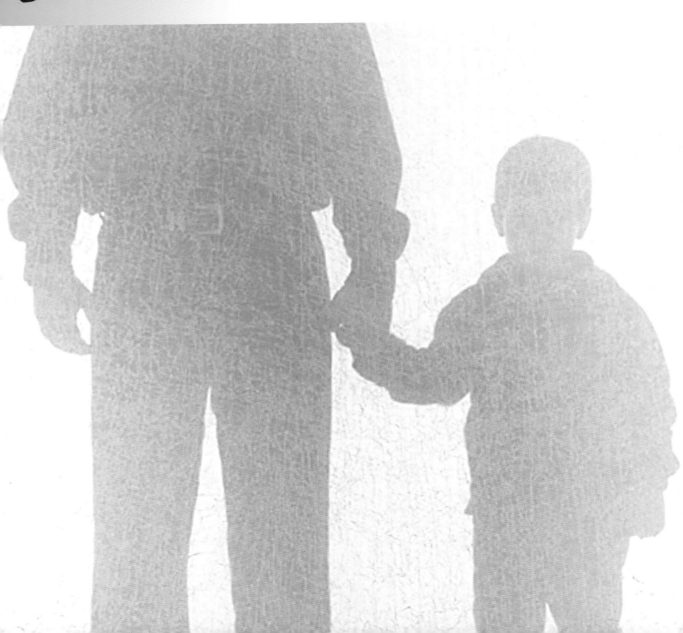

Preface

The following five chapters deal with a growing epidemic in our country: Predators stalking, molesting, injuring, and killing our children. Before we examine the dangers lurking in retail establishments (Chapter 34), churches (Chapter 35), schools (Chapter 36), the home (Chapter 37) and the Internet (Chapter 38), let us look at several global statistics and recommendation for change:

FACT:

There are over 400,000 registered sex offenders in the United States today.

FACT:

Up to one third of these known sexual predators cannot be located.

OFFENDER REGISTERATION

In addressing only the problem of known sex offenders, it is paramount that you learn your proximity to them. The location can easily be determined through the Internet: Simply do a "Google" search, and you will find the links. Type in "registered sex offenders" and the name of your state. Check often, there are daily updates. One private company, www.scanusa.com, offers email service on daily additions within your zip code. If you need help, call your local law enforcement or news media. You will be shocked to learn about your neighbors.

THE FAILURE TO REGISTER PROBLEM

You should be additionally shocked to know that one third of these registered sex offenders fail to give current addresses, as was painfully demonstrated in the 2005 case of child killer John Covey *(right)* who, over 30 years, had been arrested 24 times and was a registered sex offender. Covey lived less than 150 yards away from nine-year-old Jessica Marie Lunsford *(left)*, so it was easy for Covey to walk into Jessica's home, knowing her parents were not present, and

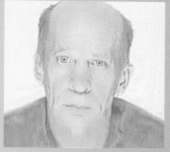

abduct her. Her body was later found, and authorities believe she was buried alive after being assaulted. Covey never registered his new home address, and no one went looking for him.

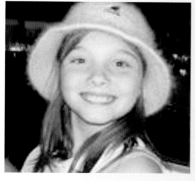

Jessica's tragedy was followed only several days later with the death of 13-year-old Sarah Michelle Lunde, also at the hands of a registered sex offender who had moved without notifying authorities.

339

What can we do about the failure of these known perverts to register? Marc Klaas is the father Polly Klaas, the victim of an infamous 1993 California abduction case in which the 12-year-old was taken from her bedroom. After his daughter's abduction, Marc formed the Klaas Kids Foundation (www.klaaskids.org) and has been a longtime advocate of common-sense solutions to the failure-to-register problem. He outlines four basic steps:

1. Force compliance by increasing penalties.

If the criminal is simply slapped on the wrist for not registering, then he has no real reason to register. Mandatory revocation of probation or parole and minimum jail time would be a start.

2. Institute a real verification policy.

The system now relies upon the perpetrators self-registering. It is the most absurd "honor system" imaginable. If the IRS can have a random audit system on our tax returns, Marc Klaas argues, why cannot law enforcement or social services have a random verification of correct home addresses for perverts? This would at least forewarn the pervert that someone could be checking. Further, if a check reveals a bum address, then a watch list can be created to be on the lookout for the perpetrator. Or even better, enact laws as did Florida in the wake of Jessica and Sarah's deaths...mandatory GPS monitors for those not reporting.

3. Break down state and local boundaries.

As the system exists now, our 50 states do not share a central database. Instead, each state has its own individual database, and therefore it is easy for the perpetrator to elude detection. There are a multitude of major cities located right at state boundary lines; virtually every state has such a city. Therefore, a centralized national database is mandatory.

4. Everyone can help.

The job is not exclusively for law enforcement or social services. All of us have a duty to know our surroundings, whether we have a child in our home or not. We also have a duty to report suspicious circumstances and odd behavior.

How many children are going to be abducted, injured or killed before we institute Marc Klaas' common-sense reforms?

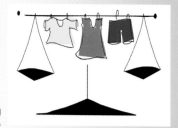

34

In Retail Establishments

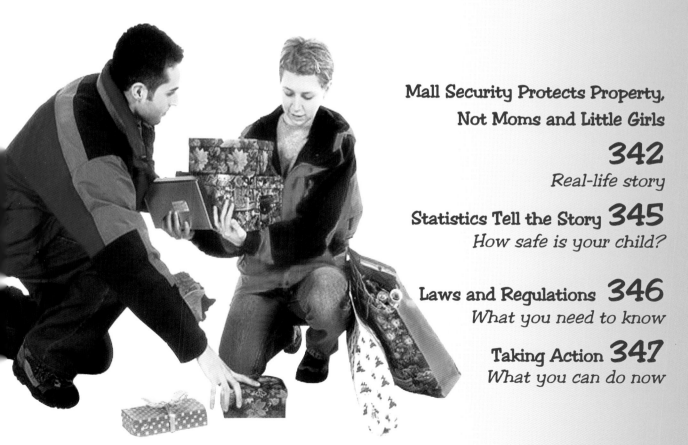

Mall Security Protects Property, Not Moms and Little Girls

One of the advantages of shopping at a luxury mall is the feeling of personal security. At the mall where Allison frequently shopped, for example, a glassed-in atrium housed a bank of over 30 television monitors, seeming to be poised to cover every inch of the interior of the mall and the outside parking lot. Several uniformed security guards watched the television monitors, instilling in shoppers a clear sense that their safety was being protected.

What Allison did not realize was that the primary purpose of the cameras and monitors was not customer safety, but rather protection against shoplifting and vandalism. In fact, the security guards were not even trained to recognize potential abductions. Allison also did not realize that there were several blind spots in the parking lot in areas that were simply out of camera range. Unlike Allison, predators knew precisely what areas of the parking lot were not visible; they had carefully studied the monitor angles to determine which areas were out of range.

With her two small children in their family minivan, Allison carefully selected a spot in the corner of the parking lot. In addition to believing that the area was being monitored by camera surveillance, Allison also took comfort that she had pulled into a parking space that had an embankment towards the front and the passenger side of the vehicle; this way no one could sneak up on her vehicle from the front or from the passenger side.

Several hours of shopping and a bundle of shopping bags later, Allison and her two children returned to the minivan. Just as she was opening the van doors on the driver's side, a dark van with heavily tinted windows stopped immediately to the rear of her minivan, with its side doors open to face the rear of Allison's van (see photo).

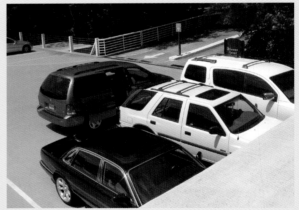

In a split second, two masked men emerged from the van. Allison could not run to the front or to the passenger side of her van because of the embankment, and she could not run away via the driver's side because of a parked car in the adjoining space. She and the girls were trapped. One masked man hit Allison with a blackjack, to stun her and then grabbed her. The other man grabbed her two little girls.

When Allison regained her senses, she reassured herself that the security personnel had viewed the abduction and were seconds away from saving them. Actually, because of the blind spot on the monitors, the security guards were oblivious to her situation. It was not until eight hours later that Allison and the little girls were dumped out at another mall parking lot, 25 miles away. In the interim, the abductors forced Allison to withdraw all of her cash from over 10 ATM machines, using her three bankcards. She was also groped and fondled by the criminals in full view of her little girls. Although the girls were physically unhurt, they were severally traumatized.

LEGAL ACTION and OUTCOME

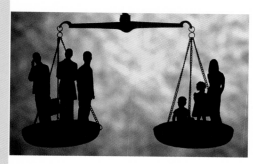

Allison's family and community were outraged that such an abduction could occur in broad daylight in a security monitored high-end shopping mall. It was not until the family hired my firm to represent them and a lawsuit was filed that the truth about the blind spot in the monitoring system became known. In fact, it was not until the criminals were apprehended that the police realized the existence of the blind spot. Although they knew of the blind spot on the day of the abduction, the mall officials had lied to the police.

During litigation, the mall and security guard service steadfastly maintained that the security was provided for the retailers ONLY and was never intended to protect the public. They said the reason they positioned the bank of TV monitors in the atrium of the mall was not so that the public would feel safe, but because "there was no other place to put the monitors."

Further investigation of the case revealed that other criminals had become knowledgeable of other blind spots at the mall: Purse snatchings and an attempted rape had already occurred in these spots due to the criminal awareness. The case was ultimately settled to the satisfaction of the family.

An added condition of settlement was that the mall remove the blind spot and guarantee that the area would be monitored. (Surprisingly, over the two years of the litigation, the blind spot continued to exist.) The mall did, in fact, fix the blind spot as a condition of settlement, and all involved in the case had believed that protection of the public had been achieved. It was not until almost a year after the lawsuit was concluded that my office received a call from a former security guard at the mall who revealed a startling fact: When the mall corrected the blind spot of Allison's abduction, they simply moved the camera, thereby creating a new blind spot. At first I could not believe this, but I remembered that the criminals detected the blind spot initially by simply watching the monitors at the mall. I therefore sent my investigator to pose as a shopper to see if this new blind spot existed. Sure enough, a new blind spot had been created.

I demanded an in-person meeting with the mall owners, security company and their lawyers. Under the threat of public disclosure, I demanded that an outside security audit be done and that all blind spots be corrected. The meeting lasted less than 15 minutes. My approach was not negotiation; it was a simple "take it or leave it" message. The mall quickly agreed to the outside audit, it was done within 60 days, and the mall parking lot then became free of blind spots.

ADDED NOTE:

Sadly, I have handled two cases of abductions and molestations in toy stores. When shoppers enter a toy store, they are in a happy frame of mind. They are also greeted with distractions of many kinds: myriad colors, noises, and activities. The last thing a caregiver is thinking about is the abduction or harm of his or her child. Perverts depend on these distractions to prey on children. Be particularly alert in toy stores.

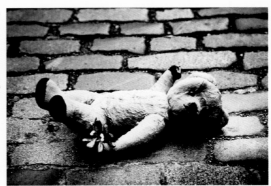

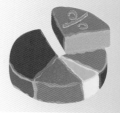

⇨Retail crime statistics are either under-reported or not reported at all. This is in stark contrast to the incidence of employee theft, which is readily available on any retail association Web site.

⇨The Department of Justice reports 58,200 children were abducted by non-family members in 1999, the most recent figures available. (Dept. of Justice,October 2002. *National Incidence Studies of Missing, Abducted, Runaway, and Thrownaway Children NISMART-2*)

The trauma that Allison and her daughters endured is repeated over and over in shopping malls throughout the country:

⇨Three-year-old Jenna was kidnapped when a man who pretended to be a good Samaritan stole her grandma's car at a Toys"R"Us store in Madison Heights, Michigan. Jenna's grandmother strapped her into a child seat outside the store, then watched in horror as a man who had just changed her tire drove off with her car and grandchild.The grandmother told police she was approached inside the Toys"R"Us toy store by the suspect, who informed her she had a flat tire and offered to change it.

⇨A suburban Illinois mother managed to thwart an unknown woman who attempted to kidnap her 15-month-old son from a Schaumburg, Illinois Toys"R"Us while shopping with the child and another son, four years old.The mother was trying to reach an item on a high shelf when she heard the screams of her youngest son, whom she had placed in a shopping cart. She heard her son yelling out and turned and saw the offender pushing the cart with her child in it. The mother ran after the woman and was able to catch her, police said.

Laws and Regulations

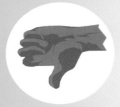

There are no laws or regulations requiring retail establishments to provide safety measures to prevent child abductions, molestations, or abuse.

Taking Action

In order to increase the safety of you and your child while you visit retail establishments, please follow the checklist below:

✔ ⚠ CHECKLIST ⚠

1	Do not rely on the retail establishment's security.
2	Always park your car with escape routes in all directions.
3	NEVER lose sight of your child.
4	Do not be distracted by the surroundings.
5	Always accompany your child to the bathroom.
6	Be aware of vulnerable/distractive times.
7	Avoid large crowds.

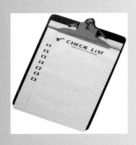

1. DO NOT RELY ON THE RETAIL ESTABLISHMENT'S SECURITY.

As is clearly evident in the tragic case outlined in this chapter, the presence of retail establishment security cameras or personnel bring no peace of mind. The sad truth is that most of the security exists to protect the retailer's property, not the safety and well-being of the customers and general public. There was one tragic case reported in the news where security guards were told not to interfere with what they perceived to be domestic dispute arguments. Thus, when a male became physical with a female, the security guards had a "hands-off" attitude; it was later discovered that the male was actually a complete stranger to the female.

2. ALWAYS PARK YOUR CAR WITH ESCAPE ROUTES IN ALL DIRECTIONS.

As we have seen in the above case example, it is necessary for you to have an escape route in all directions, so that all possibilities are open in case you are confronted. Perverts will avoid areas with escape routes. This is also true of well-illuminated areas; the criminals will try to avoid these and will prey in areas with broken lights or lower illumination.

3. NEVER LOSE SIGHT OF YOUR CHILD.

Although this sounds simple, the word "never" means never! Most abductions and kidnappings occur in a split second, during a bump in the crowd or a momentary distraction. Therefore, a child is always vulnerable and must always be in sight.

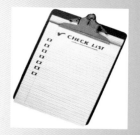

4. DO NOT BE DISTRACTED BY THE SURROUNDINGS.

There are many reported cases of children being abducted or harmed inside toy stores. (As stated earlier, my office has handled two such cases.) Toy stores typically have merchandise stacked to the ceiling, with colors, noises and visual enticements greeting shoppers in every corner. Not only are children distracted, but so are parents and caregivers. It is quite easy to become lost in the distractions of a toy store, or other retail establishment that follows a similar marketing strategy.

Another potentially dangerous place is a retail establishment that provides playgrounds. It is quite easy for a parent simply to usher a child to the play area of a restaurant or mall, for example, and then go about his or her adult business. However, pedophiles and people who want to hurt children are lured as a moth to a candle to areas such as playgrounds and toy stores. Wally Sutton was once asked why he robbed banks, and he responded, "That's where the money is." The same is true with the pedophile and toy stores and playground areas. The pedophile depends upon you or the caregiver becoming distracted.

5. ALWAYS ACCOMPANY YOUR CHILD TO THE BATHROOM.

A high number of abductions occur in bathrooms that have side doors for maintenance people. The child enters the bathroom through what the parent believes to be the only door. The parent then goes to retrieve the child after a suspicious amount of time, only to find that there is another way out of the bathroom.

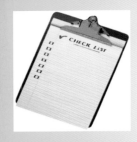

6. BE AWARE OF VULNERABLE/DISTRACTIVE TIMES.

Even though you are following rule number three (never losing sight of the child) and number four (do not be distracted by surroundings), there are certain times when you or a caregiver are particularly vulnerable. One of these times is when you are asking a question of the store employee. Often, the employee will guide you to another area of the store to engage in detailed conversation, and you may momentarily lose sight of your child. The same is true at the checkout counter, as you write a check, have a credit card processed, or dig through a wallet or purse. This is a time in which you are distracted, and pedophiles and abductors will in an instant take a child during such distractions.

7. AVOID LARGE CROWDS.

For centuries, pickpockets have preyed upon persons in large crowds with the "bump and run" technique of distraction. Pedophiles have learned this game well and have taken kids from the arms of a caregiver right in the middle of a crowd. Remember, many pedophiles and abductors are not only lured by obtaining total control over the kidnapped child, but also by the thrill, excitement and danger of the abduction. In many cases, the tougher and bolder the abduction, the more thrill the perpetrator experiences. So avoid large crowds.

On virtually every premise security case my law firm has prosecuted, we have employed the services of Larry Talley, former Vice President of Risk Management for Days Inn of America. Larry is the author of *Are You Really Safe? Protecting Yourself in America Today* (1994, Long Street Press). Recently we have been employing the services of Larry's protégé, John Harris, **www.thgconsult.com/firmoverview.htm**. Many thanks to Larry and John for their expertise in making children safe.

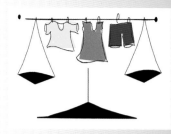

35

In Churches

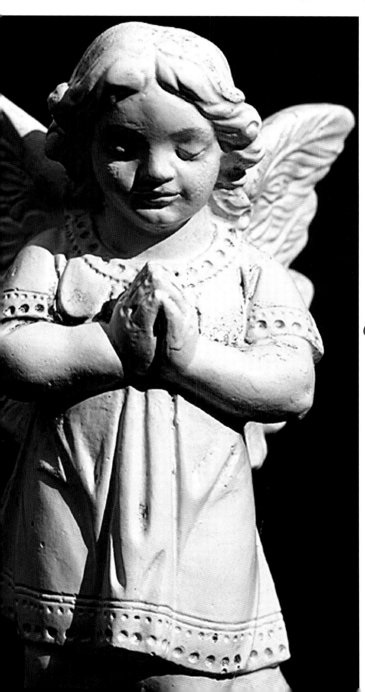

351

Church Becomes Hell for Little Boys

Of all the environments in which we place our children outside the home, none have a safer connotation than the confines of a church.

When they moved into their neighborhood, the Morelands were delighted to find that their chosen denomination had a large church less than a mile and a half away from their home. This was a growing church, with nearly 1000 members and activities pertaining to all levels of family growth. In addition to valet parking for the elderly preceding services, the church also boasted an athletic complex that would rival a small college's- complete with an Olympic-size swimming pool, a running track, two full-size basketball courts and daily exercise classes. This church athletic facility existed for the benefit of its parishioners, and it was open to the rest of the neighborhood as well. The church governing board reasoned that if it could appeal to the secular interests of the community, it would place potential members in the bosom of the church, with transition to church membership inevitable.

Peter Moreland, age six, had what his parents believed to be a self-esteem problem with his peers. So when the church offered karate lessons at the athletic center, they jumped at the chance to give Peter the opportunity to expand his friendships and his self-esteem. An article about the karate instructor appeared in the church newsletter; it outlined his prior training and experience. The man was tremendously engaging and enthusiastic about making karate not only character building, but fun as well.

Over time, the karate instructor took on almost a pied-piper persona, with most of his students engaging in hero-worshiping. In fact, Peter's parents often wished that the boy would simply stop talking about all of the exploits of his karate instructor.

Then one day, as is classic in these types of situations, the house of cards fell. One little boy told his sister about a molestation by the instructor. The sister in turn told her parent, and her parent reported the incident to a church worker. The police became involved, and, within a matter of days, 30 children came forward with recountings of pedophilia and molestation too graphic to describe here.

Ultimately, Peter revealed all of the details of his molestation, but only after defending the karate instructor's conduct as reasonable and what "tough men do with one another." As is true with many pedophilia epidemics in church settings, the tender, impressionable children accept verbatim whatever explanation is given; the church setting made their vulnerability even deeper and stronger. The church teaches rightfully that one must look to the goodness in people and accept the authority of adults.

At first the parents inflicted guilt upon themselves, believing that somehow they should have known or suspected the ongoing abuse. However, the pedophile in this case did as most do: He instilled fear in the children that prevented them from ever revealing the truth.

LEGAL ACTION and OUTCOME

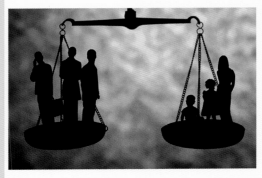

Peter's parents and other parents retained The Keenan Law Firm to hold the church accountable. While my firm has undertaken litigation against automobile manufacturers, pharmaceutical companies and toy manufacturers, the fiercest, most adversarial and mean-spirited advocate in my experience has been the church. The institution mind-set is simply incapable of accepting responsibility and believes that the litigation is focused against God and is anti-church.

The church fought this case tooth and nail. Many hearings were required to force the church to reveal that it had done nothing to investigate the background of the karate instructor. Had they done so, they would have discovered that molestation incidents and suspicion had followed this man through his last four church employments. Further, the litigation revealed that, over time, many of the children at this particular church had complained to Sunday school teachers and church personnel that the karate instructor was taking children individually into the equipment closets to play "a man's game." Yet no one followed up on these inferences.

The greatest insult to the parents came when the church alleged that it had no responsibility for the karate instructor. The activity had occurred at essentially a "community gym," they said; what happened there was not their responsibility. The facts, however, revealed that the church owned the gym, collected fees for the karate class and paid the karate instructor a salary, complete with benefits.

Equally cruel was the allegation by the church that the parents should have been the first to know of the molestations. The church said the parents had failed to pick up on the clear signs and to notify the church in time to take appropriate action.

While none of the children suffered physical damage, experts we retained to do diagnostic evaluations of the children revealed deep and, in some cases, irreversible emotional damage. While molestations can and do occur in every facet of a child's world, when they occur at a church- against the backdrop of the trust associated with the church- they can be particularly damaging. There is a whole body of psychiatric and psychological literature on the long-term effects of molestation occurring within the church setting. Each one of the children we represented, in his own way, fell into designated categories of this damage. They will each be affected for the rest of their lives.

After the church threw up every possible roadblock, filed every possible motion and delayed the trial date many times, the case was finally set for trial. At this point, the church revealed that it had depleted half of its available insurance coverage towards attorney's fees and experts in defending the case. Therefore, they claimed, they were almost out of money and offered each child mere "peanuts" to settle the lifetime of damages. We retained an asset valuation firm to determine the net worth of the church's assets. The value of their real estate holdings was shocking- even after assuming mortgages, which, in many instances, did not exist. I was further surprised to discover that the activities of the athletic center were, in fact, profit making. Compared to a YMCA, for example, the church was making a huge profit on the athletic center, mainly because volunteers supplied most of the people-power.

Knowing that this particular church was worth many millions of dollars, we held fast to what we believed would be fair justice for the children- whether or not the insurance ran out. After arduous and tenacious negotiations, full-value settlements were finally arranged for all of the children.

While I have not revealed the intricate details of the molestations, the church's ultimate negotiation ploy was to remind the parents that all of the details of the molestations would be made available at trial to the news media and the public. The church then said that it would be a sin for the parents to permit their children to go through a trial. I had practiced nearly 22 years of hard-fought law on behalf of children at that point, yet this last ploy by the church was clearly a first for me.

Please note, to dispel any inferences that I may be anti-church, I have taught Sunday school for over 12 years, been a member of my church's governing body for eight, been past chairman of our church's pulpit committee, served on the statewide governing body for my church, and have twice been a national delegate to my church's annual governing body convention.

Statistics Tell the Story

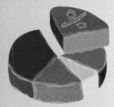

⇨ More than one million children are victims of sexual abuse each year. One in every four girls and one in every eight boys have been sexually molested before the age of 18. (*Today Show* January 15, 2004.)

⇨ Less than 35 percent of child sexual assaults are reported to authorities. (Center for Missing and Exploited Children.)

⇨ Approximately 90 percent of sexual molestation is committed by a person known to the child. They are not strangers. They are family members, teachers, coaches, babysitters, religious instructors and others who are in a position of knowing, caring for and being an authority figure for your child. (*Today Show,* Dr. Gail Saltz, New York Presbyterian Hospital.)

⇨ Statistics vary widely in the highly publicized Catholic Church molestation cases. A church-sanctioned report shows approximately 11,000 children molested by priests since 1950.(*U.S. News & World Report*, March 8, 2004). Father Andrew M. Greeley, priest, sociology professor and outspoken critic of church secrecy, reported a decade ago that the number is "well in excess of 100,000." (*America* March 20, 1993.)

⇨ A Catholic Church-sponsored report shows 150 abusive priests were quietly moved to a new church from July 2003 through January 2004. Bishops apparently did not warn police, prosecutors or parishioners. (*Bishop Accountability* January 8, 2004.)

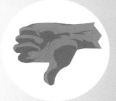

There are no laws or regulations to prevent church employee abuse/molestation of children. The only law relates to criminal prosecution of the wrongdoer and payment of damages by the wrongdoer in civil court.

Taking Action

In order to be vigilant about the harm that could occur to children in churches and religious establishments, the following checklist is provided:

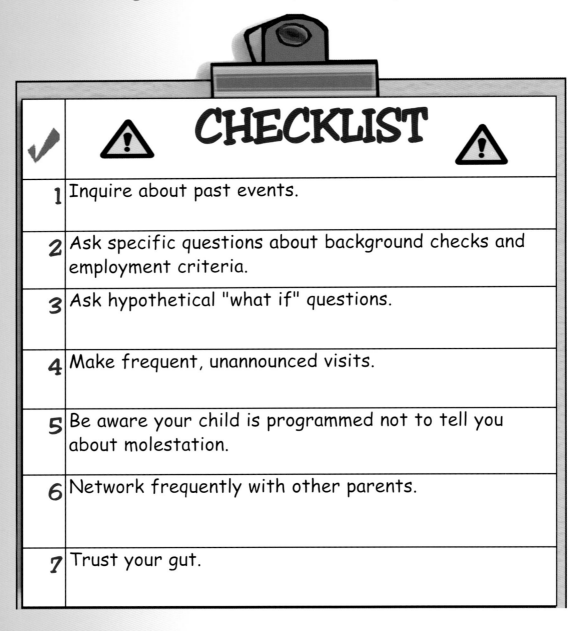

CHECKLIST

✔	⚠	⚠
1	Inquire about past events.	
2	Ask specific questions about background checks and employment criteria.	
3	Ask hypothetical "what if" questions.	
4	Make frequent, unannounced visits.	
5	Be aware your child is programmed not to tell you about molestation.	
6	Network frequently with other parents.	
7	Trust your gut.	

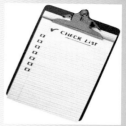

1. INQUIRE ABOUT PAST EVENTS.

There is a building in Washington, D.C. that carries the inscription "past is prologue." While a church can learn by its mistakes, history has indicated time and again that the church's response to molestation cases continues to be the same one of denial. Therefore, don't depend on the church for this valuable information. Run an Internet news check. Ask fellow parishioners about any past events dealing with pedophilia, child molestation, or other abuse of children by church employees.

The church's reaction to similar tragedies involving children will tell you a great deal about their safety awareness for children. Many Catholic churchgoers remember the subtle policy statements made by the Church concerning the need to rehabilitate molesting priests and the desire for forgiveness. These policy statements came back to haunt many churchgoers when more children were molested. Therefore, dig deep for past events and see how the church reacted.

2. ASK SPECIFIC QUESTIONS ABOUT BACKGROUND CHECKS AND EMPLOYMENT CRITERIA.

Do not simply ask whether background checks are done. Instead, inquire about the specific procedure, who implements and carries out the procedure and what items are checked. Always ask whether there is a checklist that is filled out. An absence of a checklist containing specific questions and information obtained will indicate a laissez-faire attitude towards the background check and the potential that the right questions were not asked or the answers were misinterpreted.

3. ASK HYPOTHETICAL "WHAT IF" QUESTIONS.

If the specific church or denomination has not had any pertinent past events, the parent can engage in the hypothetical "what if" questions, asking how the church would handle a situation. Specifically, "If the associate minister were caught molesting a child, what would be the church's response? Would it be to transfer the minister to another church with mandated sexual therapy?" Or, "If it is the child's word against the employee's word, what would the church's response be?" All of these "what if" questions are legitimate to ask, and answers should be forthcoming. These answers, and the forthrightness with which they are answered, will reveal a great deal about the church's attitude toward these events.

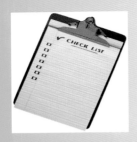

4. MAKE FREQUENT, UNANNOUNCED VISITS.

Always make frequent use of unannounced visits- at choir practice, church outings, or athletic events, for example. The molester will always pick private times to take a child off to a closet or a car or some other private place. Therefore, if there is a questionable absence of the church employee during your unannounced visit, demand further investigation.

5. BE AWARE THAT YOUR CHILD IS PROGRAMMED NOT TO TELL YOU ABOUT MOLESTATION.

Many parents naively believe that because they counseled their child many times about the need to tell about inappropriate touching, the child will be the first to reveal the abuse. Nothing could be further from the truth. In virtually all epidemic child-molesting circumstances, many, many children have remained stone silent in the face of intense questioning by suspecting parents. Therefore, inquiry of the child about potential molestation is the last and most unreliable source of information.

6. NETWORK FREQUENTLY WITH OTHER PARENTS.

Discussions with other parents may reveal collectively unusual, questionable circumstances. Therefore, constantly network and discuss events with other parents and watch out for any unusual circumstances.

7. TRUST YOUR GUT.

Last, but perhaps most importantly, if you have the slightest suspicion of an unusual occurrence, act on it immediately. In virtually all epidemic church-related child molestations, many parents would later reveal initial "gut problems" that they simply dismissed because the church was involved. It simply could not happen in the church, they believed.

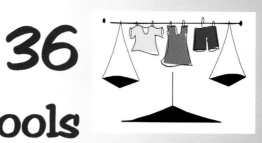

36

In Schools

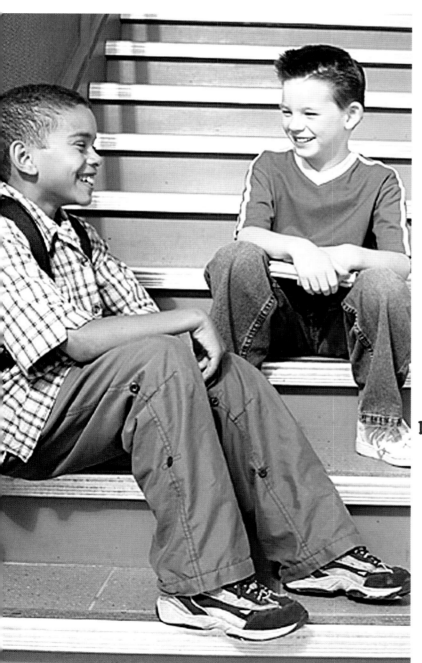

Unsafe at School

Leroy, age seven, was an introverted child. His parents were delighted when the school year came around, because then Leroy had other children to play with. One year, the school system hired a teacher's aide to assist in a number of art projects with the children. Leroy immediately took to art, and his parents were happy to see him open up, chatting almost daily about his good times with his teacher's aide, Todd. Suddenly, though, Leroy's parents noted a downward change in Leroy's disposition. Concerned, they asked him what was wrong. They even asked, pointedly, whether the aide had done anything inappropriate or touched Leroy in ways that were not proper. The child continued to say that nothing was wrong, that he just did not like school.

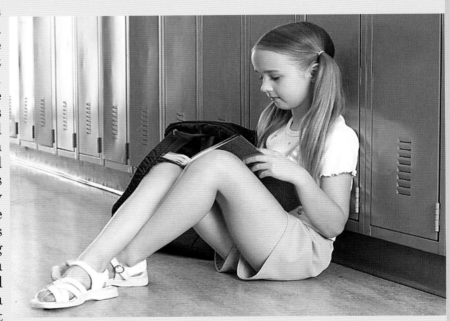

Leroy's parent's fears were realized when a detective showed up at their doorstep. Their child, he explained, was one of several who had been sexually abused by the teacher's aide over many months. The house of cards came crashing down when a teacher opened the door to a small art closet and found another little boy with his pants down and being touched by Todd.

The parents were outraged that this had occurred in their public school, a place they thought was safe for their child. Adding to their anger was the fact that this happened over many months without anyone knowing about it.

LEGAL ACTION
and
OUTCOME

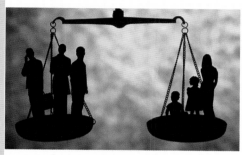

Leroy's parents requested that I bring suit to determine how the school system had failed their child. The school administration countered by alleging governmental immunity, an old legal doctrine dating back to the days of medieval kings, when, according to the law, the king could do no wrong, and therefore no recovery could be had against him. Sadly, in many states these immunity doctrines still exist. In the state in which we were litigating, there was an exception to the immunity law, however, which stated that the school could be held responsible if it had a mandatory procedure that would have prevented the harm and failed to follow it. In this case, the school did indeed have a written procedure stating that anyone working for the school had to have a criminal background check and verification of all prior employment.

The teacher's aide had been arrested twice before- once for public indecency and the other for improper actions with a minor- and both of those arrests would clearly have been shown on even a preliminary background check. Further, had the school contacted one of the aide's former employers, they would have found that he was discharged for suspicious but unproven conduct of a sexual nature towards the children he was supervising. Ironically, in his sworn testimony, Todd expressed surprise that the school system would have hired him in the first place, and he mocked the lack of supervision he had in his position.

The school also contended that since the teacher's aide was essentially a volunteer, though paid, he was technically not an employee of the school system. The school system lost all of their legal motions, however, and as the case was heading for trial, it was successfully resolved in the family's favor. The family insisted as a term of settlement that the rules of the school be amended to include that all employees have background checks, to prevent a similar occurrence in the future.

Statistics Tell the Story

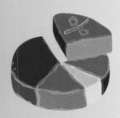

According to estimates by Carol Shakeshaft, a professor at Hofstra University who was contracted by the U.S. Congress to conduct a report on sexual abuse in public schools, seven percent of U.S. students are victims of physical sexual abuse by the time they graduate high school. She further reported, as a condition to the *No Child Left Behind Act*, that the number rises to 10 percent- four-and-a-half million students- when verbal and visual abuse are included.

In a recent interview, Shakeshaft stated that school faculty members are reluctant to report fellow teachers, because they fear ruining a teacher's career, if the suspicions are correct. Shakeshaft also noted that school officials incorrectly believe that there is some sinister profile for stereotyping sexual offenders; the reality is that sexual predators come in all shapes, sizes and backgrounds. In her report to Congress, Shakeshaft stated, "You wouldn't want to rule out someone who won 'Teacher of the Year' award if there's an allegation."

Also noted in this important report is the fact that punishment is often dangerously light. Professor Shakeshaft says, "The best that's done, although not always, is that the teacher's certificate is revoked, but that happens in very few cases. The chances that the offender will be able to teach again are high."

According to the Nevada Coalition Against Sexual Violence, school superintendents in 2003 reported that 16 percent of teachers who have lost their jobs due to charges of sexual abuse were now teaching elsewhere. The superintendents did not know the whereabouts of the other 84 percent and reported that all but one percent of the teachers had retained their teaching certificates.

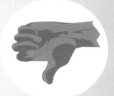

At present, there is no federal law regarding screening or investigation of potential sexual abusers in public schools. Hopefully, the end result of Dr. Shakeshaft's report will be detailed regulations, which will be mandated to any school receiving federal funds.

Many states and local school districts do have mandatory criminal checks at the time of hiring. But often, there are no follow-up checks after employment begins. Further, as noted in the tragedy recounted in the sample case, the fact that there is a policy does not mean it is followed.

Taking Action

In order to be involved in the recognition and prevention of sexual abuse in public schools, the following checklist should be followed:

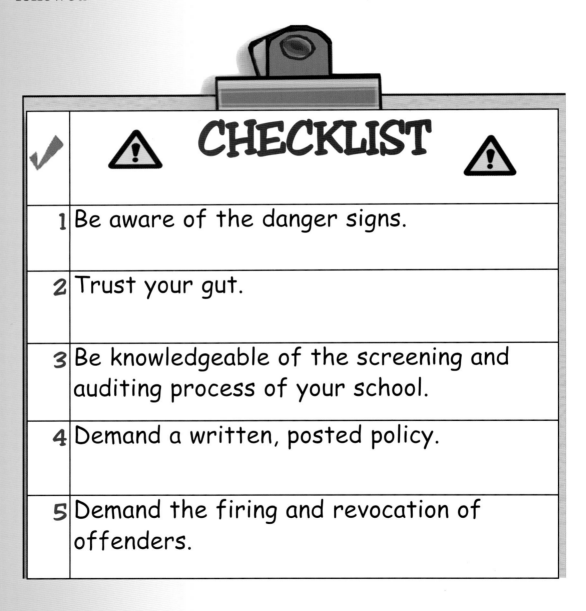

CHECKLIST

✔	⚠	
1	Be aware of the danger signs.	
2	Trust your gut.	
3	Be knowledgeable of the screening and auditing process of your school.	
4	Demand a written, posted policy.	
5	Demand the firing and revocation of offenders.	

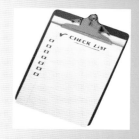

1. BE AWARE OF THE DANGER SIGNS.

While it is not always significant, a teacher or aide who spends excessive time behind closed doors or who has activities with individual students outside the school should clearly be considered as suspect.

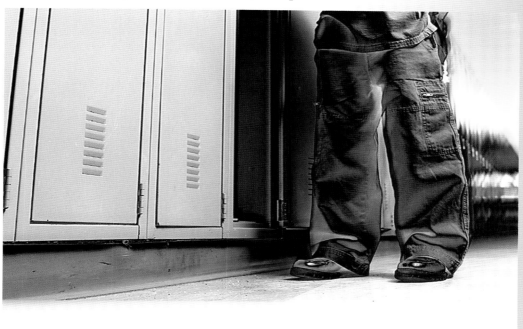

2. TRUST YOUR GUT.

If you have the slightest suspicion of foul play, follow the facts and investigate. Listen to the children talking. Often, the children have the first gut feeling- as well as the first information- and will whisper among themselves about improper conduct.

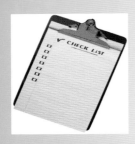

3. BE KNOWLEDGEABLE OF THE SCREENING AND AUDITING PROCESS OF YOUR SCHOOL.

Make sure that your school has both an initial hiring criminal and reference check and an annual check. There are many cases of well respected and liked principals, teachers and coaches who have been arrested for inappropriate conduct while traveling outside their cities. The truth comes to light when they are apprehended.

4. DEMAND A WRITTEN, POSTED POLICY.

If it is not in writing, the school will not do it: That's the bottom line. So make sure that there is a detailed policy that describes what will be done if an allegation is made and even what type of information will be available to the parents and caregivers in the event of an incident.

5. DEMAND THE FIRING AND REVOCATION OF OFFENDERS.

Often, school boards will permit teachers and aides to simply resign, rather than follow through with an investigation and charges. Such conduct simply sets up the next victim in the next city or state. There should not be a three-strike rule when dealing with the sexual abuse of children. One strike is enough. One proven charge of sexual abuse mandates revocation of the teacher's certificate.

37

Babysitters/ Nannies

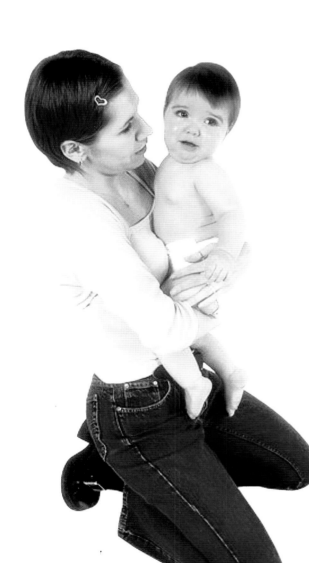

Malpractice, Accident or Murder?

During his childhood, John Stanford lost his baby brother to an untreated head trauma. As the result of the pain of growing up without his brother, John resolved early on to dedicate his life to helping children who receive severe injuries. John went to medical school and specialized in pediatric critical care, an emerging medical specialty. He worked long hours and cared deeply for the children in his care, becoming one of the nation's best critical care doctors.

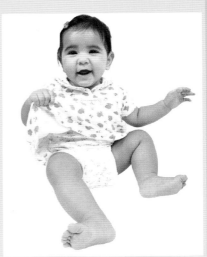

John was saddened when a two-year-old child was brought to his emergency room. The family and the child's nanny recounted that the baby had suddenly stopped breathing. The nanny, according to her version of the facts, gave mouth-to-mouth resuscitation and revived the child. John hospitalized the toddler and did a complete medical workup. He found no chronic diseases or current illnesses that could have accounted for this sudden loss of breath. He advised the parents to return to their pediatrician for ongoing care.

About three weeks later, the child once again was rushed to John's emergency room, this time completely unconscious. Despite all efforts, resuscitation was not possible, and the child died.

Once again, the nanny reported her vigilant and vigorous effort to revive the child who suddenly went lifeless. The parents, who arrived within several hours, violently confronted John, accusing him of misdiagnosing the child initially and thereby not preventing the child's ultimate death.

Most states require a medical review before a lawsuit can be filed, but John lives in a state where malpractice action can be started without an expert review or expert affidavit. The suit filed against John demanded millions of dollars in compensation for what the family called a preventable death due to John's misdiagnosis.

LEGAL ACTION and OUTCOME

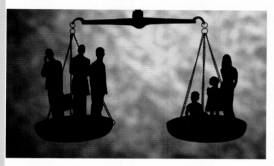

I had known John through his pioneering works in pediatric critical care and had come to admire him greatly. While most of the time I represent the parents of children who have been injured and killed, I did agree to represent John in what I believed to be a non-meritorious lawsuit brought against him.

We first requested that a detailed forensic autopsy be conducted to determine the exact cause of death. If John had misdiagnosed an ongoing disease or condition, it would clearly be seen on autopsy. The results of the autopsy indicated no ongoing condition; asphyxiation was determined to be the cause of death. Of important note were petechial hemorrhages in and around the child's eye, which to a trained forensic pathologist would indicate possible suffocation.

The question now, of course, was what caused the child to suffocate. Was it improper placement in the bed, entanglement in clothes, or intentional conduct?

On John's behalf, I hired a noted child abuse expert, one who had written the recognized textbooks in the area. After a complete workup, this expert determined that the death clearly was not accidental, but intentional.

The question then became, who was responsible? Was it someone in the immediate family or was it the nanny? A private detective was hired to research the background of the nanny, and troubling facts were revealed about her prior employment. In at least two of her earlier placements, she reported having "saved" a child-once from swallowing a toxic substance and the other from suffocation. Remarkably, while the parents of one of those children had suspicions about the nanny's involvement in the incident, they were afraid to pass along their suspicions when asked for a reference. Instead, they gave this worker a clean recommendation.

The lawyer for the parents- now faced with the clear fact that it was the nanny who caused the death-dramatically shifted gears. In court pleadings they now said that John should have suspected this on the child's first visit to the emergency room. We then retained a number of critical care emergency room pediatric experts to testify that under no circumstances should a reasonable critical care pediatrician be expected to suspect intentional criminal conducted based upon that first emergency room visit.

John and I defended the case for over three years. Finally, through a second lawyer, the family dismissed the lawsuit. No explanations were given and no apologies were extended.

John and I, and all those concerned, gained new insight into the power and responsibility held by nannies and what can occur with a nanny who is not a caregiver but a life-taker.

Statistics Tell the Story

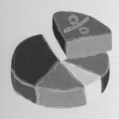

There are no statistics available for physical, sexual or emotional abuse by babysitters and nannies. But the news media report heartbreaking stories of abuse. Use the checklist to help avoid situations like these:

➩ A 23-year-old nanny, who claimed "nothing unusual happened," was convicted of mistreating a 16-month-old boy when a videotape showed her shaking, slapping and throwing the child against a wall in the home.

➩ A 62-year-old live-in nanny was caught on videotape slapping, kicking and smothering a 10-month-old baby girl.

➩ A babysitter was sentenced to four years in prison for molesting a two-year-old boy. The 31-year-old sitter was videotaped fondling, slapping, attempting to breast feed and smother the boy when she was caring for him in his grandmother's house. The grandmother had became suspicious of the woman and installed a tiny camera in an alarm clock in her home.

➩ A seven-month-old boy, who police say was shaken violently, was in a coma and not expected to survive. His babysitter, an 18-year-old male friend of the family, was charged with felony child abuse.

➩ An undocumented nanny with "good references" was charged with felony child abuse after a videotape showed her shaking a five-month-old girl so aggressively that "the baby's arms and legs whipped back and forth." In the United States illegally since 1997, the agency that placed her said "she came here with the proper identification." The agency claimed the 29-year-old nanny's references were checked.

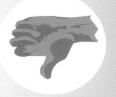

The laws and regulation vary from state to state and often from city to city, but more often than not- aside from a basic health check up- little is required of a potential caregiver.

In fact, many parents choose to entrust their children into the care of persons who are in our country illegally.

Taking Action

In order to diminish the potential for danger to your child at the hands of a nanny or babysitter, please follow the checklist below:

CHECKLIST

✔	⚠	⚠
1	Choose an older and more experienced caregiver to increase the safety index.	
2	If references are not provided, do not provide a job.	
3	Know the references, if possible.	
4	Don't depend exclusively on an agency.	
5	Role play with the caregiver.	
6	Provide the appropriate safety tools.	
7	Monitor the caregiver.	
8	Be aware of cultural differences with caregivers.	
9	Closely examine the child after the caregiver departs.	
10	Be aware that a smiling caregiver is not necessarily a happy caregiver.	

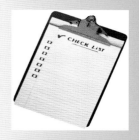

1. CHOOSE AN OLDER AND MORE EXPERIENCED CAREGIVER TO INCREASE THE SAFETY INDEX.

Many reported child abuse cases occur at the hands of very young, inexperienced caregivers. These individuals have no training in child development and will respond quite inappropriately to circumstances such as uninterrupted crying or the child not feeding properly. Experience and maturity generally brings a higher safety index.

2. IF REFERENCES ARE NOT PROVIDED, DO NOT PROVIDE A JOB.

The safety and well-being of your child is too important to be placed in the hands of someone you know nothing about. Always do a background check. This is no place for on-the-job training for someone without solid references.

In addition to references, the Internet provides a vast array of easy, checkable databases. First, most states have a registry of known sex offenders that can easily be checked. If you have been given information that your potential caregiver has resided in other states, it will be necessary to check those states as well, because the interstate transfer of information often fails. Please note that several states have followed the California model in having the Trust Line registry. For the cost of $124.00, the Trust Line will check out the proposed caregiver. Since its implementation in 1993, more than 4,000 potential caregivers have been denied clearance. This has included many convicted murderers and people with rap sheets longer than 15 pages. The Trust Line database was established at the demand of an anguished mother whose daughter was abused by a caregiver who was eventually convicted of felony child abuse but not barred from being a caregiver again.

Parents with resources may want to consider hiring a private detective. A local detective can be obtained by going to the National Association of Legal Investigators Web site, www.nalionline.org. Whether you do it yourself through a state database or hire an investigator, a complete background investigation must be done.

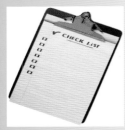

3. KNOW THE REFERENCES, IF POSSIBLE.

Unfortunately, many people give good references simply to appease the former employee in hopes of not angering them. Stress when you are talking to the reference that you want and deserve absolute candor. Ask questions like, "What's the worse thing you can say about Sally?" It is necessary to speak directly with the reference in order to gauge sincerity and credibility.

4. DON'T DEPEND EXCLUSIVELY ON AN AGENCY.

First, if you are using an agency, make sure that it is bonded. If it is not, that speaks volumes about the agency's attention to detail and professionalism. Further, review the agency's check sheet when confirming references. If possible, double-check the references to make sure that they were actually investigated, and the information is complete. Often, references are the only real information you have about the quality of the caregiver.

5. ROLE PLAY WITH THE CAREGIVER.

Engage in hypothetical questions, such as, "What do you do with a baby who won't stop crying? How would you respond to a child who refuses to feed? What is the proper way to deal with a child who has separation anxiety? If the child refuses to go to bed, how will you respond?" It is necessary to ask open-ended questions- that is, questions that do not suggest the correct answer. If you simply tell the caregiver what your expectations are when the child will not stop crying, will not feed, or will not go to bed, then you really have not examined whether the action of the caregiver will be appropriate. He or she will simply agree with you, and you will have a false sense of security.

6. PROVIDE THE APPROPRIATE SAFETY TOOLS.

Always point out the location of the fire extinguisher and how to use it. Don't just talk about the escape routes for a fire or an emergency- actually walk through the routes. Have available and point out the first-aid kit, and make sure the caregiver knows how to use its contents. And, finally, provide a detailed list of emergency phone numbers and specific reasons to call.

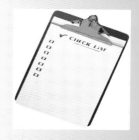

7. MONITOR THE CAREGIVER.

Nothing works better than unannounced visits. Return home early, or go back home in the middle of the time frame, saying that you forgot an item of clothing, for example. You are not going to know what goes on when you are not there if you do not make frequent, unannounced visits. Many people now use the "nanny cam" to record the nanny's interactions with a child while the parents are away, but it simply captures the abuse after it occurred, where unannounced visits could stop the abuse before it happens.

Remember: If you truly suspect abuse, don't wait until you capture it on videotape. Terminate the caregiver out of an abundance of caution and move on. It will provide you peace of mind.

8. BE AWARE OF CULTURAL DIFFERENCES WITH CAREGIVERS.

The trend in caregiving is to hire immigrants. This can provide a wonderful process of incorporating new Americans into our culture. However, cultural differences in child rearing can be a downside. Specifically, there can be wide differences in accepted discipline techniques and the level of interaction with children between our culture and those of other countries. Once again, ask the caregiver open-ended questions to determine how he or she will address certain situations. Don't simply ask the question that indicates your answer, because you are likely to simply get agreement.

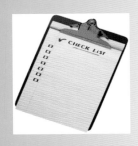

9. CLOSELY EXAMINE THE CHILD AFTER THE CAREGIVER DEPARTS.

If a child is left with an abusive caregiver, he or she will often have subtle marks or even bruising, so an examination is a good idea. Be aware, though, that most child abuse and neglect in its early stages does not leave any physical evidence. The child's disposition may change dramatically, too, so watch for subtle or obvious changes in mood after the caregiver leaves.

10. BE AWARE THAT A SMILING CAREGIVER IS NOT NECESSARILY A HAPPY CAREGIVER.

 Mountains of reported cases of child abuse by nannies and babysitters reveal deep anger and resentment towards the parents and/or the child. This anger is often taken out in the form of physical violence on the child. Often, the caregiver is considered happy and content, "a part of the family," until the moment of discovery.

There is a Web site for nannies, **www.nannynetwork.com**, which has a series of message boards. These message boards are intended to provide a venting place, but they reveal the unbelievably high degree of anger and hatred that many caregivers feel towards parents and the children in their care. They show that a smiling caregiver is not necessarily a happy caregiver.

38

On the Internet

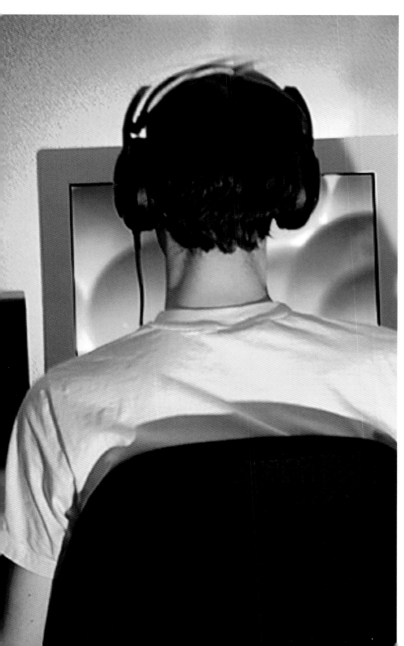

379

Caught in the Net

S amantha and Brett were very proud of their eight-year-old son, Julian. Julian gave them many reasons to be happy, but the fact that he was always striving to learn more especially pleased them. Julian was a whiz on the computer, too, far more proficient than his parents.

Aware that the Internet could present a danger as well as a great benefit for their child, Samantha and Brett installed a kiddy filter on their home computer to block pornographic material. They also considered purchasing a spy program to monitor Julian's chat room and email traffic, but they decided instead to periodically check his email box and trust him with chat room activities.

After school, Julian enjoyed going to the neighborhood recreation center. The center had basketball courts, art classes and other activities for children. Unbeknownst to Julian's parents, the center also maintained three computers with Internet access.

Late one night, Brett decided to take a peek at Julian's email box. He was shocked to find that the latest email was from an individual who was confirming a face-to-face meeting that weekend at a local park.

Julian's parents were unsure how to handle their discovery. Should they confront Julian about the intended nature of the rendezvous? Should they trust that their child exercised good judgment and would not place himself in harm's way? Samantha and Brett decided to talk with a police officer who attended their church. He advised them to take the matter extremely seriously. In fact, they agreed to set up a sting operation in which the child, without his knowledge, would be under surveillance on his trip to the park.

Two unmarked police cars and four detectives were present at the park on the day of the rendezvous. Julian believed that the person he was meeting was his age. Instead, the Internet acquaintance turned out to be a 40-year-old convicted child molester. He had two prior convictions in adjoining states and had recently moved to Julian's city.

Julian's parents were outraged that this meeting had been arranged despite all the precautions they took with their son using the Internet. They were surprised to learn that the recreation center had computers that were available to children. Julian explained that he spent time on the computer at the recreation center because he did not want his parents checking up on him.

LEGAL ACTION and OUTCOME

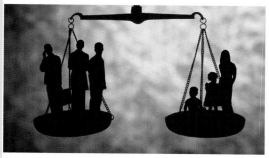

Samantha and Bret met with the directors of the recreation center and told them how close their family had come to suffering an irreversible tragedy. They requested that filters be installed on the center's computers and that all chat rooms on the center's computers be monitored. These, they felt, were reasonable requests in order to prevent a similar tragedy with another child. The recreation center's directors were unsympathetic, however. They responded that Julian's conduct was the result of bad parenting and not the center's responsibility. They remained adamant and would agree to change nothing.

The parents asked me to intervene. They were interested in finding out if an accommodation could be made without filing a lawsuit. But if a lawsuit became necessary to make the needed changes, the family was prepared to follow through so that no other family would experience a similar close call, or worse.

Face-to-face meetings and a drafting of the lawsuit followed a certified letter. The center's board of directors then overruled the on-site directors and mandated that city filters be installed immediately on the computers. They also directed that chat rooms be monitored or blocked from use. Further, the board of directors had installed spy software so that the use of the computers could be closely monitored.

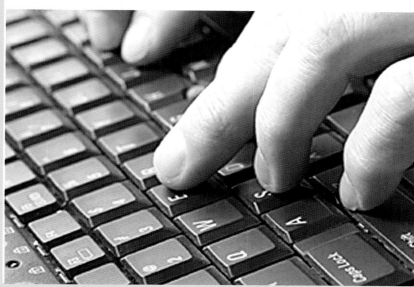

Because the center ultimately acted responsibly, no further action was required.

Statistics Tell the Story

Many of the statistics below from Protect Kids, a national Internet safety group (**www.protectkids.org**) paint an alarming picture:

⇨ More than two million American children ages six through 17 have their own personal Web sites, according to a December 2003 survey, "Children, Families and the Internet," by Grunwald Associates. This figure is 10 percent of the 23 million kids who have Internet access from home today- a threefold increase since 2000. Researchers project that more than six million American children- more than one in four of kids online from home- will have their own personal Web sites by 2005.

⇨ Only one-third of households with Internet access are proactively protecting their children with filtering or blocking software. *(Center for Missing and Exploited Children)*

⇨ Seventy-five percent of children are willing to share personal information online about themselves and their families in exchange for goods and services. *(eMarketer)*

⇨ About 25 percent of the youth who encountered a sexual approach or solicitation on the Internet told a parent. *(Youth Internet Safety Survey)*

⇨ One in five U.S. teenagers who regularly log on to the Internet say they have received an unwanted sexual solicitation via the Web. Solicitations were defined as requests to engage in sexual activities or sexual talk, or to give personal sexual information. *(Crimes Against Children Research Center)*

⇨ One in 33 youth received an aggressive sexual solicitation in the past year. This means a predator asked a young person to meet somewhere, called a young person on the phone, and/or sent the young person correspondence, money, or gifts through the U.S. Postal Service. *(Youth Internet Safety Survey)*

⇨ Seventy-seven percent of the targets for online predators are age 14 or older. Another 22 percent are ages 10 to 13. *(Crimes Against Children Research Center)*

⇨ Seventy-five percent of youth solicited online were not troubled children, 10 percent did not use chat rooms, and nine percent did not talk to strangers. *(Crimes Against Children Research Center)*

⇨ Only 17 percent of youth and 11 percent of parents could name a specific authority, such as the Federal Bureau of Investigation (FBI), CyberTipline, or an Internet service provider, to which they could report an Internet crime. *(Youth Internet Safety Survey)*

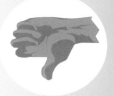

A bewildering assortment of laws have been passed recently to protect children from online pedophiles, Internet pornography and advertisers. Some laws have been challenged and overturned; others have been upheld. Much of the proposed legislation never gets past the committee stage.

The bottom line is: The government is not going to protect your child. Since the purpose of this and other chapters is prevention, I urge you to abide by the following checklist to keep your child safe from predators.

Taking Action

As Julian's parents understood, the Internet provides a valuable service for our children, but it also poses great potential for danger. Parents must take appropriate precautions to keep children safe while using the Internet. The following checklist is recommended:

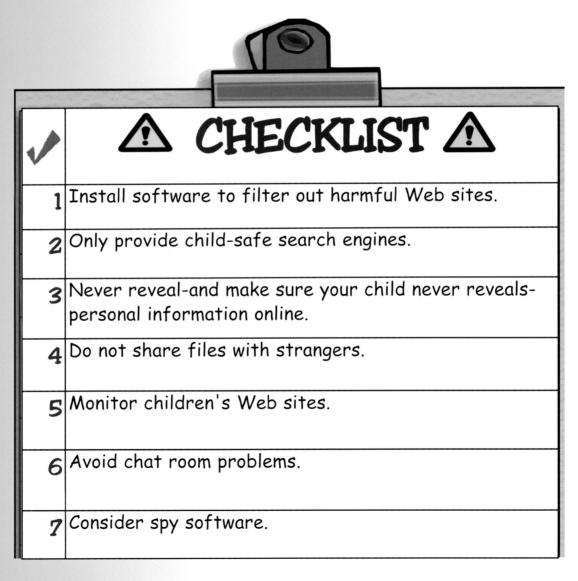

⚠️ CHECKLIST ⚠️

✔	
1	Install software to filter out harmful Web sites.
2	Only provide child-safe search engines.
3	Never reveal-and make sure your child never reveals-personal information online.
4	Do not share files with strangers.
5	Monitor children's Web sites.
6	Avoid chat room problems.
7	Consider spy software.

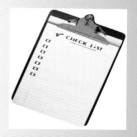

1. INSTALL SOFTWARE TO FILTER OUT HARMFUL WEB SITES.

Software to filter out harmful Web sites can be downloaded for free or purchased. The most well known of these filters for children is Net Nanny; according to most rating services, it works effectively.

Also check with your online service provider; it may offer specific tools to protect children while they are online.

The technology changes so quickly. Go online to the rating services and secure the very best. It is the first line of defense.

2. ONLY PROVIDE CHILD-SAFE SEARCH ENGINES.

There are a number of child-safe search engines, including:

> *Yahooligans*-A database with approximately 20,000 kid-safe sites, this engine has a directory that the child can easily access.

> *Education World*-This is a database with nearly 60,000 sites.

> *Ask Jeeves for Kids*-This is the *Ask Jeeves* search engine that has been filtered for children.

> *Kids Click*-Developed by librarians for children, this engine contains a number of databases.

> *Important for Google users*: Go to the *Google* preferences screen, and you will see that you can use your *Google* with a filter.

3. NEVER REVEAL- AND MAKE SURE YOUR CHILD NEVER REVEALS- PERSONAL INFORMATION ONLINE.

Adults- and most importantly children- should never disclose addresses (home or school), phone numbers, or any information that could tell a predator how to reach a child. Counsel your child not to release this information under any circumstances.

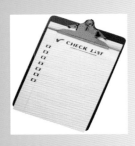

4. DO NOT SHARE FILES WITH STRANGERS.

File-sharing programs allow you to share your files with others on the Internet and vice versa. This exciting new technology is particularly attractive to children. Because file sharing can reveal identities and share intimate information regarding the family and the life of a child, no file sharing should occur with strangers.

5. MONITOR CHILDREN'S WEB SITES.

It is not uncommon for children to create their own Web sites. For the most part, this is a fun activity that bolsters self-esteem. But children may inadvertently place on their Web site information that reveals their identity and location. Such Web sites put a bull's eye on the back of the child and make him or her common prey for predators with a keyboard.

6. AVOID CHAT ROOM PROBLEMS.

An easy avenue for new friendships, chat rooms are very popular, especially among teenagers. Follow these rules to avoid chat room problems:

(a) Do not let your child chat in an unmoderated chat room. There are reputable companies that run reputable chat rooms; these are monitored at all times.

(b) Choose a screen name for your child that does not reveal either the child's email address or the child's actual identity. This can help prevent a predator from contacting your child; it can also prevent unwarranted spam mail.

(c) Consider purchasing software that blocks sensitive personal information from being transmitted through your child's chat.

UNDER NO CIRCUMSTANCES SHOULD YOUR CHILD AGREE TO A PERSONAL MEETING WITH ANYONE THEY COME IN CONTACT WITH IN A CHATROOM. THIS IS FAR TOO DANGEROUS AN ACTIVITY AND MUST BE PROHIBITED.

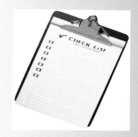

7. CONSIDER SPY SOFTWARE.

There are a number of very sophisticated spy software programs that enable a parent to monitor every keystroke of a child- from a distant email, to Web sites visited, to conversations in chat rooms. The spy software captures and transmits everything your child does on the Internet.

This type of software provides the highest level of personal security for your child. Parents must discuss whether or not to use such software with their children. Some parents have spy software loaded on the child's computer immediately, while others wait until there is a reason to be concerned. Still other parents wish after a tragedy that they had loaded it earlier, as a preventative measure. Of course, this is a very personal decision, one that is left up to the judgment of parents. However, if you believe that your child may be in harm's way when he or she is using the Internet, error on the side of safety.

Perhaps the most reliable spy software on the market now is *eBlaster*. It can be found at www.spy-software-directory.com.

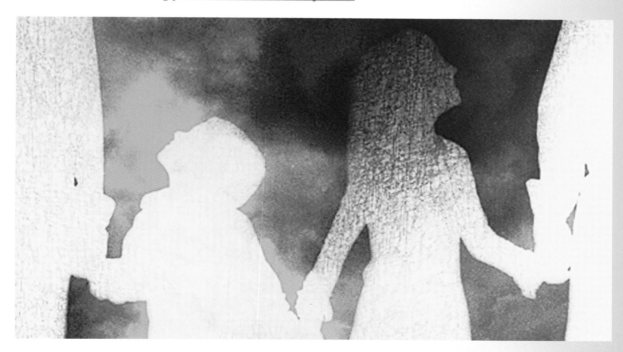

Part Seven

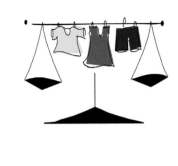

Epilogue

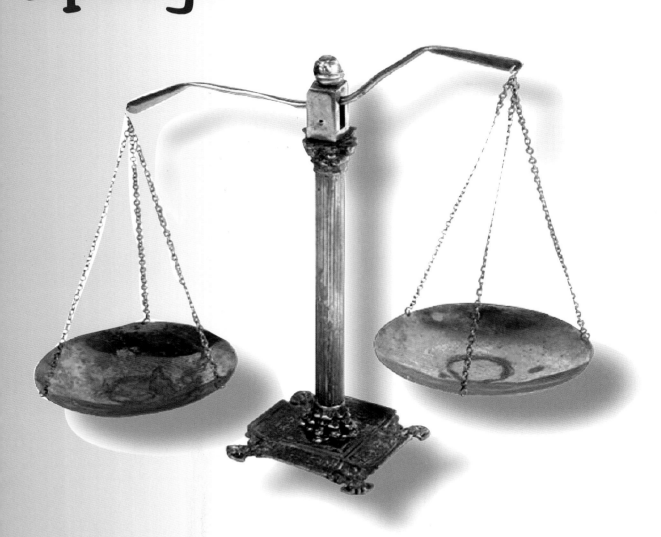

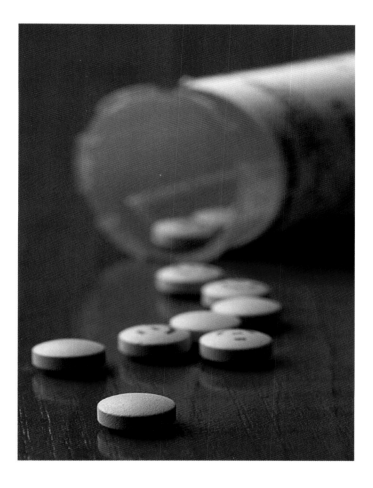

Technology, safety and the law are all evolutionary. Unfortunately, often children are harmed or die before the science establishes a clear cause and effect relationship. Often, even after the cause and effect is established, it may take years before regulations are in place that will assist in preventing injuries and deaths.

Take the case of my client Brian Lykins, a young boy who underwent elective knee surgery in November of 2001. Brian was among the 750,000 people every year who receive an inserted piece of cadaver tissue during their operation. The advantages include shorter surgery time and eliminate the need to harvest a portion of the patient's body. Virtually all knee, ankle and burn surgeries use cadaver tissue in some manner. The need for cadaver tissue created a billion dollar industry against the backdrop of no safety regulations. When Brian died of overwhelming infection, there were only two conditions that would disqualify a cadaver: an AIDS infected cadaver or Hepatitis infected cadaver. Beyond those two disqualifiers, there were no regulations concerning the safety of the industry in any manner.

Through our investigation we discovered that the cadaver from which the tissue implanted into Brian originated had been unrefrigerated for 19 hours. One does not have to be a scientist to understand the danger that decay and infectious processes create when cadavers are left unrefrigerated for long periods of time. Remarkably, when Brian died, no one suspected the cadaver insert; but because of the occurrence of Sept.11 the month before, health professionals in Minnesota suspected Anthrax. Because of the potential link to Sept.11, the CDC did a massive investigation as to the cause of Brian's death only to discover it was the unrefrigerated cadaver that had killed him.

Over the several years of litigating Brian's case, all of the failures of the cadaver industry were revealed. The absence of safety procedures was simply unbelievable. After the case was concluded, Brian's parents, Steve and Leslie, courageously walked the halls of Congress. Through their passionate efforts, *The Brian Lykins Bill* was introduced in Congress, which would mandate the FDA promulgate safety rules and regulations for this industry. In March of 2005, nearly 900 pages of regulations went into effect, making safe this previously unsafe industry.

Looking back, without Sept.11, the doctors would have never linked Brian's death to the unsafe practices of a billion dollar industry. Even today, there may be hundreds, if not thousands, of persons injured by the cadaver industry's unsafe practices, that now are safe due to the Lykins' Regulations.

Therefore, there are a number of potential causes of child injuries and death which are not yet fully established. However, out of an abundance of caution, we want to review six of the more prominent areas.

Autism Caused by Infant Vaccines

Autism is a developmental disability that generally appears between the ages of 15 months and 20 months. In most cases, the child is progressing normally, and then begins to regress, losing speech, social skills and physical abilities. While there are varying degrees of severity, most children completely withdraw into a world of their own. (**www.autismspeaks.org**)

Cause: Autism is believed to be genetic, but some strongly believe the genetic components are triggered by environmental factors. The most often "triggering" event believed by some is childhood vaccines. The manufacturers use a preservative ingredient in childhood vaccines called Thimerosal, and its key ingredient is mercury. It is believed that the mercury ingested into the infant triggers the autism.

To date, there is some, but not strong, epidemiology studies to support this cause argument. For an excellent overview of the controversy, read *New York Times* reporter David Kirby's *Evidence of Harm* 2005.

Statistics: There is no debate that autism is the fastest-growing serious developmental disability in the United States. According to the National Institutes of Health (**www.nih.gov**), there are 1.77 million cases of autism diagnosed each year. That means that every 20 minutes, there is a new case of autism diagnosed. That rate translates into 24,000 new cases a year, the bottom line being ONE IN 166 CHILDREN ARE DIAGNOSED WITH AUTISM.

Current Status: The grandchild of Bob Wright, the Chairman of General Electric and CEO of NBC, was diagnosed at the age of two and a half years old with autism. This tragic event propelled Bob and his wife, Suzanne, to launch a vigorous public awareness campaign in 2005, beginning with the cover story in the February 28, 2005 issue of *Newsweek*. Thereafter, an explosion of news stories occurred, centering on the efforts of the national organization, Autism Speaks (**www.autismspeaks.org**), which is the most comprehensive and definitive Web site on autism, including treatment centers, experts and updated medical studies.

The dedication of Bob and Suzanne is greatly appreciated, as is Bernie Marcus, the co-founder of Home Depot, who has for many years been involved in autism advocacy and research funding. A note should also be given to the Kennedy Krieger Center, which is a division of Johns Hopkins, and specifically Dr. Gary Goldstein.

Status of the vaccine cause link: In interviews, both Bob and Suzanne have said that the vaccine-linked autism is still to be determined. Lawyers have formed litigation groups, and many lawsuits have been filed. One such group alleges industry cover-up of studies. They claim that the CDC did a study which established the link, and then due to pharmaceutical industry pressure, those studies were withdrawn.

In addition to the weak evidence link, such vaccine suits are fraught with legal obstacles. There is the Vaccine Injury Compensation Program (VICP) law passed in 1986, and there has recently been proposed legislation to eliminate drug company responsibility for any damage.

In my opinion, there simply is not enough scientific evidence to support vaccine-induced autism lawsuits; thus, my firm has declined all invitations to join the ongoing lawsuits or to file new litigation. Should studies in the future reveal a stronger link, and if Congress does not grant total immunity to the pharmaceutical industry, the position of my law firm could change.

Preventative measures: Although there is not a clear evidence link between vaccines and autism to support a successful lawsuit, there are clear reasons to take all precautions so that your child does not receive the Thimerosal agent in your child's vaccines. Johns Hopkins has a complete Web site on vaccine safety, **www.vaccinesafety.edu**, and does contain a separate Thimerosal table indicating by brand name how much of the Thimerosal is present in each drug. The industry has promised to phase out Thimerosol in the future.

BOTTOM LINE: Immunizations are very important and should be done, but make sure the vaccine given to your child does not contain Thimerosol. **Very important:** Make sure you look at the label of the vaccine to satisfy yourself. I've given this advice to several friends who were told by a nurse or doctor, "there's no Thimerosol in the shot"...they demanded to see the bottle, and, clearly, the nurse or doctor was wrong. Thimerosol was on the label. They simply went to another clinic were Thimerosol was not on the label.

Cell Phone Use by Children

Today nearly all teenagers and even younger children have cell phones. Yet how dangerous are cell phones to the still developing brains of our children?

In December of 2004, there was a Swedish and Dutch research project which established a link between the radiation from cell phones and impairment of brain function.

In January of 2005, the prestigious United Kingdom's National Radiological Protection Board (*NRPB*) issued an advisory warning after conducting a number of studies. The Board indicated "a precautionary approach" to cell phone use in children. The study acknowledged that there was not firm evidence that cell phone radiation is harmful but warned that the possibility also could not be ruled out. The chairman of the committee, Sir William Stewart, stated, "I don't think we can put our hands on our hearts and say mobile phones are safe for children."

Many public health officals in our country have urged caution and suggests limiting the cell phone use of children.

BOTTOM LINE: Limit your child's cell phone use. Choose a program that has a limited number of minutes.

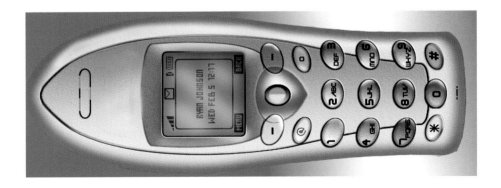

Molds are simple, microscopic organisms present virtually everywhere, indoors and outdoors. Mold is particularly prevalent in any location that has a large amount of rain and high humidity.

Although mold grows and thrives in wet, humid conditions, it is when it begins to dry out that toxic spores are produced and dispersed. It is these spores that are produced that create the next generation of mold, which can potentially be very dangerous to the developing immune systems of children. There are known tests for mold toxic levels in the blood.

Symptoms include eye irritation, coughing, nosebleeds, fatigue, muscle pains, undetermined diarrhea and loss of concentration.

The literature indicates that the danger from molds depends greatly on the mold concentration (mold counts) and the specific individual's sensitivity. With children and developing immune systems, the sensitivity can be quite high.

Over the last 10 years, there has been an explosion of mold-induced litigation. Some litigation centers on real estate values. That is non-disclosure of a mold problem to a new homeowner, and the lawsuit is then one involving the value of the real estate. There has been much litigation concerning whether existing insurance covers preexisting and newly existing mold damage. Even the TV star "The Incredible Hulk," Lou Ferrigno, brought suit for toxic mold damage at his home.

There have been several reports concerning mold damage to children while attending elementary schools. In 2002, McKinley Elementary School in Fairfield, Connecticut was closed because of mold exposure to 60 students with two requiring hospitalization. Further, South Carolina reported a case where parents sued the school system and contractors concerning a mold-induced injury to their nine-year-old son. A settlement was reached with the contracting company. However, the school board was granted governmental immunity. North Carolina reached the same result in declaring the Robeson County school system to be immune from civil lawsuits.

There is a raging debate among experts concerning the validity of mold litigation. The Internet is full of those supporting litigation and those debunking the scientific basis for such suits.

My law firm has reviewed an excess of 50 potential claims of toxic mold exposure to children and accepted only one case, which was clear and convincing. In the remaining cases, my law firm was unable to find merit because of a lack of scientific causation.

Mold litigation is clearly on the rise. The extent of future success is subject to debate.

BOTTOM LINE: Have your home tested regularly and if high levels of mold are discovered, use a professional service to remove the mold.

Coal-Burning Power Plants

There are currently hundreds of coal-burning power plants in virtually every state of the country. According to Clean The Air, an environmental advocacy group (www.cleantheair.org):

1. Fifty six percent of all U.S. power plants are fueled by coal.

2. Power plants are responsible for over 64 percent of the annual sulfur dioxide emissions in the United States.

3. Of all power plants, the coal-fired boilers generate more than 93 percent of the power industry's nitrogen oxide, 88 percent of its carbon dioxide and 99 percent of its mercury.

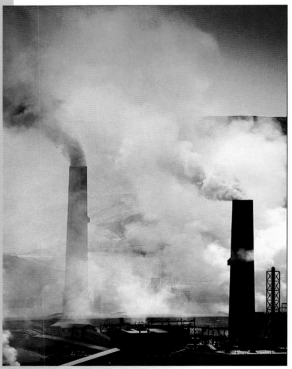

Clean The Air has on their Web site a state by state assessment of the damage done by coal-burning power plants. In the state of Georgia for example there is an epidemic of asthma cases, 409,700. According to Dr. Lorne Garrison of the Emory University School of Medicine, "We are in the midst of an epidemic of asthma among children, and air pollution is one of the triggers."

Clean The Air explains that children are more exposed to the emissions because they play outside during the summer when ozone levels are highest, and children breathe 50 percent more air per pound of body weight then adults. Also, according to Clean The Air, there are hundreds of premature deaths in Georgia annually due to power plant sulfur dioxide emissions.

Although there has been a number of successful environmental litigation cases, over the last several years, experts believe that air pollution is the most difficult to prove. In order to establish a meritorious case, one must demonstrate that the harm to the child was a direct, or as the law calls, "proximate cause" of the child's injuries. At the present time, there has not been any epidemiology studies conducted to be able to establish a clear link. Currently, there is ongoing intense investigation by a number of health professionals to establish the necessary link.

The air pollution discussed above has occurred in the spite of the 1972 *Federal Clean Air Act,* which was intended to eliminate harmful emissions. Unfortunately, all of the old coal-burning power plants were "grandfathered" and are not subject to the Act. Furthermore, during recent years, enforcement action of known violations by the Environmental Protection Agency has been withdrawn. There have been several public resignations by leading EPA officials protesting the lack of enforcement.

BOTTOM LINE: While there is not enough solid evidence to commence litigation, there is clearly enough data to alert parents of the danger to their children. Unfortunately, about the only preventative measure available is decreasing the child's time outside and exposure to outside air. However, given the explosion in childhood obesity, exercise must be encouraged. In fact, research indicates that another factor of childhood asthma is childhood obesity.

Electric Power Lines (EMF)

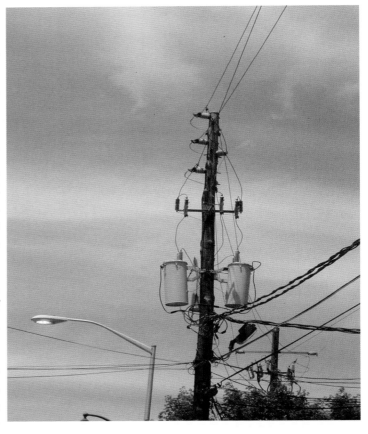

The dangers of Electro Magnetic Fields (EMF) from power lines has been hotly debated among scientists, politicians and journalists for nearly 25 years.

By 1990, there had been over 100 studies conducted world wide in an attempt to link EMFs to serious health dangers. These studies were quite contradictory and no common ground emerged.

In response to public pressure, the EPA was given the task of reviewing all literature and reaching conclusions.

In the draft report issued in March of 1990 the EPA recommended that EMFs be classified as a Class B carcinogen, a probable human carcinogen joining the ranks of formaldehyde, DDT, dioxins and PCBs.

A great deal of lobbying occurred from the utility industry, scientific community and many lobbyists such that the final EPA report deleted the notation that EMFs would be classified as a Class B carcinogen. Instead, the EPA final report indicated the following:

"At this time, such a characterization regarding the link between cancer and exposure to EMFs is not appropriate because of the basic nature of the interaction between EMFs, and biological processes leading to cancer is not understood."

The debate still rages. The Institute of Electrical and Electronic Engineers (IEEE) issued a detailed report in 1999 which can be read at **http://ewh.ieee.org/soc/embs/comar/brodeur.htm**. The report title: "*Unfounded Fears: The Great Power Line Cover-up Exposed.*"

Clearly, there is no consensus among the scientific community nor the legislatures. Any litigation concerning damage or death caused by EMFs would lack the necessary causation element and at this time would not be meritorious.

BOTTOM LINE: While there is not enough evidence to support litigation concerning an injury or death to a child, there is at least enough information to alert any potential homebuyer.

Do not buy a home within close proximity of large electrical power lines. Furthermore, do not let your children play around large electrical power lines.

Better to be safe than sorry.

Food Litigation

The poster child for frivolous lawsuits was once the McDonald's hot coffee spill case. However, recently another McDonald's case has become synonymous with frivolous litigation: The man who sued McDonald's because he got fat eating exclusively McDonald's. Fortunately, the case was tossed out of court, but not before it unleashed a multitude of state legislators banning all suits against food manufacturers on all grounds, a typical knee-jerk political reaction.

The law has always recognized that if a person understands a risk and knowingly undertakes and assumes the risk, they cannot later complain of their injury. The "McDonald's Made Me Fat" lawsuit was tossed because it's common knowledge that eating every meal at McDonalds will put anyone at risk for gaining weight. The importance is the knowledge of the risk.

In our heightened consumer age, we are all taught to read the labels and make our choices based on what we assume is true information. If we know the information and assume the risk of eating the food, then we can't hold the restaurant or food manufacturer responsible.

In the past and currently, there are a number of situations where the labels were false and deceptive, and instances where advertising was also false. Ironically, McDonald's faced a lawsuit filed by several George Washington University students because McDonald's failed to disclose and, in fact, covered up the fact they used beef fat in their French fries. McDonald's settled that lawsuit in 2002 and now makes full disclosure. Also in 2002, two successful lawsuits were filed against snack food manufacturers for fraudulently listing their fat and calorie content as low calorie. Evidence revealed that the low calorie snack actually was more unhealthy and higher in calories than the normal brand, thus causing the manufactures to settle those cases.

When the New York judge tossed the "McDonald's Made Me Fat" lawsuit, he set forth in the legal decision two ways a fast food restaurant may be responsible for a person's injuries. First, a restaurant is responsible if food additives are put in the food, which can create an addiction and are not disclosed to the general public. Second, as we saw in the cases discussed, a restaurant is at fault if the advertising is deceptive.

One of the big issues is the use of addictive additives in food by the food industries. Rachel and Richard Heller, retired doctors at the Mount Sinai School of Medicine Hospital in New York City, described in their recent text, "The Seven Day Low-Carb Rescue and Recovery Plan" (Dutton 2004), a number of foods that have addictive additives, of which the public is completely unaware.

Take the additive monosodium glutamate (MSG), used by nearly one-third of all restaurants and added to many foods. According to the Heller's, it's an additive that causes most people to consume more food or eat that food more often. Unfortunately, most restaurants don't disclose the MSG, and most labels don't disclose it either.

In the early 1990's, the use of monosodium glutamate (MSG) had reached a controversial boiling point that caused the FDA to issue a position paper, www.cfsan.fda.gov. In the position statement, the FDA concluded that MSG was "generally recognized as safe," but did detail a number of possible side-effects and indicated a growing number of people who have an allergy or reactive syndrome to MSG. Unfortunately, the FDA did not mandate labeling of MSG such that many books and guides now contain lists of foods which contain glutamates under different terms. If labeling were required, identification of MSG in our food would be easily secured. However, now those wishing to avoid MSG must carry a list of 30 names to the supermarket in order to protect against MSG ingestion. For example, a normal can of tuna, according to the Hellers, includes MSG if the label states "broth or hydrolyzed protein," even though MSG is nowhere on the can.

As our body of knowledge increases regarding food supplements, additives and addictive agents, so will the science concerning the damage that these ingredients can cause. Thus, while scientific evidence does not support lawsuits at the present time, clearly in the future deceptive advertising and deceptive labeling will be the target of lawsuits, and these suits will stop such practices, while the FDA has done nothing.

For an excellent guide to understanding food and childhood obesity, read the book, *Slim and Fit Kids; Raising Healthy Children in a Fast Food World* (HCI Publications), by John Monaco, M.D., one of our nations leading pediatricians.

BOTTOM LINE: In the meantime continue to read the labels and learn about the other words the food industry uses to cover-up bad ingredients and give your children the purest food to consume.

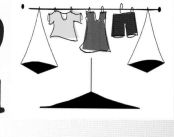

40
The Jury Has Reached a Verdict

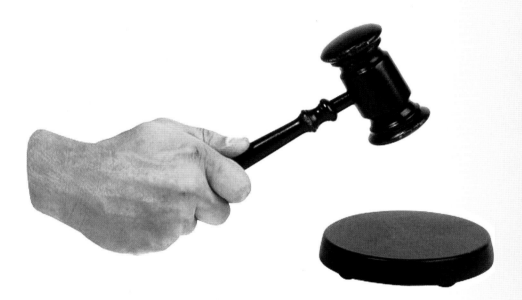

New Hazards to Eliminate

As noted in the first chapter of this final part of the book, science and the law evolve. Unlike the previous six hazards, the following two hazards now have solid evidence to demand regulation and to support litigation to make the respective industries make safer products.

Environmental Toxins in the Home

Over the last several years, my law firm has successfully handled a number of child injury and several child death cases from exposure to household or lawn care toxic substances. In fact, our first case in this area was toxic exposure to the fetus during pregnancy. The child's mother was an office worker assigned to the copy room. She worked until the last three weeks of her pregnancy and gave birth to a seriously deformed child. After retaining a team of epidemiologists and pharmacologists, we were able to establish a link between the chemicals used in the copy machine and the defect in the child.

The area of toxic exposure is a new area of law which will see a lot of activity in the coming years.

Since World War II, there have been over 80,000 new synthetic chemical compounds developed and released into the environment. Fewer than half of these have been tested for their potential toxicity to humans, and even a smaller amount has been assessed for their particular harm to children.

Researchers are now finding that some chemicals cause damage to the child's developing brain, while others cause cancer or mimic or block hormone development.

Beginning in 1993, there has been a clear recognition that children are far more vulnerable to toxic substances than adults. This was the finding of the National Academy of Sciences (NAS) and the Environmental Protection Agency (EPA).

Why are babies and children more vulnerable?

1. Their immune systems are not fully developed and, therefore, far more susceptible to the damage from toxins.

2. Children's bodies are still developing, so that the chemicals can harm and retard development.

3. Pound for pound, children breathe more air, drink more water, and eat more food than adults; thus, they are exposed to a greater "volume" of air, water pollution and pesticides.

4. On the issue of lawn products, children tend to play outdoors more than adults, increasing exposure.

5. Children often play on or near the floor and get into areas where there is dust and heavier-than-air chemicals.

6. Children have oral fixations and like to put objects in their mouths.

Unfortunately, it is impossible to cover the area of toxic exposure dangers adequately in this chapter. Fortunately, there is an outstanding national organization which can be your advocate and assist you in removing hazards in your home.

Nancy and Jim Chuda founded the Children's Health Environmental Coalition (CHEC) in 1992, (www.checnet.org). Sadly, Nancy and Jim lost their young daughter, Collette, to a cancer known as Wilm's Tumor. Later research clearly concluded that pesticide exposure caused the child's death. From this tragic recognition, Nancy and Jim, against all odds, started CHEC, which has grown to an amazing network of solid information, all set forth on their Web site. Among the information is a comprehensive review of the "state of children's health environment," which is downloadable. There is an amazing "virtual house," which is a point and click screen that will take you through all areas of the home and give you pointers on how to remove the hazards in your home. There is an extensive resource library, and should you choose to become an advocate in this area, there are several "paint by the numbers" lists to help you get started.

Hopefully, through the vision of Nancy and Jim, and your help, these dangerous toxins can be kept out of harm's way of our children.

Stevens-Johnson Syndrome: Motrin

In 2005, my law firm started receiving a surprising number of calls from parents of children who had contracted Stevens-Johnson Syndrome (SJS). SJS is an abrupt, severe injury to the eyes, skin and mouth where there are large sheets of mucosa or skin that are destroyed and then shed.

Our law firm already knew that SJS is most commonly caused by severe and adverse reactions to medication and that often the drug is a Non-Steroidal Anti-Inflammatory Drug (NSAIDs). The results can be devastating: death, blindness, lung damage, permanent loss of nail beds, scarring of the esophagus, chronic fatigue syndrome and many more.

The indications are: commonly severe rashes and blisters, persistent fever, flu-like symptoms, swelling of the eyelids and redness of the eye.

While SJS can affect persons of all ages, a large amount of its victims are children due to the overall sensitivity of children in general.

In taking these parents calls, it became apparent that the common denominator was children's Motrin, manufactured by Johnson and Johnson, and its subsidiary, McNeil Consumer and Specialty Pharmaceutics, a leading NSAID.

For years, the effective ingredients in Motrin were obtainable only by prescription. During this time, the manufacturers clearly informed the prescribing doctors and ultimately all patients of the risk that taking the drug may cause Stevens-Johnson Syndrome. However, when the drug became an over-the-counter drug accessible to the general public, the warnings were dropped. Other makers of NSAIDs did continue to provide clear warnings of SJS.

Without the warnings, none of our complaining parents had any knowledge that Motrin, one of the most common childhood over-the-counter drugs, could cause such devastation in their children.

There now have been a number of lawsuits filed against Johnson and Johnson in addition to the many filed by my office. One of them details the death of a nine year-old who took Motrin and died 20 months later from complications of SJS, that case being concluded by a confidential settlement. The other cases involve blindness and/or severe and permanent skin damage to the face and extremities of the child.

The Stevens-Johnson Foundation, started by the parents of one of the victims, Jean McCawley, reports that they are receiving two new documented cases of Motrin-induced SJS a month.

Many of the victims have banned together to ask the FDA to require warnings on Motrin. In April of 2005, the FDA announced that it now requires warnings on all NSAIDs, including Moltrin.(www.fda.gov/bbs/topics/news/2005/NEW01171.html)

Because of the severity and frequency of these injuries, we have decided to assign one lawyer to these cases and bring a lawsuit against the manufacturer, demanding justice for the families and mandating warning labels in the future.

There is one bit of good news: According to the American Academy of Ophthalmology (www.aao.org), there is now a new treatment for SJS which appears to halt the damage progression to blindness if timely instituted. No such intervention exists for the other horrible damages from SJS.

BOTTOM LINE: Motrin, other ibuprofen drugs, prescription drugs and over-the-counter drugs continue to be very important in the treatment of children. However, everyone needs to be aware of the potential side effects, including SJS, and act quickly to prevent damage.

Conclusion

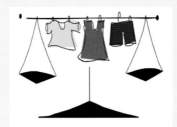

The two years that it has taken to write this text has been for me both bitter and sweet. Bitter, because it has forced me to revisit the many cases I have handled, which are contained at the beginning of each chapter. Bitter, because each of those cases were emotionally draining, depressing and heartbreaking. But my emotional despair over these tragedies pales in comparison to the daily heartbreak and tears experienced by the families of these catastrophically injured children and those who have passed away. Frankly, I wonder how these families make it through each day. Sweet, because from these tragedies, we have learned the tools of prevention. It is my sincere hope that from these tragedies, and the recognition of the prevention tools, the reader of this book will recognize the reality of what could happen and take action now to prevent similar tragedies in the future.

Catastrophic injury and deaths of children can be prevented with proper vigilance, recognition and follow-through by the caregivers of children. Observation, recognition and action is required not only by the parents and caregivers, but also by the teachers, the coaches, the next door neighbors and all those who hold the lives of children to be precious. If I am never required to represent a catastrophically injured child again, then I will be a happy man. If this book contributes to the saving of only one child, then it is well worth the effort.

I would like to open a dialogue with all readers. If you have encountered hazards in your child's world that are not contained in this book, or you have used the tools of prevention which are not detailed in this book, I would be very appreciative to hear from you. Simply contact me at my law firm at 1-800-677-2025 or email me at <u>donkeenan@keenanskidsfoundation.com</u>.

Appendix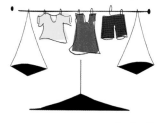

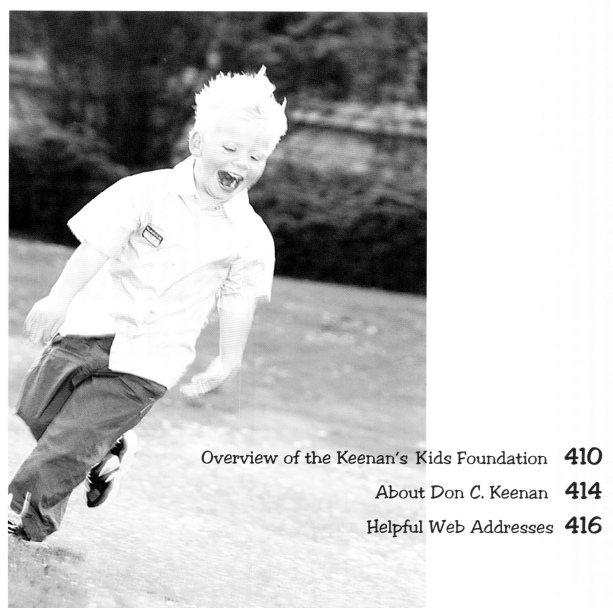

Overview of the Keenan's Kids Foundation

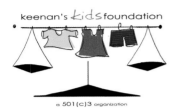

Mission Statement and Projects

Since 1993, a 501 (c)(3) Non-profit organization

Children at-risk do not vote and have neither paid lobbyists nor high-powered public relations firms. Consequently, the interests of these children are often considered unimportant and are lost in the system. Thus Keenan's Kids Foundation was formed in 1993 to address three separate needs: Community Awareness, Child Advocacy and Charity.

 Community Awareness

In keeping with Don Keenan's one-third solution philosophy, after a lawsuit has been completed, we look for ways to take the prevention lessons learned and create a safety awareness program. Here are a couple of examples:

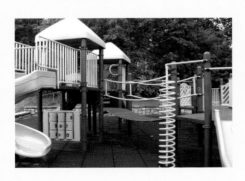

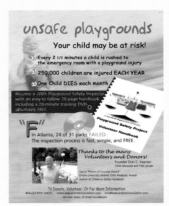

Playground Safety Project

Commenced in 2001, the project is a hands-on report card system to grade the safety of playgrounds. Noted playground safety expert, Dr. Frances Wallach, devised a simple ten-point report card and assisted in our training manual and instructional DVD. Each year, our safety project has been featured on NBC's *Today Show*. To learn more about how you can use the report card system to grade your local playgrounds, go to **www.keenanskidsplaygroundsafety.com**

As profiled in the summer 2005 issue of *Imagine* Magazine, Don Keenan has developed his one-third solution. One third of the work is devoted to achieving justice for the injured child and family. One-third of it is public awareness of the danger once the case is concluded, and one-third is effort for legislative and/or regulatory change. While the case tragedy is irreversible, the one-third solution provides a prevention program to stop the reoccurrence of the tragedy.

Toy Safety Project

Since 1993, Keenan's Kids Foundation has released, around the holiday season, a list of the ten most dangerous toys. We hold a national press conference and open our Web site with photos and descriptions of the toys. You may view the dangerous toys lists at **www.keenanskidsfoundation.com**

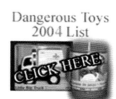

Dangerous Toys 2004 List

Additional Projects

Airbag Safety Project

Keenan's Kids Foundation was one of the first public interest groups to recognize passenger airbag dangers for children. Prior to warning labels being mandated, we conducted a number of public awareness campaigns.

School Safety Project

The majority of our nation's public schools are unprotected from the "stranger danger" problem, deranged people entering our schools to hurt children. We have conducted several public awareness and prevention campaigns.

Bio-Tissue Safety Project

Nearly a million operations each year use cadaver tissue, with a high number of these surgeries involving children. In 2003, we launched a public awareness campaign about the lack of federal regulations and also gave congressional testing, which resulted in a safe cadaver issue industry.

Gun Safety Project

Because of the high number of children who die each year from unintended gun wounds, for over five years, we have had booths in area malls and stores to distribute free gun locks.

Child Advocacy

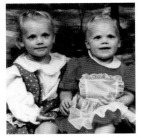

Kathy Jo v. DFACS
First U.S. case to establish
constitutional rights
for foster kids

Beginning in the early 1980s, we handled the case of Kathy Joe v. DFACS, which went to the U.S. Supreme Court, establishing for the first time that foster children had constitutional rights.

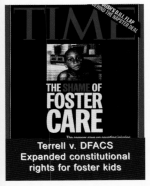

Terrell v. DFACS
Expanded constitutional
rights for foster kids

The case was followed by the late 1990's case of Terrell Peterson, a tortured six-year-old who weighed only 29 pounds when he died. *60 Minutes* and the cover of *Time* magazine were examples of the national coverage of his lawsuit which led to sweeping changes in the child prevention system.

In 2004, we successfully lobbied the passage of Georgia's first child endangerment law by using TV commercials and billboards.

Occasionally we will offer free legal help to children in need. In early 2002, we undertook the representation in New York City of a 12 year-old boy who was forced at knife point to swallow 97 condoms filled with heroin. This act occurred when the boy was in Nigeria. He surrendered himself at the New York Airport upon his arrival. We ultimately secured his release and placed him in a residential home for children with troubled pasts.

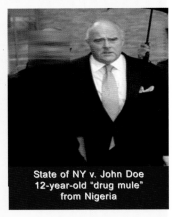

State of NY v. John Doe
12-year-old "drug mule"
from Nigeria

Charity

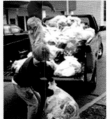

Clothing Drive for At-Risk Kids
220,000+ Items collected

Clothing Drive for Kids at Risk

Since 1993, the Keenan's Kids Foundation has collected and distributed nearly 20,000 items of clothing each year, over a quarter million items total.

Food for the Homeless

Since 1984, we have prepared between 100 and 150 bologna and cheese sandwiches per week. Several homeless shelters which service women and children are the weekly beneficiaries. Over 350,000 sandwiches have been produced.

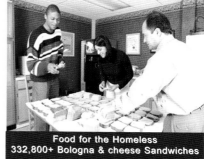

Food for the Homeless
332,800+ Bologna & cheese Sandwiches

Helping Families

Keenan's Kids Foundation periodically helps special needs families such as the Murphy and Price families. The help is in the form of buying clothes, and special outings such as

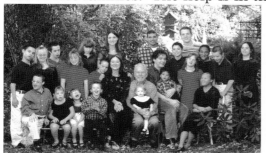

concerts, the zoo, sporting events and even hot air balloon rides. Since 1983, the Murphy's have adopted 23 Down's Syndrome children, ranging in age from 13 months to 34 years.

We are raising funds for a new home for the Murphy's; www.murphyhouseproject.com.

The Price family is also served. The family is composed of 16 children, most with severe medical needs, ventilators, wheelchairs, etc.

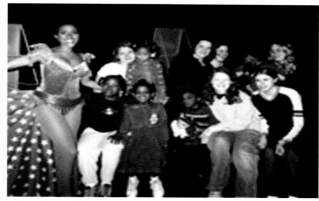

In Summary

Keenan's Kids Foundation is very proud of our accomplishments and prouder still because we employ no fundraising director. The money we raise comes from book sales, such as this book, and the generosity of the enormous donors. On a daily basis, we prove that a lot can be accomplished with just a little.

Don C. Keenan
The Keenan Law Firm

About Don C. Keenan

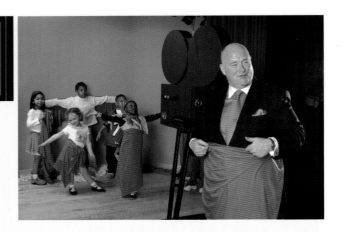

KEENAN LAW FIRM
Trial Lawyers

Don C. Keenan
The Keenan Building
148 Nassau Street, NW
Atlanta, GA 30303
www.keenanlawfirm.com
www.keenanskidsfoundation.com

Children's Lawyer

During his thirty years specializing in catastrophic injury and wrongful death cases, Mr. Keenan has secured over 100 verdicts and settlements over $1,000,000, including five over $10,000,000. Mr. Keenan has dedicated his practice to child injury and wrongful death cases arising from medical negligence, products liability, and premise liability, with the goal of making our society safer for children. He has handled cases in 44 states and on three continents.

Child Advocate

Mr. Keenan strongly believes that our duty does not end when we secure justice for the child and family. Equally important is learning from the prevention lessons of the case and formulating a public awareness campaign to help prevent future injuries and deaths and when necessary, pushing for legislation and regulations. He calls this unique approach to law the One-Third Solution: one-third litigating the case, one-third public awareness on the prevention and one-third pushing for regulations and legislation. Examples of his One-Third Solution are the Playground Safety Project being featured on the *Today Show* for the past three years, The Toy Safety Campaign profiled in *USA Today* and *Good Morning America*. The *Imagine* magazine, Summer 2005 issue, featured Don Keenan and his One-Third Solution as did *Mercedes Momentum* magazine in winter of 2004.

Don has appeared on every major national news program including: *60 Minutes*, *20/20*, *Larry King Live*, *The Oprah Winfrey Show*, *Montel*, *The O'Reilly Factor*, *The Today Show*, *Good Morning America*, CNN and *National Public Radio* (NPR), addressing children's issues.

Awards / Distinctions/Professional Accomplishments

⇨ Selected by Oprah Winfrey as one of the "People Who Have Courage," noting that Don has been fighting for the rights of abused children for 25 years

⇨ Emory University bestowed the "Career Achievement Award for Public Policy and Child Advocacy"

⇨ Named by the *National Law Journal* as one of the top three medical malpractice lawyers in the United States

⇨ Called "The Voice of the Voiceless" by *The Atlanta Globe*

⇨ "Internationally renowned child advocacy lawyer" by *Points North* magazine

⇨ "A famous advocate for children", *Business Chronicle*

⇨ "Top 100 Irish Americans" presented by *Irish America* magazine

In 1992, he became the youngest National President of the American Board of Trial Advocates, and during his tenure, led a delegation of lawyers to Czechoslovakia, and later was invited to Russia to produce the first civil trial in the history of those two emerging democracies. In 1997, he became National President of the Inner Circle of Advocates, the most exclusive group of trial lawyers in the country. In 1999, he was given the prestigious Chief Justice Award for Civility and Professionalism, the highest award possible for a lawyer in Georgia. He now serves on the Advisory Committee for the National Judicial College in Reno, Nevada, which trains the majority of new judges in the United States. In 1990 and again in 1992, he was named Trial Lawyer of The Year.

Helpful Web Addresses

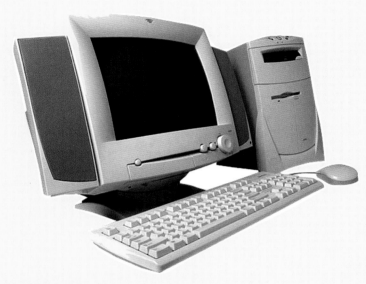

http://brands.babycatalog.com

http://ewh.ieee.org/soc/embs/comar/brodeur.htm

http://parents.berkeley.edu/recommend/where2buy/carseats/taxi.html

http://safetynet.smis.doi.gov/COhouseboats.htm

www.aaafoundation.org

www.aacca.org

www.aahperd.org/naspe

www.aao.org

www.aap.org

www.aap.org/family/carseatguide.htm

www.americancheerleader.com

www.autismspeaks.org

www.bhsi.org

www.backtobasictoys.com

www.boundlessplaygrounds.org
www.cdc.gov
www.cdc.gov/lead/qanda.htm
www.cdc.gov/ncipc/factsheets/fworks.htm
www.cfsan.fda.gov
www.checnet.org
www.childrenssafetynetwork.org
www.citizen.org
www.cleantheair.org
www.consumerreports.org
www.consumerreports.org/cro/consumer-protection/recalls/
    car-seats.htm
www.cpsafety.com
www.cpsc.gov
www.cpsc.gov/cgi-bin/recalldb/model.asp
www.cspinet.org
www.dannyfoundation.org
www.epa.gov
www.epa.gov/lead/leadinfo.htm
www.fda.gov/bbs/topics/news/2005/NEW01171.html
www.fmcsa.dot.gov
www.fmcsa.org
www.gogeisel.com
www.iihs.org
www.iihs.org/ratings/default.aspx

www.jfk-reloaded.com
www.kaboom.org
www.keenanlawfirm.com
www.keenanskidsfoundation.com
www.keenanskidsplaygroundsafety.com
www.kidsandcars.org
www.kidsource.com/cpsc/monoxide.html
www.klaaskids.org
www.knowx.com
www.livingthemoment.com
www.marshfieldclinic.org/nfmc/pages/default.aspx?page=nccra
     hs_resources_facts_sheet_4
www.medicalnewstoday.com
www.murphyhouseproject.com
www.nalionline.org
www.nannynetwork.com
www.nata.org
www.ncedl.org
www.ncsbs.org
www.nfhs.org
www.nhtsa.dot.gov
www.nhtsa.dot.gov/people/injury/airbags/airbags03/page7.html
www.nhtsa.dot.gov/people/injury/airbags/airbags03/page9.html
www.nhtsa.dot.gov/cps/safetycheck/typeseats/index.htm
www.nhtsa.dot.gov/people/injury/enforce/protecting
     children/protecting%20children.pdf
www.nhtsa.dot.gov/cars/testing

www.nih.gov

www.nocsae.org

www-odi.nhtsa.dot.gov/cars/problems/recalls/childseat.cfm

www.pbs.org/wgbh/pages/frontline/shows/teenbrain/etc/script.html

www.pwcwatch.org

www.poison.org

www.preventinjury.org

www.preventthebite.com

www.protectkids.org

www.riddell.com

www.safercar.gov

www.safekids.org

www.safekidssafedogs.com

www.scanusa.com

www.schoolbusinfo.org

www.smf.org/stds

www.spy-software-directory.com

www.statefarm.com/consumer/dogbite.htm

www.thgconsult.com/firmoverview.htm

www.toysafety.net

www.toysafety.org

www.usgovinfo.about.com/od/consumerawareness/a/toy
     recalls2004.htm

www.vaccinesafety.edu

www.windowcoverings.org

www.windowcoverings.org/howtorepair.html

Index